Body Mass Index in Clinical Practice

Edited by Samy I. McFarlane

Published in London, United Kingdom

Body Mass Index in Clinical Practice
http://dx.doi.org/10.5772/intechopen.1008605
Edited by Samy I. McFarlane

Contributors
Adam Green, Andreea-Consuela Timnea-Florescu, Andrew Chambers, Angel Martin Castellanos, Bogdana Virgolici, Daciana Costina Andrada Stefan, Dheeraj Kattula, Donghui Liu, Esen Öksüzoğlu Makbule, Gavril Gheorghievici, Hannah Kim, Heewon Kim, Jiangbo Ye, John Badylak, John T. Riehl, Ken Kiyono, Lachlan F. Anderson, Madhur Mangalam, Maria-Zinaida Dobre, McKenna W. Box, Michael Muncy, Mohamed Aly Elsherif, Naira Elsherif, Olivia Timnea, Oya Gökmen, Qian Du, Roxana Nartea, Stephen Amarjeet Jiwanmall, Tuğba Gürbüz, Wansu Yu, Yassmin Salaheldin Ibrahim, Yiting Zhao

First published in London, United Kingdom, 2026 by IntechOpen
IntechOpen is the global imprint of INTECHOPEN LIMITED, registered in England and Wales, registration number: 11086078, 167-169 Great Portland Street, London, W1W 5PF, United Kingdom

For EU product safety concerns: IN TECH d.o.o., Prolaz Marije Krucifikse Kozulić 3, 51000 Rijeka, Croatia, info@intechopen.com or visit our website at intechopen.com.

British Library Cataloguing-in-Publication Data
A catalogue record for this book is available from the British Library

Body Mass Index in Clinical Practice
Edited by Samy I. McFarlane
p. cm.
Print ISBN 978-1-83635-926-5
Online ISBN 978-1-83635-925-8
eBook (PDF) ISBN 978-1-83635-927-2

If disposing of this product, please recycle the paper responsibly.

Meet the editor

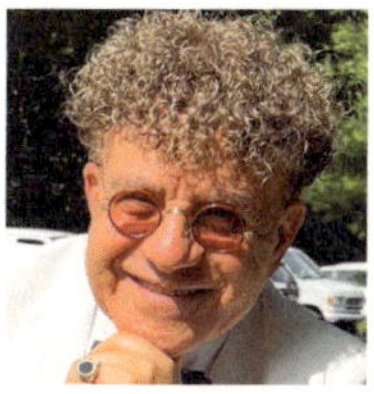

Dr. McFarlane is Distinguished Teaching Professor of Medicine/Endocrinology and Associate Dean at Downstate-Health Sciences University, Brooklyn, New York, USA. He has extensive experience in clinical and translational research, with over 600 publications, more than 26,000 citations, an h-index of 70, and an i10-index of 217 (Google Scholar). Among his citations are those appearing in major guidelines by the American Heart Association (AHA), such as stroke guidelines (2018 and 2019), the Scientific Statement from the AHA on Lifestyle and Risk Factor Modification for Reduction of Atrial Fibrillation 2020, and the 2021 SHNE/HRS/EHRA/APHRS Expert Collaborative Statement. Dr. McFarlane's work extensively explored thc intersection of obesity with diabetes, cardiovascular disease, sleep disorders, and cancer. It also addressed the obesity paradox and the complex metabolic pathways leading to chronic illnesses in obese populations. His work in this area was cited hundreds of times, including the WHO-European Regional Obesity Report 2022. Furthermore, Dr. McFarlane's work significantly influenced modern nutritional guidelines on dietary carbohydrate restriction; his collaborative work with national and international scholars provided support for the "Upside-Down" food pyramid, a major shift in the 2025-2030 US Dietary Guidelines. Dr. McFarlane edited several books on diabetes, hypertension, Renin Angiotensin Aldosterone System, dyslipidemia, obesity, cardiovascular disease, and related topics. He also edited the popular study guide, *The First Aid for the Medicine Clerkship*, by McGraw-Hill and Co.®, and the Resident Inpatient Selective Educational (RISE) Manual (2020 and 2022). Dr. McFarlane served three 4-year terms as a member of the National Institutes of Health's National Institute of Diabetes and Digestive and Kidney Diseases (NIH-NIDDK), and twice as chairman of NIH-NIDDK U01 committees and as Co-Chair of the NIH NIDDK DPPOS review committee. He also served as a consultant to the NIH special panels on multiple occasions, including the NIH-NIDDK Board of Scientific Counselors (BSC) in 2026. At the National Kidney Foundation (NKF), Dr. McFarlane served as Chair of the Clinical Subcommittee of the Kidney Early Evaluation Program (KEEP). Locally, he held several leadership positions, including Medical Director of Clinical Research, Program Director, and Chief of the Division of Endocrinology, Diabetes, and Metabolism. He also served as Brooklyn District President of the American College of Physicians (ACP) from 2014 to 2016. Dr. McFarlane served as the founding Associate Editor for Endocrine Today, and a founding Editor-In-Chief, Associate Editor, Section Editor, Lead Guest Editor, and Editorial Board Member for several PubMed-indexed journals such as *Clinical Practice, Current Diabetes Reports, Current Hypertension Reports, Current Cardiovascular Reports,* and *International Journal of Hypertension*, in addition to several open-access journals. He is the recipient of numerous awards and honors, including recognition from the United States Army, the US House of Representatives, Pioneer in Public Health, the Alpha Omega Alpha Medical Honor Society, and the Gold Foundation for Humanism in Medicine.

Contents

Preface

Body Mass Index (BMI) has been widely used for the past few decades as a measure of obesity and is highly used in epidemiological studies, classification, major interventional trials, and various guidelines related to obesity definitions and management. It is also used in risk assessment for multiple health conditions. However, several limitations and major concerns emerged regarding the use of BMI in clinical practice. These limitations include its inability to differentiate between muscle mass and fat, as seen in athletes with high muscle mass or in elderly populations with sarcopenia. Using only body weight and height in its calculation, BMI also fails to reflect body fat distribution, including central obesity, that has serious cardiometabolic implications. Furthermore, BMI has been derived mainly from data on White, non-Hispanic populations and therefore, it does not account for racial and ethnic differences in the cardiometabolic risk assessment at a given BMI, such as the case with the Asian population, for example. It also has other limitations, such as its inability to read gender and age.

These serious limitations have been the focus of concern of major organizations such as the American Medical Association, in 2023, adopting a new policy on the use of BMI and its problematic historical harm, and potential use for racial exclusion. Considering these many limitations of BMI, a group of 58 international experts in the field of obesity, in their attempt to move away from BMI as the sole defining measure in obesity, published an expert report in the January 2025 issue of the Lancet Diabetes and Endocrinology Journal. This report provides a more useful classification of obesity for practicing clinicians and introduces two new diagnostic categories of pre-clinical and clinical obesity. Persons with clinical obesity, according to the new classification, will have evidence of end-organ damage resulting from excessive body weight, such as liver disease, chronic kidney disease, heart disease, diabetes, and hypertension, as well as chronic lower extremity joint diseases. This timely and rather revolutionary definition of obesity will reshape the field, with specific diagnostic and therapeutic interventions that will be highly individualized, including lifestyle interventions as well as pharmacological and non-pharmacological options for obesity management.

In this volume, *Body Mass Index in Clinical Practice*, we assembled a group of internationally recognized scholars in the field of obesity to address the changing landscape of obesity, highlighting the implications of these new classifications on the epidemiology, clinical, and therapeutic guidelines, with emphasis on the potential betterment of the health of various minority groups. We also discuss the current approaches to obesity in this new era that is heralded by innovative thinking regarding clinical and pre-clinical obesity that reached pandemic proportions, affecting nearly 1 billion individuals worldwide.

This book provides readers with essential knowledge ranging from epidemiology and biology to modern, sophisticated tools for obesity measurement, as they relate to special populations such as growing children and adolescents, pregnant and menopausal women, and other populations commonly encountered in clinical practice.

Samy I. McFarlane
Division of Endocrinology,
Department of Medicine,
Downstate Health-Sciences University,
Brooklyn, New York, USA

Section 1

BMI from Basic Biological Concepts to Mathematical Bias

Chapter 1

From BMI to Biology: Advancing the Science of Obesity

Mohamed Aly Elsherif, Yassmin Salaheldin Ibrahim and Naira Elsherif

Abstract

Body Mass Index (BMI) has been the main tool used to define and classify obesity in clinical practice. It links weight and health risk in a simple and reproducible manner. However, the current understanding of obesity recognizes it as a complex interplay of genetic, biological, metabolic, and psychosocial factors. This chapter aims to trace the chronological evolution of BMI over the years. It was initially developed by Quetelet in the 19th-century and later modified to be utilized by global health authorities. Through a couple of clinical vignettes, we will highlight how individuals with similar BMI values may differ significantly in metabolic health. Additionally, we will emphasize BMI's inability to distinguish between lean and fat mass or delineate fat distribution. This chapter further explores the biology of obesity, including genetic predisposition, hormonal appetite regulation, adipose tissue function, and environmental factors. Furthermore, it addresses additional or alternative assessment tools, such as waist circumference, dual-energy X-ray absorptiometry (DXA), and bioelectrical impedance analysis (BIA), all of which provide a precise assessment of body composition and cardiometabolic risk. The Edmonton Obesity Staging System (EOSS) has been established as a measure of staging obesity, keeping in consideration metabolic, functional, and psychological disease toll. Finally, this chapter recommends shifting from a weight-centric to a health-focused, patient-centered approach, emphasizing continuous monitoring, multidisciplinary care, and precision medicine. BMI remains an important starting point, but comprehensive assessment based on metabolic risk, functionality, and health outcomes represents the future of obesity management.

Keywords: Body Mass Index (BMI), obesity assessment, adiposity, body composition, Edmonton Obesity Staging System (EOSS), clinical obesity guidelines, Patient-Centered care, obesity management, metabolic health, precision medicine

1. Introduction

For decades, body mass index (BMI) has been the primary tool by which obesity is defined and managed, offering a simple and practical measure that links weight to health risk [1]. However, as we deepen our understanding of obesity and recognize it as a complex chronic disease, it becomes increasingly clear that BMI alone fails to reflect the biological, metabolic, and psychosocial complexity of this disease. Two individuals with the same BMI can have significantly different health statuses, highlighting the limitations of this exclusively weight-based approach. This chapter aims to explore the shift from BMI to biology and redefine obesity beyond body size, toward a clearer, health-focused understanding that can better guide how we treat and care for our patients.

2. Clinical vignettes

At a tertiary care center specialized in obesity management, two patients walk into the clinic, both with a body mass index of 32 kg/m^2. Although both are classified as having obesity by WHO BMI guidelines, their health conditions may differ significantly [2].

Mrs. L is a 52-year-old office worker who has struggled with progressive weight gain since her adolescence. She has been diagnosed with type 2 diabetes, hypertension, obstructive sleep apnea, and early osteoarthritis of both knees. Her waist circumference is 110 cm, and liver sonography shows a large fatty liver. She feels fatigued, complains of limited mobility, and overall poor quality of life. This scenario delineates an example of obesity-related metabolic and functional complications.

Mr. J, in contrast, is a 29-year-old professional bodybuilder with a BMI of 32 kg/m^2. However, his physical and metabolic profiles are significantly different from those of Mrs. L. Years of intensive training and strict nutrition have built a body composed predominantly of muscle, with very little adiposity. His waist circumference is 82 cm, his metabolic profile is normal, and his exercise tolerance is exceptional. Despite having the same BMI, Mr. J does not have obesity as a disease. Instead, he is metabolically and functionally healthy.

These two patient presentations highlight the fundamental limitation of BMI: it cannot distinguish between fat and muscle, between subcutaneous and visceral adiposity, or between health and disease. While BMI remains a useful clinical assessment tool for patients with obesity, it fails to address the biological complexity and heterogeneity of this disease [3]. To advance our understanding and treatment of this condition, we must move beyond the basics of BMI and dive deeper into the biology of obesity as a complex and multifactorial disease.

Over the next few sections of this chapter, we will shed some light on the history of BMI in the clinical assessment of obesity, the clinical utilization and limitations of BMI as an assessment tool. Moreover, we will discuss some existing and emerging future alternative methods for evaluating and categorizing patients with obesity to better reflect their metabolic and functional health.

First, it is valuable to reflect on the historical origins of BMI and trace its evolution over the last two centuries prior to its adoption in contemporary medical practice.

3. Evolution of BMI throughout the years

The evolution of the BMI began nearly two centuries ago with the Belgian mathematician and statistician Adolphe Quetelet. In the 1830s, Quetelet attempted to define the characteristics of "the average man". Through his observations, he concluded that human body weight tended to increase in proportion to the square of height [4]. Thereafter, he proposed that the correlation between weight and stature is equal to weight divided by height squared (kg/m^2). Initially, this measure was not designed for clinical use but rather for population-based and epidemiological studies [4, 5].

During the late 19th and early 20th centuries, life insurance companies developed height–weight tables to estimate mortality risk, recognizing that heavier individuals often faced higher rates of chronic disease and premature death. These tables were unrelated to Quetelet's equation; however, they reflected a similar conclusion that body size correlated with health condition and wellbeing [6]. Despite that, this equation had not yet been utilized in clinical practice.

In 1972, the Quetelet Index was revised and renamed the Body Mass Index by the American physiologist Ancel Keys, who published an influential *Nature* article titled *"Indices of Relative Weight and Obesity."* Keys and his colleagues compared various weight-for-height formulas across multiple populations and demonstrated that the Quetelet Index correlated most strongly with body fat and was, therefore, the most reliable and practical indicator of weight [7]. Afterward, Keys coined the term *"Body Mass Index"* and suggested using it as a simple measure in obesity research [8].

Over the following decades, BMI was adopted as a practical and cost-effective tool for large-scale epidemiological studies. By the 1980s and 1990s, international health authorities formalized its use for clinical purposes. In 1995, the World Health Organization (WHO) introduced standardized BMI cutoffs to classify underweight, normal weight, overweight, and obesity [9]. This provided a universal framework that could be applied across populations, allowing for comparisons and global surveillance of obesity. Around the same time, the U.S. National Institutes of Health (NIH) and Centers for Disease Control and Prevention (CDC) also incorporated BMI into their clinical and public health guidelines [10].

With these changes taking place, BMI became widely accepted and utilized in medical practice, research, and clinical practice guidelines. It is currently used to define and classify obesity, guide clinical interventions, and track the global epidemiology of weight-related disorders. However, as the 21st century progressed, the limitations of BMI have become more evident [11]. The use of BMI is limited by its inability to distinguish between fat mass and lean mass, leading to confusion and possible misclassification of muscular individuals as overweight or obese. In addition to that, BMI alone does not account for ethnic differences in body composition, fat distribution, or risk of cardiometabolic disease. As we can see from the examples in the clinical scenarios above, two people with identical BMI values may have vastly different health profiles. One has high muscle mass and excellent metabolic health, while the other has significant visceral adiposity and insulin resistance, in addition to other possible cardiometabolic complications [11, 12].

As of today, the scientific understanding of obesity is evolving beyond this single numerical index. Researchers and clinicians are shifting toward more precise assessments of fat distribution, body composition, and metabolic parameters. Modern tools such as waist circumference, waist-to-hip ratio, dual-energy X-ray absorptiometry (DXA), MRI, and metabolic biomarkers provide deeper insights into morbidity risk and disease pathology than BMI alone could [13-15].

To understand the complexity of obesity assessment, it is crucial to dive deeper into the biology of obesity as a disease. In the next section, we will be looking into obesity pathophysiology, identifying genetic, hormonal, neurological, and gut-related contributors to this complex disease.

4. Understanding the biology and science behind obesity

Obesity is not simply an excess of weight; it is a chronic, relapsing, multifactorial disease surrounded by a complex interplay of biology, behavior, and environment. To move beyond BMI, we must examine the biological fundamentals that govern body weight and energy balance.

4.1 Genetics and epigenetics

Obesity is a strongly heritable disease. Multiple family and twin studies have demonstrated that 40–70% of the variation in body weight can be attributed to genetic components [16]. Monogenic obesity is caused by rare single-gene mutations that affect the leptin- melanocortin. It is characterized by severe, early-onset obesity, sometimes in association with severe hyperphagia and the early onset of obesity-related comorbid conditions. Polygenic obesity, in contrast, is an interplay of hundreds of genetic variants, each contributing differently to weight gain and energy regulation [17].

In addition to the genetic component, epigenetic modifications play a significant role in weight changes. Exposure to certain modifiers, such as maternal nutritional state, stress, or metabolic changes during pregnancy, can modify gene expression and lead to a strong predisposition to obesity long before lifestyle and environmental factors contribute [18].

4.2 Neurotransmitters and appetite regulation

Adipose tissue storage and weight changes are regulated by a finely tuned neurobiological system that balances energy intake and expenditure [19]. The hypothalamus, specifically the arcuate nucleus and the paraventricular hypothalamic nucleus, acts as the chief appetite brain center, integrating signals from peripheral hormones and nutritional input [20].

Leptin, an adipokine secreted by adipose tissue, signals energy sufficiency and is involved in long-term energy regulation. In the overfed or obese state, the abundance of leptin signals to suppress appetite and increase energy expenditure [19].

Ghrelin is a gastric hormone produced by the gastric fundus and is the only known hormone that stimulates hunger. The signaling of ghrelin in the brain stimulates the hypothalamic nuclei to increase appetite and reduce energy expenditure. In addition, it has mechano- and chemoreceptors on the vagal nerve, aiding in the stretching of the stomach in preparation for food ingestion [21].

Gastrointestinal hormones such as GLP-1, PYY, and CCK are secreted by different parts of the gastrointestinal tract and work to stimulate satiety and slow gastric emptying. These hormones are involved in short-term energy regulation, as their secretion is governed by direct components of the ingested meal and signal satiety as the meal arrives at the small intestine [22, 23].

In obesity, this system becomes dysregulated. Many individuals develop leptin resistance, blunting the satiety signal despite high circulating levels of leptin [24]. Moreover, the brain's reward pathways, driven by dopamine, can override the homeostatic control of energy, driving hedonic eating in response to highly palatable foods [25]. Obesity, therefore, is not simply a failure of willpower but a disruption of the neural circuitry that evolved to defend body weight [24].

4.3 Endocrine and metabolic pathways

Adipose tissue is not a passive fat depot but an active endocrine organ. Visceral adipose tissue, located around internal organs, is metabolically active and strongly linked to cardiometabolic complications [26, 27]. It produces a wide variety of adipokines, including leptin, TNF-α, IL-6, and resistin, among others. Such markers are involved in chronic low-grade inflammation, insulin resistance, and further cardiometabolic complications. Dysregulated lipid metabolism leads to ectopic fat deposition in the liver, pancreas, and muscle, impairing their function and worsening insulin resistance. Thus, the metabolic complications of obesity are determined not only by the amount of fat but by its distribution and metabolic activity as well [27, 28]. On the contrary, adiponectin, another adipose tissue product, has emerged as a protective adipokine. Adiponectin enhances insulin sensitivity via AMP-activated protein kinase (AMPK) and peroxisome proliferator-activated receptor α (PPARα) signaling, promoting fatty acid oxidation and suppressing inflammation. Therefore, it protects against endothelial dysfunction and atherosclerotic processes and promotes healthy adipose tissue remodeling in the liver, skeletal muscle, vascular endothelium, and the immune system. **Table 1** below shows a summary of some adipokines and their functions [27, 28].

4.4 The gut microbiome

Recent evidence suggests that the gut microbiome plays a role in obesity by influencing nutrient absorption, energy regulation, and systemic inflammation [29]. Studies have shown differences in the gut microbiota of individuals with obesity compared to lean individuals, with certain bacterial types promoting more efficient calorie extraction from food. In addition, certain microbial metabolites, such as short-chain fatty acids, interact with host metabolism and influence appetite regulation [30]. There is still plenty of room

Adipokine	Physiological function	Clinical significance
Adiponectin	↑ Insulin sensitivity, ↑ fatty acid oxidation, anti-inflammatory, anti-atherogenic	Protective against cardiovascular risk, low in obesity
Leptin	Regulates appetite and energy expenditure	High obesity leads to leptin resistance
TNF-α/IL-6	Pro-inflammatory markers, worsen insulin resistance	High in obesity, marking adipose inflammation
Resistin	Induces insulin resistance and promotes chronic inflammation	High in obesity, linked to cardiometabolic risk
MCP-1	Attracts inflammatory monocytes and macrophages, promoting adipose chronic inflammation	Reflects adipose tissue immune activation

MCP-1 Monocyte Chemoattractant Protein-1

Table 1.
Adipokines and their functions.

for research on gut microbiomes, possibly aiding in the prevention or management of obesity.

4.5 The environment

In addition to the complex interplay of factors explained above, the environmental factors play a major role in weight changes. Environmental influencers include early life events, exposure to certain chemicals, sedentary lifestyles, and the ready availability of calorie-dense foods lacking nutritional value [31]. The biological systems that once conferred a survival advantage in environments of scarcity now contribute to weight gain in an environment of energy abundance [32].

Taken together, these factors reveal obesity as a heterogeneous disease with diverse biological changes. Two individuals with the same BMI may carry vastly different risks depending on their genetic profile, fat distribution, and cardiometabolic health. While BMI is convenient to use, it remains too simple to reflect the complexity of obesity. Biology reveals a richer and more comprehensive picture, one that calls for precision medicine approaches tailored to the individual rather than a one-size-fits-all approach [32].

5. BMI as a diagnostic tool for obesity

BMI is the most practical and widely used anthropometric tool for categorizing patients by weight in both clinical and research settings. It is defined as weight in kilograms divided by the square of height in meters (kg/m^2). BMI provides a simple, cost-effective, and reproducible measure of obesity that can be applied universally [1]. **Table 2** below shows BMI categories for adults as standardized by the WHO [2]. These categories were established through epidemiological studies linking higher BMI levels to greater risks of morbidity and mortality.

The adoption of BMI as a clinical assessment tool has been reinforced by several international guidelines, recognizing it as a strong predictor of multiple chronic diseases [33, 34]. Numerous studies have demonstrated that higher BMI categories correlate with increased risks of cardiovascular disease, type 2 diabetes, certain types of cancer, and overall mortality. BMI enables governments and health agencies to track obesity prevalence, monitor long-term trends in weight, and guide public health interventions [35].

Category	BMI range (kg/m^2)	Clinical description
Underweight	< 18.5	May indicate a nutritional deficiency or another condition
Healthy weight	18.5 – 24.9	Associated with the lowest cardiometabolic risk
Overweight	25.0 – 29.9	Increased risk for cardiometabolic disease
Obesity Class I	30.0 – 34.9	Moderate obesity may have early metabolic complications
Obesity Class II	35.0 – 39.9	Severe obesity, high risk of comorbidities
Obesity Class III	≥ 40.0	Very severe obesity is often associated with multiple complications

Table 2.
WHO BMI categories for adults.

6. Utility and strengths of BMI in clinical practice

In clinical practice, BMI is an important first-line screening tool that directly correlates with a patient's weight [3]. It is quick to obtain or calculate and only requires basic equipment. It is strongly associated with cardiometabolic risk and is recommended to be performed annually in adults, along with waist circumference, when possible, blood pressure, and basic laboratory tests [1, 35]. It is important to note that an elevated BMI is not considered diagnostic of obesity-related disease; rather, it serves as a red flag to initiate a more comprehensive evaluation. This evaluation typically includes laboratory assessment (lipids, fasting glucose, liver enzymes), screening for metabolic syndrome, and evaluation for conditions such as sleep apnea, osteoarthritis, and depression [35].

BMI is used in the pediatric population as well, but with some adjustments. In children and adolescents, growth and development considerably affect body composition [36]. Therefore, BMI is plotted on age- and sex-specific growth charts, with obesity defined as a BMI at or above the 95th percentile for age and sex. This percentile-based approach allows clinicians to differentiate between normal growth variation and clinically significant overweight [2].

The strength of BMI lies in its feasibility and reproducibility. It requires no specialized equipment or technical training, making it practical and suitable in both resource-rich and resource-limited settings. BMI is very practical in contrast to other advanced body composition measures, such as dual-energy X-ray absorptiometry (DXA) or magnetic resonance imaging (MRI), which require technical training and may be operator-dependent. Furthermore, BMI categories are familiar to both clinicians and the public, facilitating communication and patient education. Taken together, these features have established BMI as a cornerstone of both population-level assessments and clinical screening for obesity [37].

7. Challenges and limitations of BMI

BMI remains essential for population health and the initial screening of obesity; however, its clinical utility has several significant limitations that have become increasingly recognized as obesity research has advanced and as precision medicine has been developed to ensure individualized care [38, 39]. Some of these limitations are listed below.

7.1 Lack of distinction between fat and lean mass

One of the most significant limitations is that BMI does not distinguish between lean body mass (muscle, bone, organ tissue) and adipose tissue. As a result, an athlete with high muscle mass may have a BMI in the overweight or even obesity range, despite having a very low percentage of body fat and minimal cardio-metabolic risk [38]. Conversely, older adults may develop muscle or bone mass loss (sarcopenia or osteopenia) while gaining fat mass, and still have a "normal" BMI. This scenario is not uncommon and may impose significant health risks that BMI alone fails to detect [38].

7.2 Failure to assess fat distribution

Regardless of body fat percentage, the location of fat storage plays a critical role in metabolic risk. Visceral fat, stored within the abdominal cavity and around organs, is strongly associated with insulin resistance, dyslipidemia, and cardiovascular disease since it is metabolically active, secreting several inflammatory adipokines (IL-6, TNF-alpha, etc.) [40], while subcutaneous fat is less likely associated with chronic metabolic complications [39]. BMI provides no information on fat distribution; consequently, waist circumference is now recommended as an additional measurement in clinical practice. Indeed, large studies have shown that waist circumference predicts cardiometabolic risk and mortality more accurately than BMI alone. A patient with a normal BMI but elevated waist circumference may have a higher risk profile than a patient with elevated BMI but low central adiposity [39].

7.3 Age and sex variability

BMI does not adjust for differences across the lifespan or between sexes [41]. As an example, some elderly people may experience a decline in muscle mass or bone density, leading to lower body weight despite increases in body fat percentage. In such a scenario, BMI alone may underestimate obesity-related risks in this age group [41]. Similarly, women generally have a higher proportion of body fat than men at the same BMI, which may underrate cardiometabolic risk if BMI is used solely [42]. These discrepancies indicate that BMI cut-offs do not carry the same implications across all populations [41, 42].

7.4 Ethnic and population differences

Another significant limitation of BMI is its inability to account for ethnic variability. At a given BMI, body fat percentage and risk for developing metabolic comorbidities differ markedly across populations [43]. For example, Asian populations have higher body fat and greater metabolic risk at lower BMI thresholds compared to Europeans. For this reason, WHO has suggested lower BMI cutoffs for Asian populations ($\geq$23 kg/m^2 for overweight, $\geq$ 27.5 kg/m^2 for obesity) [44]. To date, there are no region-specific BMI cutoff values for defining overweight or obesity in Middle Eastern populations. Such variability underscores the need for population-specific cutoffs or the integration of additional measures into clinical assessment.

Because of these limitations, BMI is best regarded as a screening tool rather than a definitive diagnostic measure. It is useful for labeling individuals at risk but must be interpreted in the context of other clinical and biochemical data [36].

This multimodal approach in obesity management recognizes the complexity of obesity as a chronic disease that extends far beyond a single number. While BMI remains a useful and cost-effective measure in obesity screening, it should not be used alone. Clinicians and researchers must integrate it with complementary tools and consider the context of patients' overall health profile.

8. Bridging the gap: Advanced methods in body composition assessment

To avoid excessive dependence on BMI as a sole measure for patients with obesity, multiple advanced modalities of body composition have evolved and are currently being utilized in clinical practice to ensure a comprehensive assessment. **Table 3** below shows a summary of advanced body composition analysis modalities.

Method	Principle	Accuracy	Advantages	Limitations	Clinical use
BMI	Weight/height^2	Low for body composition analysis	Simple, universal, cheap, well-validated cut-offs	Does not distinguish between fat and lean mass, ignores fat distribution, ethnicity, and age	Screening for overweight/obesity in all settings
Waist circumference, WHR, WHtR	Anthropometric measures of central adiposity	Moderate	Cheap, quick, reflects visceral risk better than BMI	Measurement error, ethnic variation, cut-offs variable	Routine use alongside BMI for cardiometabolic risk
BAI, BRI, ABSI	Derived anthropometric formulas	Variable	Non-invasive, attempts to reflect body shape	Validation inconsistent, less used in clinics	Research and selected risk stratification
Hydrostatic weighing	Body density by underwater weighing	High (research standard)	Historically used, accurate	Not patient-friendly, poor feasibility	Research reference
Air displacement plethysmography (ADP)	Body volume by air displacement	High	Non-invasive, suitable for all ages	Sensitive to hydration, cost, and not widely available	Specialty centers, research
DXA	X-ray attenuation differentiates fat, lean, bone	High	Relatively quick, reproducible, widely studied	Size/weight limits, radiation, inter-device variability	Clinical research, osteoporosis, obesity
CT	X-ray imaging with cross-sectional quantification	Very high (gold standard)	Precise quantification of visceral vs. subcutaneous fat, muscle	Radiation, costly, size limitations	Oncology, sarcopenia
MRI	Magnetic resonance imaging	Very high (gold standard)	Excellent soft tissue detail; no radiation	High cost, limited availability, and long scan times	Research, sarcopenia, fat distribution
Ultrasound	Sound wave reflection	Variable	Portable, radiation-free, muscle/fat depth	Operator-dependent, poor visceral resolution	Bedside muscle/fat assessment

Method	Principle	Accuracy	Advantages	Limitations	Clinical use
Single-frequency BIA	Electrical conductivity estimates TBW → lean/fat	Low-moderate	Portable, cheap, simple	Inaccurate in severe obesity and edema, hydration-dependent	Community/ clinical screening
Multifrequency BIA	Impedance at multiple frequencies, regional	Moderate-high	Better for hydration	Limited by calibration	Weight management, clinics
AI-based/3D optical methods	Computer vision and imaging algorithms	Emerging, promising	Non-invasive, scalable, inexpensive	Requires validation, device/ software limits	Future large-scale monitoring

BMI Body Mass Index, WHR Waist-Hip Ratio, WHtR Waist-Height Ratio, BAI Body Adiposity Index, BRI Body Roundness Index, ABSI Body Shape Index, DXA Dual X-ray Absorptiometry, CT Computed Tomography, MRI Magnetic Resonance Imaging, BIA Bioelectrical Impedance Analysis, AI Artificial Intelligence.

Table 3.
Body composition analysis modalities.

8.1 Anthropometric indices and derived metrics

In routine clinical care, simple anthropometric measures can be used to enhance BMI utilization. Waist circumference (WC), waist-to-hip ratio (WHR), and waist-to-height ratio (WHtR) are established measures of central adiposity and are stronger predictors of cardiometabolic risk than BMI alone. Among these, WHtR has been recognized as the most valid method across populations, with a universal cut-off of 0.5, making it easy to apply in diverse clinical settings [45]. A tiered approach, using BMI together with WC or WHtR in all patients, represents a reasonable clinical solution.

8.2 Volume-based methods

Volume-based techniques are used to assess body density and estimate body fat percentage using multi-compartment models. Hydrostatic weighing is limited by its overwhelming procedure and poor patient compliance. Air displacement plethysmography (ADP), represented by the BodPod, provides a user-friendly alternative, offering quick, non-invasive measures [46]. These methods are most valuable in highly specialized or research settings, where they can serve as standardization models for validating simpler clinical tools. However, they heavily rely on calculations of tissue density and hydration. Moreover, they are costly and not widely available, limiting their practical use in clinical settings [47].

8.3 Imaging-based modalities: DXA, CT, MRI, and ultrasound

Imaging has transformed body composition analysis by allowing the direct assessment of fat, lean mass, and bone, as well as the differentiation of fat depots. Below are some examples of these modalities.

8.3.1 Dual-energy X-ray absorptiometry (DXA)

DXA produces accurate measurements of fat and lean mass with relatively low risk of radiation and is widely used in clinical research. However, limited scanner size and higher weight reduce its applicability in severe obesity [48, 49].

8.3.2 Computed tomography (CT) and magnetic resonance imaging (MRI)

These imaging modalities provide gold-standard assessments of visceral and subcutaneous fat and skeletal muscle. CT involves radiation exposure, while MRI is costly and time-consuming. Both can be challenging to achieve in patients with severe obesity [50].

8.3.3 Ultrasound

Ultrasound is a lower-cost option for measuring subcutaneous fat and muscle thickness. It avoids radiation but is highly operator-dependent and less accurate for visceral adiposity [51].

8.4 Bioelectrical impedance analysis (BIA)

BIA estimates body composition by measuring the body's resistance to electrical currents. Being portable and simple to use makes it widely employed in clinical and community settings. Unlike single-frequency BIA, which has limited accuracy in cases of edema or altered hydration states, multifrequency BIA devices provide greater accuracy by differentiating intracellular and extracellular water content [52].

Although the results of BIA may vary, it is still useful in patients' follow-up during their weight-loss journeys, given that machine standardization has been performed [52, 53].

8.5 Emerging technologies: AI and optical imaging

Recent novel techniques provide noninvasive modalities for obesity assessment. CT scans analyzed by AI enable precise measurement of fat and muscle masses. Smartphone-based applications and 3D optical scanning tools are under development to estimate fat percentage and distribution, with results comparable to DXA. These techniques may provide better patients' accessibility and more accurate results [54].

Integration of these assessment tools into clinical practice should follow a stepwise, need-based strategy. Clinicians can begin with anthropometric indicators for baseline screening and risk stratification, then progress to BIA for monitoring body composition changes over time. In patients with complex metabolic profiles or unclear findings, densitometry or advanced imaging modalities (DXA, CT, MRI, ultrasound) can provide deeper evaluation into fat distribution and muscle mass. AI-assisted and optical imaging technologies can further enhance accuracy and enable personalized treatment planning. This tiered approach ensures that assessments are both clinically relevant and cost-efficient [50]. **Table 4** below provides a suggested stepwise approach to utilizing different modalities in clinical practice based on the patient's condition and management context.

Clinical context	Recommended method (s)	Rationale
General screening (primary care, public health)	BMI + WC/WHtR	Simple, inexpensive, better cardiometabolic risk stratification than BMI alone
Obesity management (secondary and tertiary clinic)	BMI + WC/WHtR + BIA or DXA	Track body composition changes during therapy; identify sarcopenia
Cardiometabolic risk stratification	WC, WHtR, CT/MRI (for visceral fat)	Central adiposity is strongest predictor of risk
Bariatric surgery candidates	DXA, BIA, CT (if available)	Baseline body composition, risk stratification, surgical planning
Renal/hepatic disease	Multifrequency BIA, DXA	Fluid shifts affect accuracy; need careful evaluation and clinical correlation
Sarcopenia/cachexia (geriatrics, oncology)	DXA, CT, MRI (where available), Ultrasound (muscle thickness)	Quantify muscle mass and body composition
Community/public health monitoring	BMI + WHtR, AI tools	Cost-effective, accessible for population
Pediatrics	BMI for age + WC/WHtR + DXA	Growth charts and accurate fat vs. lean estimates for early obesity detection

BMI Body Mass Index, WC Waist Circumference, WHR Waist-Hip Ratio, WHtR Waist-Height Ratio, DXA Dual Xray Absorptiometry, CT Computed Tomography, MRI Magnetic Resonance Imaging, BIA Bio-Impedance Analysis.

Table 4.
Suggested clinical contexts for body composition modalities.

BMI is a useful and practical tool for detecting obesity due to its simplicity and strong association with morbidity and mortality. However, it should be used as a screening tool rather than the sole measure for obesity diagnosis. Combining BMI with other measures like WC, laboratory investigations, comorbidity screening, and body composition analysis gives a more comprehensive picture of a patient's health profile.

9. Integrating evidence-based guidelines into clinical assessment of obesity

To avoid incorrect labeling of patients with obesity based solely on body shape or size, it is crucial to incorporate other measures in clinical assessment. A comprehensive obesity evaluation requires a systematic assessment inclusive of anthropometric parameters, related comorbid conditions, physical functionality, and psychosocial well-being. Such a multidimensional approach provides a more accurate picture of the patient's health and allows clinicians to better stratify risk and guide personalized management interventions [55, 56].

9.1 Anthropometric measurements

For comprehensive obesity assessment, WC and WHtR should be obtained in addition to BMI due to their better correlation with central adiposity and cardiometabolic risk [45]. Cut-off values of WC ≥ 102 cm in men and ≥ 88 cm in women are widely accepted, with varying thresholds among different ethnicities [1].

Body composition assessment adds depth to obesity evaluation and should be routinely incorporated into the assessment of the disease.

9.2 Clinical evaluation of obesity complications

Full obesity assessment must be integrated with a systematic clinical evaluation of obesity-related complications, including, but not limited to:

- **Metabolic:** Type 2 diabetes, dyslipidemia, metabolic dysfunction-associated steatotic liver disease (MASLD) [57].
- **Cardiovascular:** Hypertension, heart failure with preserved ejection fraction, atherosclerotic cardiovascular disease [58].
- **Respiratory:** Obstructive sleep apnea, obesity hypoventilation syndrome, asthma [59].
- **Musculoskeletal:** Osteoarthritis, back pain, mobility impairment [60].
- **Reproductive:** Polycystic ovary syndrome, infertility, pregnancy complications [61].

9.3 Routine laboratory investigations

These include fasting blood glucose or glycated hemoglobin (HbA1C), lipid profile, hepatic and renal function tests. A hormonal panel, including thyroid function tests, sex hormones, and cortisol levels, should be evaluated based on the patient's presentation and clinical picture. In addition, a basic profile of vitamin and mineral levels is preferred based on the patient's symptoms [62]. A sleep study and echocardiography can be considered when symptoms suggest cardiopulmonary involvement or in cases of severe obesity [63].

9.4 Functional and physical assessment

Functional health is an important component of obesity assessment, despite being frequently overlooked. Tools such as the 6-minute walk test, grip strength measurement, or mobility assessment can provide some understanding of the impact of obesity on activities of daily living. In older individuals, it is highly recommended to screen for lean mass loss using tools such as the SARC-F questionnaire and muscle strength testing [64].

9.5 Psychosocial and behavioral evaluation

Psychosocial and behavioral factors are integral components of obesity assessment. Screening for depression, anxiety, and eating disorders can be achieved using tools such as the PHQ-9 and the Binge Eating Scale [65, 66]. A full dietary history, physical activity assessment, and evaluation of sleep patterns provide a clear view of lifestyle interventions. Motivational interviewing techniques are valuable for assessing readiness to change and setting realistic goals [66, 67].

10. Clinical staging of obesity

Obesity clinical staging systems were developed to provide a more individualized risk stratification than BMI categories alone. The Edmonton Obesity Staging System (EOSS) was proposed by Sharma and Kushner in 2009 and aims to classify obesity by clinical and functional impact rather than weight alone **Figure 1** [68]. Due to its strong association with mortality and cardiovascular risk, it was validated and used in combination with BMI to guide treatment intensity [68, 69]. The EOSS classifies patients with obesity according to the metabolic, functional, and psychological impact of the disease, ranging from Stage 0 (no risk factors) to Stage 4 (end-stage disability) [68]. It was also adapted for the pediatric population (EOSS-P) since it demonstrated superior predictability of health risk and individualized patient needs compared to BMI [70].

Figure 1 below shows the components of the Edmonton Obesity Staging System. **Table 5** below shows the stepwise approach to obesity management based on the patient's EOSS.

10.1 EOSS in clinical practice

EOSS stage provides risk stratification and patient prognosis as it correlates with all-cause and cardiovascular mortality outcomes, regardless of the BMI, in cohort studies. Patients with EOSS stage ≥ 2 have shown higher mortality rates compared with lower stages. Clinicians can use this to identify high-risk patients who need urgent or intensive intervention [71].

EOSS is used to identify patients who may potentially benefit from conservative management versus pharmacotherapy versus bariatric surgery earlier in the

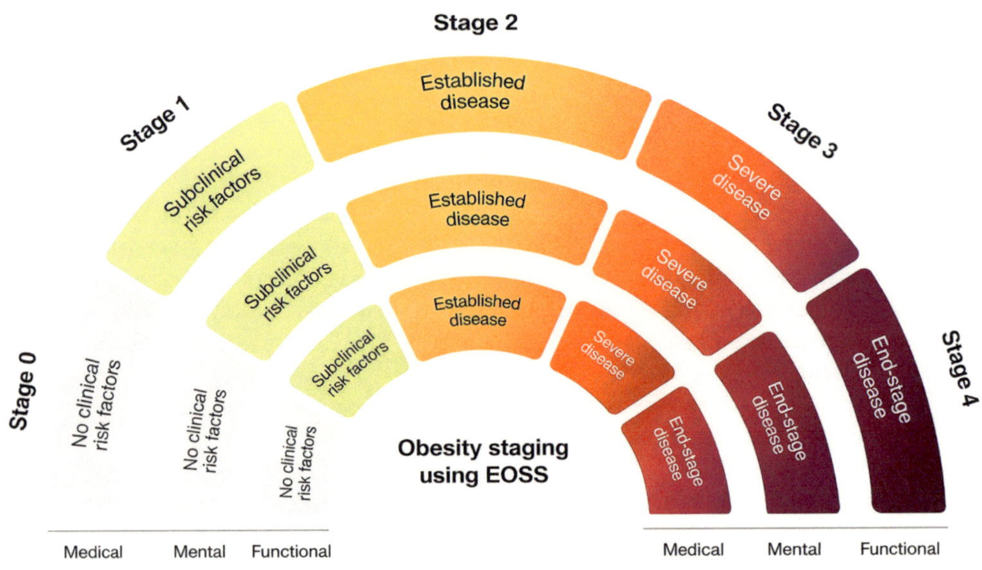

Figure 1.
Edmonton obesity staging system. https://pmc.ncbi.nlm.nih.gov/articles/pmc8673483/.

Stage	Management approach
0	a) Identify weight-gain-promoting factors. b) Advise lifestyle modifications.
1	a) Intensify lifestyle interventions. b) Risk factor monitoring and follow-up.
2	a) Start obesity management, including behavioral, pharmacological, and surgical interventions. b) Monitor obesity-related complications.
3	a) Intensify the obesity treatment plan. b) Promptly manage comorbidities.
4	a) Intensify the obesity treatment plan. b) Consider additional management, such as occupational therapy, pain management, and psychosocial support.

Table 5.
Management of patients based on Edmonton Obesity Staging System (EOSS).

management. For example, a patient with a BMI of 33 but EOSS stage 2 may be prioritized for more intensive therapy than a patient with a BMI of 36 who is EOSS stage 0–1 [72].

When it comes to research and outcome measurements, EOSS provides clinically meaningful results, surpassing weight changes. These results can be used to create a database for research purposes and to track patients' treatment progress longitudinally, to obtain clinical outcomes [72].

MDCalc and several other available staging checklists and calculators help clinicians record patients' stages systematically during a consultation. These tools determine the classification of comorbidities, mental-health issues, and functional limitations under each stage [73].

10.2 EOSS strengths

EOSS helps in aligning treatment decisions with patient morbidity by directly measuring the health burden associated with obesity, focusing on metabolic, physical, and psychological complications rather than weight or BMI alone [68]. Moreover, multiple cohort studies and reviews highlight the ability of EOSS to predict mortality and adverse outcomes. In addition, EOSS allows for a more patient-centered approach, assisting clinicians in determining treatment intensity based on the individual's level of morbidity, ensuring more efficient and directed care [68, 69, 71].

10.3 Limitations and practical caveat

EOSS has a few limitations despite being useful in clinical care. Different studies use slightly different ways to define the stages, making it harder to compare results and ensure consistency. Detailed medical information, such as laboratory testing, sleep studies, and mental or physical assessments, which are not available in all settings, are required to fulfill the EOSS system. Finally, EOSS is meant to complement, not replace, BMI. While BMI is still needed for public health tracking, EOSS helps guide clinical decisions and personalized care [68, 69, 71].

10.4 Our practical recommendations

1. Include a standardized EOSS checklist in patients' assessment forms.

2. Offer staff training on linking medical, functional, and psychological issues to EOSS stages for better consistency.

3. Record both BMI for body measurements and EOSS for clinical decision-making.

4. Define the criteria used in research or quality improvement projects, including lab values, diagnoses, and functional measures.

11. Monitoring and follow-up

Given that obesity is a chronic, relapsing condition requiring ongoing assessment and monitoring, follow-up of patients with this disease is a cornerstone of efficient management. Follow-up frequency and duration should be determined on an individual basis, depending on disease severity, comorbidities, and treatment intervention. Generally, initial follow-up is advised every 1–3 months during the active intervention phase to monitor treatment progress, adjust therapy, and provide behavioral support. After treatment stabilization, clinicians can space follow-up encounters to every 3–6 months for long-term maintenance. Additionally, in case of rising complications or unmet treatment goals, clinicians can offer appointment flexibility for earlier review of the patient's condition [74].

Practical measures during follow-up include [74, 75]:

- Tracking anthropometric measures and body composition, if available.

- Evaluating clinical outcomes (e.g., blood pressure, glucose levels, lipid profile, liver function parameters) and functional status.

- Assessing psychosocial aspects of health, including mood, stress, sleep, and quality of life.

- Reviewing medications that may contribute to weight gain or interfere with weight loss.

- Reinforcing behavioral lifestyle interventions, including dietary habits and regular physical activity goals.

- Adjusting treatment plans based on response and comorbidity status, including pharmacotherapy or consideration of bariatric surgery or procedures.

- Integrate telehealth options to improve patient compliance and enhance follow-up.
- Encourage multidisciplinary collaboration, including dietitians, psychologists, and exercise specialists.
- Develop patient education resources highlighting the chronic nature of obesity and the importance of long-term patient commitment.

12. Shifting from a weight-centric to a health-focused model and future directives in obesity management

To provide personalized and holistic care for patients with obesity, treatment strategies should be tailored to obesity phenotype, behavioral patterns, clinical comorbidities, and patient preferences rather than weight or BMI targets. Adipokines, metabolomic signatures, and microbiome profiles are recent biomarkers that enable clinicians to perform more precise risk stratification and apply personalized therapies. In addition, digital health tools are becoming widely used in providing real-time feedback and long-term support. When combining these advanced tools, clinicians can merge obesity care with the principles of precision medicine. These modalities include:

Holistic, multidisciplinary, patient-centered care team including **an** obesity physician or specialist, dietitian, psychologist, exercise physiotherapist, pharmacist, as well as a bariatric surgeon whenever possible [76].

Novel biomarkers could improve diagnosis, prognosis, and treatment through measuring fasting or postprandial metabolite panels. This will help to stratify metabolic risk and predict liability for weight-gain or response to certain interventions [77]. Adipokines, such as leptin and adiponectin, can provide information on adipose tissue dysfunction and appetite signaling, which could assist in risk stratification and tracking response [78]. On the other hand, microbiome profiles and bile-acid signaling are associated with differential responses to diet, bariatric procedures, and some drugs [77].

12.1 Precision medicine

Phenotyping can classify patients by dominant drivers to predict treatment responsiveness. As an example, some patients may be appetite-driven, have insulin resistance, or exhibit hedonic eating patterns. Others may have low energy expenditure or hormonal dysregulation contributing to weight gain. In cases of early-onset severe obesity with evident hyperphagia or atypical features, genetic testing is valuable to detect rare monogenic obesity, and pharmacogenomics can guide drug or surgical options. Individualized management options, including pharmacotherapy and behavioral strategies aligned to phenotype and biomarker profiles, will lead to enhanced response and minimal side effects [79].

12.2 eHealth interventions for weight loss and weight maintenance

Remote monitoring and wearable devices have been used to track activity, sleep, and weight to provide objective behavioral data and trigger immediate interventions.

Mobile apps can provide scalable behavioral changes, including goal setting, self-monitoring, and problem-solving, all of which have been shown to be comparable to face-to-face interventions [80]. Telehealth and online coaching can improve access, support maintenance, and allow multidisciplinary virtual visits, overcoming geographic limitations [81]. Recent studies showed that when combining AI applications with pharmacotherapy, clinical outcomes are substantially improved. Furthermore, the integration of biomarkers with real-time digital data can be valuable in predicting relapse risk, recommending medication adjustments, and prompting clinician outreach [82].

13. Implementation challenges and safeguards

Despite the promising effects of the proposed future modalities for diagnosis and management, each comes with challenges limiting their practical applications. These include, but are not limited to:

a) Biomarker testing and digital tools may widen inter-patient disparities, leading to inequity and potential bias in resource allocation [83].

b) Data privacy should be protected by keeping all information in secure records that clinicians can access and by obtaining informed consent before using any digital data [83, 84].

c) Clinician workflow should include decision-support tools within electronic health records to reduce extra work, and teams should be trained to understand biomarkers and digital data [83].

14. Ideal model of obesity management

An ideal model for obesity management has not yet been achieved; however, integrating evolving approaches, such as multi-omics, precision medicine, digital health, and AI assistance, represents a crucial step toward developing a more effective and personalized model of care [79, 80].

A health-focused approach also plays an essential ethical and psychosocial role by encouraging the reduction of weight bias and stigma. It shifts the view of obesity care from a weight reduction focus to improving the overall health of the patient. By concentrating on "health gain" instead of "kilograms lost," clinicians can help patients stay more engaged, confident, and committed to their treatment, resulting in better health outcomes for individuals and the wider community [76, 77].

15. Clinical versus preclinical obesity: A functional re-definition debate

The 2025 Lancet Diabetes & Endocrinology Commission's statement distinguishes between clinical and preclinical obesity, where clinical obesity is defined as excess adiposity leading to considerable metabolic and organ dysfunction, while preclinical obesity denotes excess adiposity with preserved physiological function. According to the statement, the diagnosis of obesity requires quantification of fat mass through DXA, MRI, CT, or validated BIA, or at least one anthropometric marker such as WC, WHR, or WHtR, rather than relying on BMI alone [85].

The new redefinition has policy and public health implications and could expand insurance coverage for anti-obesity medications and multidisciplinary care. Data from the All of Us cohort showed that the application of the new definitive criteria increased obesity prevalence from 42.9% to 68.6%, accounting for patients with preclinical obesity and early risk of organ dysfunction. Individuals with preclinical obesity exhibited a 3.3-fold higher diabetes risk and a 1.4-fold higher cardiovascular risk compared to metabolically healthy, non-obese individuals, reinforcing the need for early risk-stratified prevention [86].

Proponents of this new definition emphasize better diagnostic precision and aim to eliminate stigma by identifying obesity as a pathophysiological disorder rather than merely a body size description. However, critics argue that the surveillance of obesity may be complicated by this newly proposed definition and that reimbursement systems are still reliant on BMI [85, 86].

Implementation of this proposed concept of clinical and preclinical obesity poses a few challenges in clinical practice, including accessibility limitations and the high cost of imaging modalities, in addition to the inaccuracy of BIA due to hydration and sex differences. In alignment with that, the KDIGO conference noted the poor reproducibility of adiposity measures in patients with chronic conditions associated with fluid retention. Furthermore, functional assessment limitations include time constraints, training deficiencies, and persistent obesity stigma [87].

To overcome these limitations, the American College of Cardiology (ACC) and the American Heart Association (AHA) proposed the following stepwise diagnostic approach:

a. Waist-based indices for screening

b. DXA or BIA for those with BMI < $35\,kg/m^2$ or diagnostic uncertainty

c. Practical and cost-effective functional tests, including gait speed, six-minute walk, and handgrip strength.

d. Integration of adiposity and functional data into patients' electronic health records allows for better monitoring and reimbursement decisions [88].

We recommend the combination of the new Lancet adiposity framework with EOSS staging to enable better disease stratification and to guide tailored intervention, keeping in consideration an individual's functional capacity [85, 89]. This integration supports individualized intervention, including lifestyle and behavioral therapy, in addition to pharmacologic or surgical interventions. It also allows for early detection of individuals with organ vulnerability and enables adiposity disease prevention. Additionally, this integration supports a more reasonable health policy framework across all disease spectrums [90].

16. From willpower to biology

In conclusion, obesity is not a disease of willpower or personal failure, it's rather a complex, chronic disease driven by a congress of biological, environmental, psychological, and social factors. Modern understanding of biology has revealed that body weight regulation is influenced by multiple neurohormonal and metabolic mechanisms that resist weight loss. Therefore, the simple concept of "eat less, move more" as a treatment for obesity is never sufficient. Managing obesity as a multifactorial and relapsing chronic illness shifts the focus from blame to evidence-based care, emphasizing prevention, individualized treatment, and long-term support. This understanding encourages both clinicians and patients to move beyond weight stigma and toward compassionate, effective obesity management that prioritizes health over judgment.

Nomenclature

BMI	Body Mass Index
GLP-1	Glucagon Like Peptide-1
PYY	Peptide YY
CCK	Cholecystokinin
WC	Waist Circumference
WHR	Waist-to-Hip Ratio
WHtR	Waist-to-Height Ration
EOSS	Edmonton Obesity Staging System
BIA	Bioelectrical Impedance Analysis
DXA	Dual Energy X-ray Absorptiometry
CT	Computed Tomography
MRI	Magnetic Resonance Imaging

Acknowledgments

The authors acknowledge the ethical use of artificial intelligence (AI) assistance, specifically "ChatGPT," in the preparation of this chapter. AI was applied to support language enhancement, reference formatting, and summarization of non-sensitive scientific content. All content, interpretations, and conclusions were manually written, reviewed, and validated by the authors. The authors hold full accountability for this chapter's scientific content.

Conflict of Interest

The authors declare no actual or potential conflicts of interest, including any financial, personal, or other relationships with other people or organizations. No financial support has been provided for the manuscript being submitted. All authors approved the contents of the manuscript and validated the accuracy of the data.

DOI: http://dx.doi.org/10.5772/intechopen.1014540

Author details

Mohamed Aly Elsherif[1,2]*, Yassmin Salaheldin Ibrahim[1,2] and Naira Elsherif[3]

1 National Bariatric Center, Qatar Metabolic Institute, Hamad Medical Corporation, Doha, Qatar

2 Weill Cornell Medicine- Qatar, Doha, Qatar

3 School of Medicine, New Giza University, Cairo, Egypt

*Address all correspondence to: drmlll.endocrine@gmail.com

References

[1] World Health Organization. Obesity and overweight. 2025, May 7; World Health Organization. Available from: https://www.who.int/news-room/fact-sheets/detail/obesity-and-overweight [Accessed: 2025-October-01]

[2] World Health Organization. Body Mass Index (BMI). World Health Organization. Available from: https://www.who.int/data/gho/data/themes/topics/topic-details/GHO/body-mass-index [Accessed: 2025-October-01]

[3] Wu Y, Li D, Vermund SH. Advantages and limitations of the Body Mass Index (BMI) to assess adult obesity. International Journal of Environmental Research and Public Health. 2024;**21**(6):757. DOI: 10.3390/ijerph21060757

[4] Eknoyan G. Adolphe Quetelet (1796-1874). The average man and indices of obesity. Nephrology, Dialysis, Transplantation: Official Publication of the European Dialysis and Transplant Association. European Renal Association. 2008;**23**(1):47–51. DOI: 10.1093/ndt/gfm517

[5] Heymsfield SB, Sorkin JD, Thomas DM, Yang S, Heo M, McCarthy C, Brown J, Pietrobelli A. Weight/Height2: Mathematical overview of the world's most widely used adiposity index. Obesity Reviews: an Official Journal of the International Association for the Study of Obesity. 2025;**26**(1):e13842. DOI: 10.1111/obr.13842

[6] Czerniawski AM. From average to ideal: The evolution of the height and weight table in the United States, 1836-1943. Social Science History. 2016;**31**(2):273–296. DOI: 10.1017/S0145553200013754

[7] Keys A, Fidanza F, Karvonen MJ, Kimura N, Taylor HL. Indices of relative weight and obesity. Journal of Chronic Diseases. 1972;**25**(6–7):329–343. DOI: 10.1016/0021-9681(72)90027-6

[8] Keys A, Fidanza F, Karvonen MJ, Kimura N, Taylor HL. Indices of relative weight and obesity. International Journal of Epidemiology. 2014;**43**(3):655–665. DOI: 10.1093/ije/dyu058

[9] World Health Organization. Physical status: The use of and interpretation of anthropometry, report of a WHO expert committee. World Health Organization; 1995. Available from: https://www.who.int/publications/i/item/9241208546

[10] Clinical guidelines on the identification, evaluation, and treatment of overweight and obesity in adults: Executive summary. Expert panel on the identification, evaluation, and treatment of overweight in adults. The American Journal of Clinical Nutrition. 1998, **68** (4), 899–917. DOI: 10.1093/ajcn/68.4.899

[11] Pray R, Riskin S. The history and faults of the Body Mass Index and where to look next: A literature review. Cureus. 2023;**15**(11):e48230. DOI: 10.7759/cureus.48230

[12] Bray GA. Beyond BMI. Nutrients. 2023;**15**(10):2254. DOI: 10.3390/nu15102254

[13] Ashwell M, Gunn P, Gibson S. Waist-to-height ratio is a better screening tool than waist circumference

and BMI for adult cardiometabolic risk factors: Systematic review and meta-analysis. Obesity Reviews: an Official Journal of the International Association for the Study of Obesity. 2012;**13**(3):275–286. DOI: 10.1111/j.1467-789X.2011.00952.x

[14] Messina C, Albano D, Gitto S, Tofanelli L, Bazzocchi A, Ulivieri FM, Guglielmi G, Sconfienza LM. Body composition with Dual Energy X-ray absorptiometry: From basics to new tools. Quantitative Imaging in Medicine and Surgery. 2020;**10** (8):1687–1698. DOI: 10.21037/qims.2020.03.02

[15] Bennett JP, Lim S. The critical role of body composition assessment in advancing research and clinical health risk assessment across the lifespan. Journal of Obesity & Metabolic Syndrome. 2025;**34**(2):120–137. DOI: 10.7570/jomes25010

[16] Naukkarinen J, Rissanen A, Kaprio J, Pietiläinen KH. Causes and consequences of obesity: The contribution of recent twin studies. International Journal of Obesity. 2012;**36**(8):1017–1024. DOI: 10.1038/ijo.2011.192

[17] Loos RJF, Yeo GSH. The genetics of obesity: From discovery to biology. Nature Reviews Genetics. 2022;**23** (2):120–133. DOI: 10.1038/s41576-021-00414-z

[18] King SE, Skinner MK. Epigenetic transgenerational inheritance of obesity susceptibility. Trends in Endocrinology and Metabolism TEM. 2020;**31**(7): 478–494. DOI: 10.1016/j.tem.2020.02.009

[19] Kershaw EE, Flier JS. Adipose tissue as an endocrine organ. The Journal of Clinical Endocrinology and Metabolism. 2004;**89**(6):2548–2556. DOI: 10.1210/jc.2004-0395

[20] Timper K, Brüning JC. Hypothalamic circuits regulating appetite and Energy Homeostasis: Pathways to obesity. Disease Models & Mechanisms. 2017;**10**(6):679–689. DOI: 10.1242/dmm.026609

[21] Diéguez C, Da Boit K, Novelle MG, Martínez de Morentin PB, Nogueiras R, López M. New insights in ghrelin orexigenic effect. Frontiers of Hormone Research. 2010;**38**:196–205. DOI: 10.1159/000318511

[22] Martin AM, Sun EW, Keating DJ. Mechanisms controlling hormone secretion in human gut and its relevance to metabolism. The Journal of Endocrinology. 2019;**244**(1):R1–R15. DOI: 10.1530/JOE-19-0399

[23] Smarkusz-Zarzecka J, Ostrowska L, Radziszewska M. The impact of environmental factors on the secretion of gastrointestinal hormones. Nutrients. 2025;**17**(15):2544. DOI: 10.3390/nu17152544

[24] Izquierdo AG, Crujeiras AB, Casanueva FF, Carreira MC. Leptin, obesity, and leptin resistance: Where are we 25 years later? Nutrients. 2019;**11**(11):2704. DOI: 10.3390/nu11112704

[25] Berthoud HR, Münzberg H, Morrison CD. Blaming the brain for obesity: Integration of hedonic and homeostatic mechanisms. Gastroenterology. 2017;**152**(7): 1728–1738. DOI: 10.1053/j.gastro.2016.12.050

[26] Zwick RK, Guerrero-Juarez CF, Horsley V, Plikus MV. Anatomical,

physiological, and functional diversity of adipose tissue. Cell Metabolism. 2018;**27**(1):68–83. DOI: 10.1016/j.cmet.2017.12.002

[27] Oikonomou EK, Antoniades C. The role of adipose tissue in cardiovascular health and disease. Nature Reviews. Cardiology. 2019;**16**(2):83–99. DOI: 10.1038/s41569-018-0097-6

[28] Xu S, Lu F, Gao J, Yuan Y. Inflammation-mediated metabolic regulation in adipose tissue. Obesity Reviews: an Official Journal of the International Association for the Study of Obesity. 2024;**25**(6):e13724. DOI: 10.1111/obr.13724

[29] Lee CJ, Sears CL, Maruthur N. Gut microbiome and its role in obesity and insulin resistance. Annals of the New York Academy of Sciences. 2020;**1461**(1):37–52. DOI: 10.1111/nyas.14107

[30] Sankararaman S, Noriega K, Velayuthan S, Sferra T, Martindale R. Gut microbiome and its impact on obesity and obesity-related disorders. Current Gastroenterology Reports. 2023;**25**(2):31–44. DOI: 10.1007/s11894-022-00859-0

[31] Meldrum DR, Morris MA, Gambone JC. Obesity pandemic: Causes, consequences, and solutions-but do we have the will? Fertility and Sterility. 2017;**107**(4):833–839. DOI: 10.1016/j.fertnstert.2017.02.104

[32] Danesh Doost H, Jounaghani MN, Riahi R, Heidari-Beni M, Hosseini M, Sharifianjazi F, Kelishadi R. Association of genetic, environmental, and nutritional factors with metabolic phenotypes of obesity: A scoping review. Journal of Obesity. 2025;8472196. DOI: 10.1155/job e/8472196

[33] World Health Organization. Obesity: Preventing and managing the global epidemic. Report of a WHO consultation. WHO Technical Report Series 894. Geneva: WHO; 2000

[34] National Institutes of Health. Clinical guidelines on the identification, evaluation, and treatment of overweight and obesity in adults: The evidence report. Obes Res. 1998;**6**(Suppl 2): 51S–209S

[35] Dicker D, Karpati T, Promislow S, Reges O. Implications of the European Association for the Study of Obesity's New Framework Definition of Obesity: Prevalence and Association With All-Cause Mortality. Annals of internal medicine. 2025;**178**(8):1065–1072. DOI: 10.7326/ANNALS-24-02547

[36] Kyle UG, Earthman CP, Pichard C, Coss-Bu JA. Body composition during growth in children: Limitations and perspectives of bioelectrical impedance analysis. European Journal of Clinical Nutrition. 2015;**69**(12):1298–1305. DOI: 10.1038/ejcn.2015.86

[37] de Gonzalez A B, Hartge P, Cerhan JR, et al. Body-mass index and mortality among 1.46 million white adults. New England Journal of Medicine 2010;**363**:2211–2219

[38] Romero-Corral A, Somers VK, Sierra-Johnson J, et al. Accuracy of body mass index in diagnosing obesity in the adult general population. International Journal of Obesity (London) 2008;**32**:959–966

[39] Janssen I, Katzmarzyk PT, Ross R.Waist circumference and not Body Mass Index explains obesity-related health risk. American Journal of Clinical Nutrition. 2004;**79**(3):379–384

[40] Kolb H. Obese visceral fat tissue inflammation: From protective to detrimental? BMC Medicine. 2022;**20**(1):494. DOI: 10.1186/s12916-022-02672-y

[41] National Academies of Sciences, Engineering, and Medicine; Health and medicine; division; food and nutrition board; roundtable on obesity solutions; Callahan EA, editor. Translating Knowledge of Foundational Drivers of Obesity into Practice: Proceedings of a Workshop Series. Washington (DC): National Academies Press (US); 2023. **10**, The Science, Strengths, and Limitations of Body Mass Index. Available from: https://www.ncbi.nlm.nih.gov/books/NBK594362/

[42] AMA adopts new policy clarifying role of BMI as a measure in medicine. American Medical Association. 2023, June 14. Available from: https://www.ama-assn.org/press-center/ama-press-releases/ama-adopts-new-policy-clarifying-role-bmi-measure-medicine

[43] Heymsfield SB, Peterson CM, Thomas DM, Heo M, Schuna Jr JM. Why are there race/ethnic differences in adult body mass index-adiposity relationships? A quantitative critical review. Obesity Reviews: an Official Journal of the International Association for the Study of Obesity. 2016;**17**(3):262–275. DOI: 10.1111/obr.12358

[44] Li Z, Daniel S, Fujioka K, Umashanker D. Obesity among Asian American People in the United States: A review. Obesity (Silver Spring Md.). 2023;**31**(2):316–328. DOI: 10.1002/oby.23639

[45] Ashwell M, Gunn P, Gibson S. Waist-to-height ratio is a better screening tool than waist circumference and BMI for adult cardiometabolic risk factors: Systematic review and meta-analysis. Obes Rev. 2012;**13**(3):275–286

[46] Fields DA, Goran MI, McCrory MA.Body-composition assessment via air-displacement plethysmography in adults and children: A review. American Journal of Clinical Nutrition. 2002;**75**(3):453–467

[47] Wells JC, Fewtrell MS. Measuring body composition. Archives of Disease in Childhood. 2006;**91**(7):612–617. DOI: 10.1136/adc.2005.085522

[48] Kaul S, Rothney MP, Peters DM, Wacker WK, Davis CE, Shapiro MD, Ergun DL. Dual-energy X-ray absorptiometry for quantification of visceral fat. Obesity (Silver Spring, Md.). 2012;**20**(6):1313–1318. DOI: 10.1038/oby.2011.393

[49] Nana A, et al. DXA: Technical considerations for accurate assessment in humans. Eur J Clin Nutr 2015; **69**:730–741

[50] Prado CM, Heymsfield SB.Lean tissue imaging: A new era for nutritional assessment and intervention. Journal of Parenteral and Enteral Nutrition. 2014;**38**(8):940–953

[51] Lee SY, Gallagher D. Assessment methods in human body composition. Current Opinion Clinical Nutrition and Metabolic Care. 2017;**20**(5):452–457

[52] Kyle UG, et al. Bioelectrical impedance analysis—part I: Review of principles and methods. Clinical Nutrition 2004;**23**:1226–1243

[53] Earthman CP. Body composition tools for assessment of adult malnutrition at the bedside: A tutorial on research considerations and clinical

applications. Journal of Parenteral and Enteral Nutrition. 2015;**39**(7):787–822

[54] Ng BK, et al. Detailed 3D body shape features predict adiposity and body fat distribution better than traditional anthropometric measures. American Journal of Clinical Nutrition 2020;**112**:406–416

[55] Kyle TK, Dhurandhar EJ, Allison DB.Regarding obesity as a disease: Evolving policies and their implications. Endocrinol Metab Clin North Am. 2016;**45**(3):511–520

[56] Sharma AM, Kushner RF. A proposed clinical staging system for obesity. Int J Obes. 2009;**33**(3):289–295

[57] Zhang X, Ha S, Lau HC, Yu J. Excess body weight: Novel insights into its roles in obesity comorbidities. Seminars in Cancer Biology. 2023;**92**:16–27. DOI: 10.1016/j.semcancer.2023.03.008

[58] Powell-Wiley TM, Poirier P, Burke LE, Després JP, Gordon-Larsen P, Lavie CJ, Lear SA, Ndumele CE, Neeland IJ, Sanders P, St-Onge MP; American Heart Association Council on Lifestyle and Cardiometabolic Health; Council on Cardiovascular and Stroke Nursing; Council on Clinical Cardiology; Council on Epidemiology and Prevention; and Stroke Council. Obesity and cardiovascular disease: A scientific statement from the American Heart Association. Circulation. 2021;**143**(21):e984–e1010. DOI: 10.1161/CIR.0000000000000973

[59] Reyes-Angel J, Kaviany P, Rastogi D, Forno E. Obesity-related asthma in children and adolescents. The Lancet. Child & Adolescent Health. 2022;**6**(10):713–724. DOI: 10.1016/S2352-4642(22)00185-7

[60] Nedunchezhiyan U, Varughese I, Sun AR, Wu X, Crawford R, Prasadam I. Obesity, inflammation, and immune system in osteoarthritis. Frontiers in Immunology. 2022;**13**:907750. DOI: 10.3389/fimmu.2022.907750

[61] Ennab F, Atiomo W. Obesity and female infertility. Best practice & research. Clinical Obstetrics & Gynaecology. 2023;**89**:102336. DOI: 10.1016/j.bpobgyn.2023.102336

[62] Adult clinical practice guideline. Obesity Canada. (2025, September 18). https://obesitycanada.ca/healthcare-professionals/adult-clinical-practice-guideline/

[63] Pedersen S, Manjoo P, Dash S, Jain A, Pearce N, Poddar M. Pharmacotherapy for obesity management in adults: 2025 clinical practice guideline update. Canadian Medical Association Journal. 2025. Available from: https://www.cmaj.ca/content/197/27/E797 [Accessed: 2025-November]

[64] Nishikawa H, Asai A, Fukunishi S, Takeuchi T, Goto M, Ogura T, Nakamura S, Kakimoto K, Miyazaki T, Nishiguchi S, Higuchi K. Screening tools for sarcopenia. Vivo (Athens, Greece). 2021;**35**(6):3001–3009. DOI: 10.21873/invivo.12595

[65] Dębski J, Przybyłowski J, Skibiak K, Czerwińska M, Walędziak M, Różańska-Walędziak A. Depression and obesity-do we know everything about it? A narrative review. Nutrients. 2024;**16**(19):3383. DOI: 10.3390/nu16193383

[66] Liu H, Dong H, Zhou Y, Jin M, Hao H, Yuan Y, Jia H. The association between metabolic score for visceral fat and depression in overweight or obese

individuals: Evidence from NHANES. Frontiers in Endocrinology. 2024;**15**:1482003. DOI: 10.3389/fendo.2024.1482003

[67] Moizé V, Graham Y, Salas XR, Balcells M. Motivational interviewing (MI) in obesity care: Cultivating person-centered and supportive clinical conversations to reduce stigma: A narrative review. Obesity Science & Practice. 2025;**11**(1): e70057. DOI: 10.1002/osp4.70057

[68] Sharma AM, Kushner RF. A proposed clinical staging system for obesity. International Journal of Obesity. Nature 2009;**33**(3):289–295. DOI: 10.1038/ijo.2009.2

[69] Swaleh R, McGuckin T, Myroniuk TW, Manca D, Lee K, Sharma AM, Campbell-Scherer D, Yeung RO. Using the Edmonton obesity staging system in the real world: A feasibility study based on cross-sectional data. CMAJ Open. 2021;**9**(4):E1141–E1148. DOI: 10.9778/cmajo.20200231

[70] Grammatikopoulou MG, Chourdakis M, Gkiouras K, Roumeli P, Poulimeneas D, Apostolidou E, Chountalas I, Tirodimos I, Filippou O, Papadakou-Lagogianni S, Dardavessis T. Edmonton obesity staging system among pediatric patients: A validation and obesogenic risk factor analysis. Journal of Endocrinological Investigation. 2018;**41**(8):947–957. DOI: 10.1007/s40618-017-0821-9

[71] Kuk JL, Ardern CI, Church TS, Sharma AM, Padwal R, Sui X, Blair SN. Edmonton obesity staging system: Association with weight history and mortality risk. Applied Physiology, Nutrition, and Metabolism = Physiologie Appliquee, Nutrition Et Metabolisme. 2011;**36**(4):570–576. DOI: 10.1139/h11-058

[72] Kodsi R, Chimoriya R, Medveczky D, Grudzinskas K, Atlantis E, Tahrani AA, Kormas N, Piya MK. Clinical use of the Edmonton obesity staging system for the assessment of weight management outcomes in people with class 3 obesity. Nutrients. 2022;**14**(5):967. DOI: 10.3390/nu14050967

[73] Edmonton Obesity Staging System (EOSS). MDCalc. n d. https://www.mdcalc.com/calc/10536/edmonton-obesity-staging-system-eoss [Accessed: 2025-November]

[74] O'Shea D, Kahan S, Lennon L, Breen C. Practical approaches to treating obesity: Patient and healthcare professional perspectives. Advances in Therapy. 2021;**38**(7):4138–4150. DOI: 10.1007/s12325-021-01748-0

[75] Kaplan LM, Golden A, Jinnett K, Kolotkin RL, Kyle TK, Look M, Nadglowski J, O'Neil PM, Parry T, Tomaszewski KJ, Stevenin B, Lilleøre SK, Dhurandhar NV. Perceptions of barriers to effective obesity care: Results from the National Action study. Obesity (Silver Spring, Md.). 2018;**26**(1):61–69. DOI: 10.1002/oby.22054

[76] Yumuk V, Tsigos C, Fried M, Schindler K, Busetto L, Micic D, Toplak H; Obesity Management Task Force of the European Association for the Study of Obesity. European guidelines for obesity management in adults. Obesity Facts. 2015;**8**(6): 402–424. DOI: 10.1159/000442721

[77] Vo DK, Trinh KTL. Emerging biomarkers in metabolomics: Advancements in precision health and disease diagnosis. International Journal of Molecular Sciences. 2024;**25**(23):13190. DOI: 10.3390/ijms252313190

[78] Clemente-Suárez VJ, Redondo-Flórez L, Beltrán-Velasco AI, Martín-Rodríguez A, Martínez-Guardado I, Navarro-Jiménez E, Laborde-Cárdenas CC, Tornero-Aguilera JF. The role of adipokines in health and disease. Biomedicines. 2023;**11**(5):1290. DOI: 10.3390/biomedicines11051290

[79] Ulusoy-Gezer HG, Rakıcıoğlu N, The future of obesity management through precision nutrition: Putting the individual at the center. Curr Nutr Rep. 2024;**13**:455–477. DOI: 10.1007/s13668-024-00550-y

[80] Kupila SKE, Joki A, Suojanen LU, Pietiläinen KH. The effectiveness of eHealth interventions for weight loss and weight loss maintenance in adults with overweight or obesity: A systematic review of systematic reviews. Current Obesity Reports. 2023;**12**(3):371–394. DOI: 10.1007/s13679-023-00515-2

[81] Fløl o TN, Tørris C, Riiser K, Almendingen K, Chew HSJ, Fosså A, Albertini Früh E, Hennessy E, Leung MM, Misvær N, Pavel N, Sundar TKB, Sæterstrand TM, Torbjørnsen A, Løyland B, Holmen H. Digital health interventions to treat overweight and obesity in children and adolescents: An umbrella review. Obesity Reviews: an Official Journal of the International Association for the Study of Obesity. 2025;**26**(6):e13905. DOI: 10.1111/obr.13905

[82] Johnson H, Huang D, Liu V, Ammouri MA, Jacobs C, El-Osta A. Impact of digital engagement on weight loss outcomes in obesity management among individuals using GLP-1 and dual GLP-1/GIP receptor agonist therapy: Retrospective cohort service evaluation study. Journal of Medical Internet Research. 2025;**27**: e69466. DOI: 10.2196/69466

[83] Whitehall JM, Cook EJ, Vseteckova J, Jones K, Pappas Y, Donald L, Chater AM. A systematic review of influences on engagement with remote health interventions targeting weight management for individuals living with excess weight. International Journal of Obesity. 2005;**49**(8):1427–1468. DOI: 10.1038/s41366-025-01811-8

[84] Donnelly JE, Smith BK, Dunn L, Mayo MM, Jacobsen DJ, Stewart EE, Gibson C, Sullivan DK. Comparison of a phone vs clinic approach to achieve 10% weight loss. International Journal of Obesity. 2007;**31**(8):1270–1276. DOI: 10.1038/sj.ijo.0803568

[85] Rubino F, Cummings DE, Eckel RH, Cohen RV, Wilding JPH, Brown WA, Stanford FC, Batterham RL, Farooqi IS, Farpour-Lambert NJ, le Roux CW, Sattar N, Baur LA, Morrison KM, Misra A, Kadowaki T, Tham KW, Sumithran P, Garvey WT, Kirwan JP, Mingrone G. Definition and diagnostic criteria of clinical obesity. The Lancet: Diabetes & Endocrinology. 2025;**13**(3):221–262. DOI: 10.1016/S2213-8587(24)00316-4

[86] Fourman LT, Awwad A, Gutiérrez-Sacristán A, Dash CA, Johnson JE, Thistle AK, Chahal N, Stockman SL, Toribio M, Anekwe C, Gattu AK, Grinspoon SK. Implications of a new obesity definition among the all of us cohort. JAMA Network Open. 2025;**8**(10):e2537619. DOI: 10.1001/jamanetworkopen.2025.376191

[87] Furth SL, Colhoun HM, Kanbay M, Kukla A, Lim LL, MacLaughlin HL, Navaneethan SD, Shroff R, Stenvinkel P, Cheung M, King JM, Grams ME, Jadoul M, Rossing P; Conference Participants. The relationship between obesity and chronic kidney disease: Conclusions from a Kidney Disease: Improving Global Outcomes (KDIGO) controversies conference. Kidney International. 2025;**S0085-2538** (25):00771 4. DOI: 10.1016/j.kint.2025.09.019

[88] Kittleson MM, Benjamin EJ, Blumer V, Harrington J, Januzzi JL, McMurray JJV, Vest AR. 2025 ACC scientific statement on the management of obesity in adults with heart failure: A report of the American College of Cardiology. Journal of the American College of Cardiology. 2025;**86** (20):1953–1975. DOI: 10.1016/j.jacc.2025.05.008

[89] Hong S, Park CY. From old to new: A comprehensive review of obesity diagnostic criteria and their implications. Endocrinology and Metabolism (Seoul Korea). 2025;**40** (4):517–522. DOI: 10.3803/EnM.2025.2590

[90] Dicker D, Karpati T, Promislow S, Reges O. Implications of the European Association for the Study of Obesity's new framework definition of obesity: Prevalence and association with All-Cause mortality. Annals of Internal Medicine. 2025;**178**(8):1065–1072. DOI: 10.7326/ANNALS-24-02547

Chapter 2

The Impact of Body Mass Index on All-Cause Mortality Worldwide: A Mathematical Demonstration of Clinical Bias Regarding Causal Risk from Body Composition Measures

Angel Martin Castellanos

Abstract

Body mass index (BMI) defined obesity as characterized by excess fat mass (FM). In associating BMI with mortality, different J-shaped curve patterns have been repeatedly observed. However, BMI refers not only to FM but also to fat-free mass (FFM). We aimed to demonstrate that differences between FM and FFM can mask the use of any mean BMI. Novel mathematical and anthropometric considerations about relationships between FM and FFM were explored. A review of studies on millions of participants associating BMI and newer variables, such as the ratios and mean differences between the two components, with all-cause mortality was conducted. The means of all variables were newly pooled in each of six BMI categories, separately by sex. If, after checking for associations, systematic differences between FM and FFM remained, this indicated that body components differed, and causality could not be assumed. A linear dose–response analysis of FM and FFM with all-cause mortality was found. A significant difference in all associations was demonstrated (p <0.001). A risk equivalence between BMI and FFM only in underweight was demonstrated in either sex (FFM >90%; FM <10%; p <0.001). In women with class III obesity, the same sensitivity for BMI and excess FM was proven (FM% > FFM%; p < 0.001). In all means of BMI for the associations FM and FFM were significantly different (p <0.001). In any BMI-associated risk, a protective overestimate of FFM over FM consistently occurred. In all BMI cut-offs repeatedly observed for defining population risk, the true causal risk always appeared biased confusing clinicians for a long time.

Keywords: anthropometric, bias, body composition, body mass index, obesity, mortality risk.

1. Introduction

Obesity is a well-recognized major risk factor for cardiovascular disease (CVD) and several health conditions that involve clinical practice and impact both all-cause mortality and morbidity. Body mass index (BMI) has been widely used over the past decades as a measure of obesity [1], related to excessive fat deposits that can impair health. It is highly utilized in epidemiological studies, classification, as well as international guidelines related to obesity definitions and management. Of importance, a BMI in overweight/obesity ranges is associated with an increased risk of CVD and other noncommunicable diseases such as diabetes, musculoskeletal disorders, specific cancers, and even cardiovascular and cause-specific mortality [1–15]. Moreover, being underweight is also associated with adverse health outcomes, including diabetes, specific cancers, and other types of cause-specific mortality [5–13]. Thus, a nadir of mortality has been shown in individuals within normal weight (>20 to <25 kg/m^2) or in overweight (≥25 to <30 kg/m^2) ranges [1–13]. Consequently, since last century, the relationship between BMI and mortality in many epidemiological studies follows an unexpected U- or J-shaped curve ("obesity paradox") [1–15] that directly complicates the clinical application of BMI to control holistic health. In other words, undernutrition statuses and overweight/obesity have been associated with adverse mortality outcomes and different causes of death, which may be visualized on the left and right branches of the different curve patterns [1–17]. However, the excess mortality linked to normal–low or high values of BMI may be considered a biased causal association if high-risk body composition and real adiposity are not well compared beyond BMI [18, 19]. In this approach, knowledge about human body composition turns out to be essential because total body weight may be organized at a tissue-system level where the adipose tissue or fat mass (FM) is a component, and the fat-free mass (FFM), which includes muscle and bone masses as well as visceral organs and other tissues, corresponds to the rest of body weight, constituting the other metabolically opposite component [16–20]. From this insight, it is obvious that BMI includes two distinct components relative to stature in squared meters. Expressed in this manner, BMI is equal to weight in kilograms (i.e., FM + FFM) divided by height squared in meters. Thus, FM index (FMI; i.e., FM/height (m)^2) and FFM index (FFMI; i.e., FFM/height (m)^2) make up two indices that contribute to total BMI in unequal proportions (FFMI ≠ FMI), either in healthy adults or in categories below class II and III obesity (<40 kg/m^2), in which FFMI is always higher than FMI [16–20]. In addition, it is well known that BMI does not discriminate between FM and FFM (and their distribution), nor does it distinguish between visceral and subcutaneous fat, or reflect body shape or a risk volume per unit of height.

From another perspective, the relationships between body components, rather than BMI, will ultimately shed the most light on this issue of mortality and health risk [16–19]. Evidence supports that a high FM (within a moderate–high BMI) and reduced FFM (within a low BMI and undernutrition) may be independently associated with increased mortality, with both body components showing opposite joint effects on all-cause mortality [10, 16–28]. It is clear that body composition is highly variable among individuals identified with the same risk exposure level based on their BMI [16–20]. Thus, regarding causal risk association, a more serious clinical problem is that individuals with the same BMI can have widely differing amounts of FM and FFM, with both factors conferring opposite health outcomes

[16–20, 22–31]. In this issue, the mathematical relation of equivalence between the two concerned components is a key concept for specifying whether FM and FFM within BMI are the same with respect to a given risk when defining different BMI categories. This is important because the concept of treating overweight or obesity categories to reduce the risk of cardiovascular complications is becoming established in clinical practice, irrespective of treating other obesity-related cardiovascular risk factors, such as dyslipidemia, hypertension, and diabetes. Clinically, it is not the same to lose weight and decrease FM percentage as it is to decrease weight and BMI, especially when accompanied by a reduced total musculoskeletal component (i.e., the FFM component being decreased, and yet the total FFM percentage increasing).

To date, different studies have examined mortality risk in relation to body composition measured directly (e.g., by using dual-energy X-ray absorptiometry or imaging technologies) or indirectly (e.g., by using anthropometric prediction equations or bioelectrical impedance), with research findings not entirely consistent [16, 22–31]. Overall, although the relationships between FM and FFM with mortality are still inconclusive, since BMI conceals the proportions of FM and FFM, it is impossible to ensure any causal risk from a mean BMI used as the nominal difference of a pre-post difference within a parallel group analysis, whether both components present differences in the risk consideration between groups (or categories) in a paired analysis being compared [18, 19]. Hence, only a rigorous interpretation of the real risk expressed by BMI and the two intrinsically related body components could avoid confusing or paradoxical information. An excessive FFM component in individuals who have a high BMI and normal FM percentage should never justify an increased health risk. Conversely, weight loss due to reducing FFM may lead to a lower range of BMI and less proportional FM loss, and thus, mean or median values of FFM and FM may show opposing associations with all-cause mortality [16–18, 20, 22, 24–30]. The fact that being overweight may be associated with a higher cardiometabolic risk and simultaneously show a lower all-cause mortality risk might indicate methodological flaws due to between-group comparisons for different high-risk body compositions [13, 18, 19, 32–34]. This is because the balance and anthropometric risk consideration for the two body components within each BMI category turn out to be key beyond traditional risk factors [16–19].

From mathematical observations in anthropometrically healthy adults and in those with overweight and class I obesity, it is possible to say that anthropometrically or technologicallymeasured FM and FFM always presented inequality [1, 16–24, 29, 32–34]. Thus, mathematically, FFM is usually higher than FM within BMI, and then, any FM-to-FFM ratio (FMFFMR) is <1 (a proper abstract fraction, where the numerator and the fraction never refer to a whole) [33]. So, BMI should not have a univocal biological risk concept when assessing health outcomes, at least without balancing the two components between groups being compared [18, 19, 32–34]. In fact, the health risk depends on total body composition rather than any component in isolation, which may or may not be statistically associated with the overall risk. This is because each component is an inseparable part of the body's structure, but participates in the body composition of risk in a different way. This means that FM and FFM may independently be associated with any health risk, while any BMI cut-off may or may not indicate a true high-risk body composition.

We aimed to mathematically demonstrate that differences in body composition from each BMI risk category can mask the use of any BMI cut-off when evaluated in relation to all-cause mortality.

2. Mathematical and anthropometric considerations regarding FM and FFM within BMI

After the advancement of knowledge, by using weight, waist circumference, and height, it is possible to predict FM [26, 27] for determining relationships with body composition. Thus, predicted FM may be calculated using the validated sex-specific anthropometric prediction equations developed by the NHANES [27]: For women: FM (kg) = 11.817 + 0.041 × age (years) – 0.199 × height (cm) + 0.610 × weight (kg) + 0.044 × WC (cm) + 0.388 (if Mexican) + 0.073 (if Hispanic) – 1.187 (if Black) + 0.325 (if other race). For men: FM (kg) = –18.592 – 0.009 × age (years) – 0.080 × height (cm) + 0.226 × weight (kg) + 0.387 × WC (cm) + 0.080 (if Mexican) – 0.188 (if Hispanic) – 0.483 (if Black) + 1.050 (if other race). Similarly, waist circumference and height may be used for calculating a relative abdominal volume from the waist-to-height ratio [19, 32–35] or, after validation by dual-energy X-ray absorptiometry, these simple measurements may be used for estimating a relative FM [36], with both abdominal volume and FM being linked to a high-risk body composition. Relative FM can be obtained in agreement with the formula: 64 – (20 × height [m]/WC [m]) + (12 × sex); sex = 0 and 1 for male and female, respectively [36]. FFM can be calculated by subtracting FM from weight.

Of particular importance is the FMFFMR as well as its inverse (i.e., 1 divided by FMFFMR = the FFM-to-FM ratio) because, in anthropometrically healthy adults, both ratios mathematically are always <1 and >1, respectively, without it involving any putative risk or protective effect, either by age, sex, or ethnicity. Additionally, FM and FFM percentages never express equality for a whole as a mathematical object, at least before class II–III obesity, where FM percentage is always <50% of weight [16, 18, 33, 34]. Thereby, FFM > FM is a natural inequality that responds to a linear equation as a true premise: FFM = FM + x (in kg), where subtracting FFM by FM allows us to calculate "x" as a unit of mass (x = FFM – FM: $x > 0$), with its standard value always being higher in men than in women [16–20]. On this basis, only when "x" is mathematically zero is there equality (i.e., FFM = FM; FMFFMR = 1; FFM-to-FM ratio = 1), and only then are FM and BMI risk equivalent for representing a whole as a true conclusion [18]. This means that in any population study pointing out a BMI risk cut-off above the underweight category, only those individuals having an FMFFMR ≥ 1 and FFM-to-FM ratio ≤ 1 may present the same overall risk as being a true premise. This is because at-risk individuals from a given mean BMI may have an FMFFMR < 1 and FFM-to-FM ratio > 1, while being false positives, and then, its BMI cut-off of reference appears with clinical misinformation.

FM and FFM values with respect to total weight represent the same as FMI and FFMI, respectively, with respect to total BMI. Thus, FM versus FFM, and FMI versus FFMI, in kg and kg/m^2, respectively, represent a corresponding percentage with respect to 100% of weight and BMI, as appropriate. In addition, an "x" value, as the difference between FFM and FM, corresponds to an "x" percentage as the difference between FM and FFM percentages. In this approach, values, percentages, and ratios for the corresponding variables express the same concept when assessing risk from total weight or BMI, as appropriate; however, different "x" values may correspond to equal "x" percentages, and vice versa. This is because initial "x" values and percentages may or may not vary, respectively, with respect to different final weights and BMIs. Thus, FM and FFM values may vary without it meaning the same variation in the final percentages, on which the true joint risk depends. Hence, different beneficial or harmful pathophysiological variations for FFM and FM values on health depend on genetic and acquired body composition, but any variation in the FFM percentage mathematically affects the percentage of FM, and vice versa, and thus, the causal risk measured from equal–different BMIs may correspond to different–equal body compositions.

Epidemiologically, FM and FFM percentages are intrinsically related factors, while being complementary and metabolically opposite parts integrating a unique risk indicator, such as BMI, which does not differentiate the body composition of risk that affects the entire organism. Moreover, variations in the values of one component may or may not affect the percentages of both components. Mathematically, we may have two situations at both ends of the BMI range (i.e., in underweight [BMI < 18.5] and beyond class II–III obesity [BMI > 35 to > 40]), where "x" values and percentages may be negative ($x < 0$), (i.e. a reduced FFM contributing to the highest percentage of weight in underweight range or an increased FM being higher than FFM in severe obesity) [1, 18]. First, in underweight ranges, weight loss leads to reduced musculoeskeletal mass, and FFM mathematically must take a negative sign, irrespective of FM being low or even zero. In this situation, FFM percentage is always higher than 50% of weight, and FMFFMR and its inverse are < 1 and > 1, respectively; in mathematical terms: "x" = (−FFM) − (±FM): "x" = $-x$: "x" < 0. This is because toward underweight ranges FFM usually decreases, while being the largest contributor to final total weight; and FM hardly increases as being low and the lowest contributor to final weight. Second, beyond class II/III obesity, weight gain might lead to excess FM beyond 50% of weight, and the inequality between FM and FFM (i.e., FMFFMR > 1 and FFM-to-FM ratio < 1) would be fulfilled, but only then, in mathematical terms: "x" = FFM − FM: "x" = $-x$: "x" < 0 [18],. In this situation, high FM is directly associated with mortality and probably largely causal, irrespective of FFM. Thus, any conclusion for the overall risk from BMI and high adiposity may hold true in all individuals who meet that mathematical criterion. In contrast, when in underweight range "x" is negative and FMFFMR < 1, we find a low FM and reduced FFM (with a FFM-to-FM ratio > 1), which biologically justifies that FFM may inversely be associated with mortality and probably largely causal, irrespective of FM. Moreover, in underweight, FM and BMI may never be risk equivalent from an FMFFMR < 1 [18]. In fact, only in collated underweight ranges with an FM close to zero, FFM and BMI may mathematically be risk equivalent for the same causal risk, and any conclusion for an overall risk from a mean BMI lower than 18.5 kg/m^2 (and low FFM) may hold true in all individuals, irrespective of FM [17, 18].

Biologically, if in the risk assessment by excess FM an adjustment for FFM is uncontrolled, any BMI cut-off could be prone to the generation of bias because of between-group or between-risk category comparisons never accounting for the same high-risk body compositions [18, 19, 32–34]. Of course, only in large studies including enough participants and deaths at both ends of the BMI spectrum could a demonstration of bias be completely verified. That way, causal association criteria such as biological plausibility, consistency, sensitivity, specificity, and anthropometric coherence from the body components within BMI would appear fulfilled.

Unfortunately, the statistical models and outcomes of associating BMI with all-cause mortality never captured this dynamic of causal risk, and the normal differences between FM and FFM were always omitted in all positive or negative pathophysiological variations for BMI [18, 19, 33].

3. Theoretical causal risk from the relationships between FM and FFM percentages within BMI across the entire risk spectrum

Despite FM and FFM being significantly different in anthropometrically healthy individuals [18, 19, 33], a theoretical causal risk between zero (minimum) and 100 as a whole (maximum) for FM and FFM percentages moving in opposite directions would make it possible to capture a dynamic of mortality risk. As opposed to the universal U- or J-shaped curve pattern for the association of BMI and all-cause mortality, it is mathematically and epidemiologically possible to draw a linear function (mortality risk line) for the ratios between FM and FFM within BMI, where FM and FFM percentages show opposing causal associations across the entire risk spectrum (i.e., as FM percentage increases, FFM percentage decreases and vice versa) (see **Figure 1**) [17–19, 21–33]. In mathematics, from a linear equation ($y = mx + b$), the "m" slope can measure the change in FMFFMR (as the y variable) per unit in BMI (as the x variable). That way, values for FMFFMR may be described in an increasing line that goes from left to right between a minimum (value of zero) and a maximum of risk (value of ≥1). In reverse, the FFM-to-FM ratio would quantify a minimum (value of ≤1) at the top and a maximum risk (value of 100) at the bottom in a decreasing line that goes from right to left, while BMI decreases (see **Figure 1**). Thus, any line between two Cartesian points will always draw an "m" slope that depends on the variations of FM and FFM (y-axis) within the variations of BMI (x-axis) (i.e., $m = \Delta y/\Delta x$).

From this novel insight, in the underweight range after weight loss and having a reduced FFM (FFM minus FM = "x" = –x), FM percentage would show the minimum risk (FM = 0% – 1% of the weight) with an FMFFMR value of approximately 0.0 or 0.01. At the opposite extreme, a maximum risk of 100 for FM percentage as a whole would quantify an FMFFMR value of ≥1 (i.e., FM ≥ 50%; FFM ≤ 50%), with this ratio being an improper fraction, and BMI directly depending on the numerator (FM), while "x" is equal to zero or even negative if FM > FFM [18]. Of note, when FMFFMR = 1 (FM [50%] + FFM [50%] = 100% of weight), FM percentage captures 100% of the risk for having the same sensitivity as BMI, and any "x" value is always located in severe obesity. Similarly, when FMFFMR = 1, the "m" slope in the linear equation is a squared diagonal with a value of 1, where the y variable = x variable (i.e., FM and FFM within BMI have the same percentage and the same risk consideration, and FMFFMR and BMI also have the same sensitivity).

As described here, at the end of the underweight range, FFM percentage would quantify an FFM-to-FM ratio value close to 100 (maximum risk for FFM percentage as a whole: FFM ≈ 100% of weight), whereas at the opposite end, the risk is minimized by quantifying an FFM-to-FM ratio value of ≥ 1 (FFM ≥ 50%; FM ≤ 50%), with the FFM-to-FM ratio still being an improper fraction. BMI is then directly dependent on the numerator (FFM). Of note, when the FFM-to-FM ratio = 100 (FM = 0%), FFM percentage captures 100% of the risk, having the same sensitivity as BMI. Mathematically, the minimum risk exposure level from FMFFMR, being between 0.0 and 0.01, coincides with the maximum difference between FM and FFM percentages (i.e., the highest "x" percentage being located in the

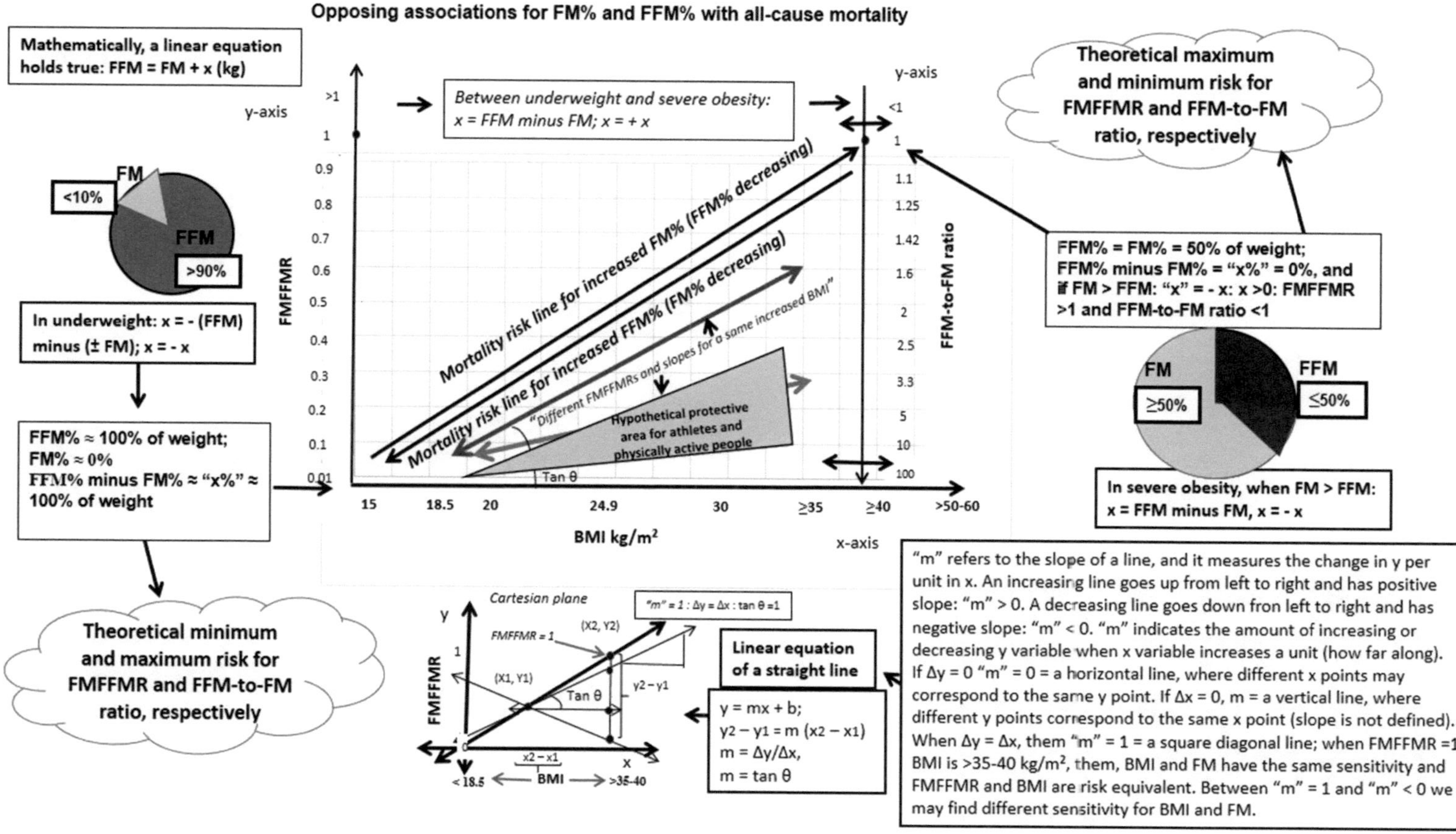

Figure 1.
*Theoretical causal risk for the association of FM and FFM percentages with all-cause mortality. Positive and negative linear functions for FMFFMR and FFM-to-FM ratio, respectively, across the entire risk spectrum from BMI. Mathematical explanations about the linear equations. BMI: body mass index; FM: fat mass; FMFFMR: fat mass-to-fat-free mass ratio; FFM: fat-free mass. * Any BMI category may be found in the overall population and across the entire risk spectrum. Until the maximum risk exposure level can be demonstrated, both ratios and the slope of the respective linear equations depend on the final variations for both FM% and FFM% in each BMI-defined range. ** To demonstrate a theoretical minimum and maximum risk level for both FMFFMR and FFM-to-FM ratio within BMI, a significant number of participants at both ends of the risk spectrum must be included in any population study. *** While any BMI value may or may not be invariably in the same category, the value of the ratios and the "m" slope of a segment of line may vary. This depends on the body compositions of the selected population, which must be differentiated by body size and sex. **** In mathematics, the point–slope formula or the slope–intercept formula may be described on a Cartesian plane. By analogy, change in FMFFMR (as the y-axis) and change in BMI (as the x-axis) may be applied in each segment of line for understanding the different slopes that can be found from the different variations in the two body components. Source: This theoretical graphic was created by the author, who has the copyright.*

underweight range). On the contrary, the maximum risk level from an FMFFMR value of ≥ 1 coincides with the minimum difference between FM and FFM percentages (i.e., "*x*" percentage being approximately equal to zero or even negative if FM > FFM), with their "*x*" values always located in severe obesity. In this approach, it is possible to find different body compositions of risk across the entire risk spectrum, where causality depends on the joint effect of FM and FFM percentages. Thus, only from equal ratios would it be possible to accept the same causal risk measured from different BMIs, irrespective of age, ethnicity, and sex. In light of this, under any segment of an epidemiological risk line for all-cause mortality defined from a mean FMFFMR, either in normoweight or in high overweight/obesity, it is possible to find a protective area for athletes and physically active people, who may present healthier ratios by decreasing FM and increasing FFM percentages, respectively, despite having high BMIs of theoretical epidemiologic risk. Clearly, different FMFFMR values within the same or different BMI ranges can modify any "*m*" slope of a segment of the line, where "*m*" may positively be > 0 (FMFFMR increasing in its variation), become horizontal ("*m*" = 0: FMFFMR without experiencing variation), or even negative ("*m*" < 0: FMFFMR decreasing in their variation; see **Figure 1**). Thus, in healthy adults from BMI > 18.5 up to BMI ≥ 30 being included, a higher final FFM percentage can involve a lower final FMFFMR, and therefore, the linear function in that segment of the line describes a protective area of lower risk and better prognosis. This means that from equal or different BMIs, healthier FMFFMRs than those of the general mortality line might be demonstrated in any population subcategory.

4. Methods of identifying sources and studies, and adding new variables

4.1 Study design

From a new insight, a research work was carried out focusing on a selection of pertinent studies conducted over the last three decades to elucidate the relationships between BMI and body composition measures with all-cause mortality in either sex. Included studies for this investigation were identified through searches of PubMed, Web of Science, Google Scholar, academic social networking sites, and references from relevant articles. Searches included terms such as BMI and direct or indirect measures of body composition and all-cause mortality, which were combined (last search on June 25, 2025). A sufficiently large sample size was required, with preference given to studies investigating ≥1,000 individuals, although studies with smaller samples were not excluded. The investigation encompasses various study types, with a particular focus on cohort studies aimed at exploring the mathematical relationship of BMI and body composition measures with all-cause mortality. Thus, the mathematical relations between FM and FFM within BMI were analyzed as an original research from mathematically defined newer variables. This study was designed to ensure a rigorous evaluation of the relationship between BMI and all-cause mortality because of the mathematical issue described herein may itself be an crucial factor that deserves greater attention.

On the contrary, while being an objective of mathematical demonstration that operates with numbers, neither a structured review/meta-analysis nor higher statistical power seems necessary. Thus, any study not seen in this research could be included in the method if any population mean BMI was associated with mortality, or the body components could be associated and distributed by BMI categories. In the analysis of the literature, some extensive reviews of the associations between body composition measures and mortality [29, 34] showed that the majority of studies found counterintuitive associations with the different body components. Many studies have investigated the relationship of FM and measures of FFM with mortality, with the majority of them reporting disparate associations. No study has investigated the impact of the ratios and the differences between FM and FFM, yet total weight/BMI change is associated with complementary changes in both components (i.e., the higher the FM percentage, the lower the FFM percentage, and vice versa). Thus, equal–different variations in both components may result in different–equal FMFFMRs and "x" values, and subsequently in differentiated causal risks.

A synthesis of more than 25 relevant epidemiological studies, comprising more than 1 million participants, was summarized in supplementary **Table S1**. From the dataset and anthropometric characteristics reported in each study, the new variables were mathematically extracted/calculated as appropriate. In this approach, each study was reproduced, but with the addition of new pertinent variables that were originally omitted.

4.2 Variables

From scientific information published elsewhere [1–27], all variables were established in either sex. Six BMI categories were considered according to the international consensus statement [1]. Similarly, six corresponding theoretical risk exposure levels were established. From all studies associating BMI and body composition measures with mortality risk, their means ± standard deviation (SD) or medians were newly pooled for calculating the corresponding mean of means in each BMI category. Thus, means or medians were distributed in each category from their association level and classification into percentiles, tertiles, quartiles, quintiles, or means and medians when available. From some studies, technologically measured variables of body composition (e.g., by using bioimpedance, dual-energy X-ray absorptiometry, or imaging technologies) were used in the pooled dataset [10, 16, 17, 21–30]. From other studies, FM and respective percentages were extracted from their dataset or reproduced and calculated from validated anthropometric prediction equations [26, 27, 36]. For calculation, all values were subsumed to any race and average age. Values for FM percentages were taken from the dataset or calculated from the transformation from unit of mass to FM percentage: FM% = FM × 100/mean weight (kg). Values for FFM were taken from the dataset or reproduced and calculated by subtracting FM from mean total weight: FFM = mean weight − mean FM. Similarly, mean FFM percentages were taken or calculated by subtracting FM percentages from 100% as a whole. FMI and FFMI variables were directly taken from studies or calculated from mean, median, or BMI cut-offs once weight/height and FM/FFM or respective percentages were known [22]. Mean FFMI was calculated by subtracting FMI from mean BMI as a whole or 100%. Mathematically, a standard difference exceeding 0.5 kg/m^2 or $p < 0.05$ was taken to indicate a significant difference between the total mean FMI and FFMI within any category or between categories.

Among the new variables, mean FMFFMR and FFM-to-FM ratio were calculated from the mean values of FM and FFM. In this approach, if FMFFMR increased and decreased between zero and a value of 1 (proper fraction) in the respective directions across the entire spectrum of BMI, similarly, the FFM-to-FM ratio (while being an improper fraction) decreased and increased between 100 and 1 as appropriate. Then, FM and FFM percentages showed opposing relationships with the causal risk [18, 33]. A specific modulus $|x|$ was described as another new variable derived from the absolute difference in means between FM and FFM. The total mean $|x|$ measures the difference resulting from subtracting the total mean FM from FFM in any BMI category [18, 19, 32–34]. Mathematically, a non-zero difference in means (i.e., a total mean $|x|$ value of >0: "x" > ± 0.5 kg, or "x" exceeding 1% of weight, or $p < 0.05$) would indicate an unbalanced distribution for total mean FM and FFM within any BMI category or when comparing between two or all categories. By deduction, if and only if the total means of differences in two categories take the same value and different signs, the total mean $|x|$ of both categories equals zero ($|x| = 0$), validating its pooling in the same body composition, despite having different BMI categories. Likewise, if two categories take significantly different non-zero $|x|$ values, both categories present different body compositions. Thus, any significant difference from a non-zero mean indicates that different $|x|$ values were compared between two groups or categories, and therefore, there is no equivalence in their body compositions and risk exposure levels [18, 19].

From all reviewed studies, all risk associations for BMI and different body components were established from different measures of association, such as Cox proportional hazard ratio models, sensitivity/specificity analysis, or other statistical models. If, after checking the cut-off points for associations and comparing inter and intragroups, systematic differences between FM and FFM remained, this indicated that the high-risk body compositions between the groups and categories compared differed consistently. Similarly, if ratios and $|x|$ values or percentages appeared to be associated with inequality between components, an over- or underestimation of one measurement over another indicated a biased causal association from any population mean BMI. By deduction, if in any BMI cut-off or nadir of mortality lying from normoweight to class II/III obesity there was a clear significant difference between both components in favor of the musculoskeletal component, the overall causal risk was not assumed. Conversely, only in categories with a total mean FMFFMR < 1 and $|x| = -x$ or with a total mean FMFFMR >of 1 and $|x| = -x$ would we meet risk criteria to link low or high mean BMI, respectively, with causality, and results showing opposing relations of FM and FFM to mortality.

4.3 Statistical analysis

All participants were pooled into the corresponding BMI category and risk exposure level based on means, medians, or cut-offs from all studies. In the pooled dataset, categorized by body composition measures, descriptive analyses for all variables of interest were performed using analysis of variance (ANOVA) and comparison of means with Bonferroni post hoc tests. The Student's t-test was used to compare the means of the variables between two continuous categories or even within the same category. When comparing means within the same category or between two continuous categories, other standard differences were also considered (i.e., a mean $|x|$ modulus >0.5 kg or exceeding 1% of weight would be considered a variable significantly different when comparing means between FM and FFM). All variables were tested for normality using the Kolmogorov–Smirnov test. Based on differences in body size, men and women were analyzed separately. Variables are described in quantities, ratios, ranges, and percentages; quantitative variables are summarized with both the mean and SD. In hypothesis testing, the maximum rate of type I error was set to less than 5%. The confidence interval (CI) was calculated for each relevant variable. Data were analyzed using SPSS for Windows (IBM SPSS Statistics 20).

5. Results

5.1 Participant characteristics

In the review of studies with more than 30 million participants worldwide, all mortality nadirs were found between normoweight (BMI > 18.5–20) and overweight/obesity (BMI ≤ 30) for describing different U- or J-shaped curve patterns, which have been repeatedly observed and published elsewhere [2–15, 17]. Generalized cut-off points for the association of BMI and the body composition variables with all-cause mortality are shown in **Table 1**. All BMI cut-offs were located in normoweight or overweight ranges. All variables showed inequalities significantly different between FM and FFM when comparing both categories (p <0.05). In any nadir of mortality for BMI, whether at normoweight or overweight, a mean FFM > 50.5% and FM < 49.5% (i.e., a difference exceeding 1% of weight: $|x|$ >1%), mean FFMI > 15.25 and FMI < 14.75 (i.e., any difference exceeding 0.5 kg/m^2), mean FMFFMR <1, mean FFM-to-FM ratio > 1, and mean $|x|$ > 0 (i.e., the absolute difference exceeding 0.5 kg) may universally be endorsed from scientific knowledge and our method [2–19, 33].

Variables	Men	Women	Findings
BMI (kg/m^2)	22.6 (1.2)–27.1 (0.7)*	22.2 (1.6)–26.5 (1.1)*	Positive
FM (%)	25 (5.4)–29.8 (3.1)*	31.4 (4.9)–37.2 (4.3)*	Positive
FFM (%)	76.1 (7)–69.9 (4.3)*	68.1 (4.4)–63.3 (4.5)*	Inverse
FM/FFM ratio	0.34–0.42; <1*	0.46–0.59; <1*	Positive
FFM-to-FM ratio	3.1–2.3; > 1*	2.1–1.6; > 1*	Inverse
FFM - FM = $|x|$ (kg)	33.6 (5.9)–32.1 (5.1)*	25.4 (3.3)–17.9 (7)*	Inverse
FMI (kg/m^2)	5.8 (1.5)–8.0 (0.7)*	6.8 (1.6)–9.3 (1.1)*	Positive
FFMI (kg/m^2)	16.7 (1.2)–19.0 (0.9)*	15.5 (0.5)–17.0 (1.2)*	Inverse
|FFM% – FM%| (%)	50.3 (12)–40.0 (6.4)*	36.7 (9)–26.0 (9.6)*	Inverse

BMI: body mass index; FFM: fat-free mass; FFMI: fat-free mass index; FM: fat mass; FMI: fat mass index; FMFFMR: fat-mass-to-fat-free-mass ratio; $|x|$: modulus as the absolute difference between FFM and FM, which may mathematically be +x or −x (±x).
**Values are presented as total means (standard deviation) for each variable. Significance level at p < 0.05 between both categories. Other standard differences here considered: $|x|$ > 0.5 kg or > 1% of weight; differences between FMI and FFMI exceeding 0.5 kg/m^2 of BMI.*
a. Measures of association through Cox proportional hazard ratio models and sensitivity/specificity analysis or other statistical models were used in all studies to indicate which type of association was found to be appropriate.
b. BMI cut-offs in normoweight category are found in the nadirs of all-cause mortality, where FM versus FFM and FMI versus FFMI are also significantly different.
c. Ethnically specific risk cut-offs are included in each range.

Table 1.
Generalized means in normoweight and in overweight categories for the associations of BMI and other newer variables with all-cause mortality worldwide.

Regarding body composition measures and BMI categories on more than 1 million participants, results after adding the new variables are shown in **Table 2.** Only a few studies included data belonging to a few hundred subjects in the underweight range. In most studies, subjects in the underweight range were

Variables	UW: <18.5	NW: 18.5– <25	OW: ≥25– <30	IO: ≥30– <35	IIO: ≥35–39.9	IIIO: ≥40
TREL	High	Minimum	Moderate	High	Very high	Maximum
BMI (kg/m^2)	M: 15.4 (1.2)* W: 15.4 (1.4)*	M: 22.6 (1.2)* W: 22.9 (1.6)*	M: 27.1 (0.7)* W: 26.5 (1.1)*	M: 32.1 (1.2)* W: 32.1 (2.5)*	M: 35.0 (3.5)* W: 35.3 (2.4)*	M: 50.5 (4.8)* W: 53.8 (7.6)*
FM (%)*	M: 7.4 (3.3)* W: 8.0 (3.5)*	M: 25 (5.4)* W: 31.4 (5)*	M: 29.8 (3.1)* W: 37.2 (4.3)*	M: 35.2 (3.4)* W: 44.3 (3.1)*	M: 33.5 (1.2)* W: 48.7 (3.2)*	M: 45.9 (7.6)* W: 59.3 (3.9)*
FFM (%)	M: 92.8 (3.2)* W: 92.0 (3.9)*	M: 76.1 (7)* W: 68.1 (4)*	M: 69.9 (4.3)* W: 63.3 (5.5)*	M: 65.8 (5.4)* W: 55.5 (3.1)*	M: 66.5 (1.2)* W: 51.2 (3.3)*	M: 54.0 (7.6)* W: 40.6 (3.8)*
FMFFMR	M: 0.07 (0.03)* W: 0.08 (0.04)*	M: 0.34 (0.1)* W: 0.46 (0.1)*	M: 0.42 (0.06)* W: 0.59 (0.11)*	M: 0.54 (0.09)* W: 0.80 (0.09)*	M: 0.50 (0.1)* W: 0.95 (1.3)*	M: 0.87 (0.2)* W: 1.4 (0.2)*
FFM/FM	M: 17.8 (13)* W: 15.5 (7.7)*	M: 3.1 (0.9)* W: 2.1*	M: 2.3 (0.3)* W: 1.6*	M: 1.8 (0.3)* W: 1.2 (0.1)*	M: 2 (0.3)* W: 1.0 (0.1)*	M: 1.2 (0.3)* W: 0.7 (0.1)*
$\|x\|$ (%)	M: 85.6 (6.6)* W: 84.0 (7.8)*	M: 50.3 (12)* W: 36.7 (9.3)*	M: 40.0 (6.4)* W: 26.0 (9.6)*	M: 28.7 (7)* W: 10.0 (6.7)*	M: 33 (2.4)* W: 2.4 (6.6)*	M: 8.1 (15.3)* W: -18.7 (7.7)*
FMI (kg/m^2)	M: 1.1 (0.4)* W: 1.2 (0.9)*	M: 5.8 (1.5)* W: 6.8 (1.6)*	M: 8.0 (0.7)* W: 9.3 (1.1)*	M: 11.4 (1.2)* W: 13.8 (0.6)*	M: 11.7 (1.2)* W: 17.2 (2)*	M: 23.4 (5.8)* W: 32.0 (4.7)*
FFMI (kg/m^2)	M: 14.2 (1.3)* W: 13.7 (1.5)*	M: 16.7 (1.2)* W: 15.5 (0.5)*	M: 19.0 (0.9)* W: 17.0 (1.2)*	M: 20.9 (1.2)* W: 18.4 (2)*	M: 23.3 (2.3)* W: 21.4 (5)*	M: 27.1 (1.2)* W: 25.2 (3.4)*
FM (kg)	M: 3.6 (1.4)* W: 3.7 (1.2)*	M: 17.1 (4.3)* W: 20.2 (3.3)*	M: 24.8 (3.8)* W: 26.3 (2.8)*	M: 33.1 (3.1)* W: 36.6 (3.2)*	M: 35.0 (6)* W: 44.3 (6.6)*	M: 72.9 (18.2)* W: 84.6 (11.7)*
FFM (kg)	M: 46.6 (4.6)* W: 44.4 (8.7)*	M: 50.8 (12)* W: 45.6 (6.7)*	M: 57.0 (3.9)* W: 46.5 (8)*	M: 62.7 (5.2)* W: 46.0 (8.1)*	M: 69.5 (10)* W: 45.0 (3)*	M: 84.3 (4.3)* W: 58.1 (12.1)*
$\|x\|$ (kg)	M: -42.5 (4)* W: -40.3 (9)*	M: 33.6 (5.9)* W: 25.4 (3.3)*	M: 32.1 (5.1)* W: 17.9 (7.2)*	M: 31.1 (7)* W: 9.4 (6.9)*	M: 34.5 (5.2)* W: 0.7 (9.6)*	M: 11.3 (21.8)* W: - 26.4 (11.7)*

BMI: body mass index; FFM: fat-free mass; FFMI: fat-free mass index; FM: fat mass; FMI: fat mass index; FMFFMR: fat-mass-to-fat-free-mass ratio; IO: class I obesity; IIO: class II obesity; IIIO: class III obesity; M: men; NW: normoweight; TREL: theoretical risk exposure level from BMI; UW: underweight; W: women; |x|: absolute difference between FFM and FM in kg or in percentages, which may mathematically be + x or −x (±x).

a. Values are presented as total means (standard deviation) for each variable, derived from the pooled analysis of means or medians in all studies. Values were extracted or calculated by measuring the body composition of adults using different anthropometric or technological formulas published elsewhere.

b. From some studies, FM versus FFM and FMI versus FFMI in underweight and in class II/III obesity may coincide with the lowest and the highest percentiles-quintiles, respectively, while several thousand subjects were included in the respective BMI categories.

c. Sums of differences in the percentages may not be 100% because of rounding.

Table 2.

Baseline characteristics of the variables in the pooled dataset by BMI category and TREL.

excluded or not reported. Nevertheless, from the dataset or from data in their figures, an approximate average for FM/FMI and FFM/FFMI in each study was established, and the total mean for the difference between means of FM/FMI versus FFM/FFMI was higher than 80% of weight/BMI in favor of FFM/FFMI in either sex: Total mean FM <10% in men and 8% in women; total mean $|x|$ percentage of 85.6% in men and 84% in women: $|x| > 0$ in either sex: $|x| = -x$; all $p < 0.001$ in either sex. In this issue, if the left branches of the U- or J-shaped curves worldwide were plotted over thousands of subjects in correlation with increased mortality risk; then, thousands of cases of cause-especific mortality were distributed in the same underweight range. Millions of subjects in all studies belonged to normoweight category. From studies that reported body composition measures, a few hundred thousand participants were included in the normoweight range; the total mean $|x|$ percentage was of 50.3% and 36.7% for men and women, respectively ($|x| > 0$: $|x| = +x$; $p < 0.001$), and being always in favor of FFM/FFMI. Similarly, a total mean for FM percentage (25% for men and 31.4% for women) and for FFM percentage (76.1% and 68.1% for men and women, respectively) were reported with a significantly difference ($p < 0.001$ in both sexes). From here, a total mean FMFFMR of 0.34 for men and of 0.46 for women in the normoweight range was established. In overweight and class I obesity were contained millions of subjects who predicted all-cause, CVD and cause-specific mortality from the different nadirs of BMI. From studies about body composition, subjects in overweight/class I obesity showed a significant difference between FM/FMI and FFM/FFMI ($p < 0.001$), and the total mean for FM percentage was between 29.8% and 34.5% in men and between 37.2% and 44.3% in women. From here, the total mean FMFFMR was between 0.42 and 0.52 in men, and from 0.59 upto 0.80 in women. The total mean $|x|$ percentage was between 40.0% and 29.9% in men, and between 26% and 10% in women (all > 0: $|x| = +x$; FFM% > FM%, all $p < 0.001$). In class II and III obesity, thousands of individuals belonged to all-cause, CVD and cause-specific mortality from BMI studies. A few thousands of participants with class II obesity and several thousands with class III obesity were included among studies with body composition measures, and the majority presented significant differences for the total mean values of FM and FFM percentages in both sexes ($p < 0.001$). Between class I and II obesity in men, there was a gap in the partial trend line due to a decrease in the mean FMFFMR and FM percentage ($p \leq 0.05$) and increase in the FFM percentage ($p = 0.07$) in class II with respect to class I obesity. In class III obesity, the total mean $|x|$ percentage was significantly different between men and women, with a value of 8.1% for men (FFM% > FM%: $|x| > 0$: $|x| = +x$) and of −18.7% for women (FM% > FFM%: $|x| > 0$: $|x| = -x$), and with total mean FMFFMR values of 0.87 (<1) and 1.4 (>1) for men and women, respectively (all $p < 0.001$).

5.2 Relationships between variables and all-cause mortality

Relationships between variables and BMI risk categories were plotted in **Figures 2** and **3**. Scatterplots showing relationships between FMFFMR and $|x|$ percentage with BMI categories, separately by sex, were used. The position of dots showed a linear dose–response analysis with a high R-squared value in all the diagrams. The trend line for FMFFMR showed a strong positive correlation,

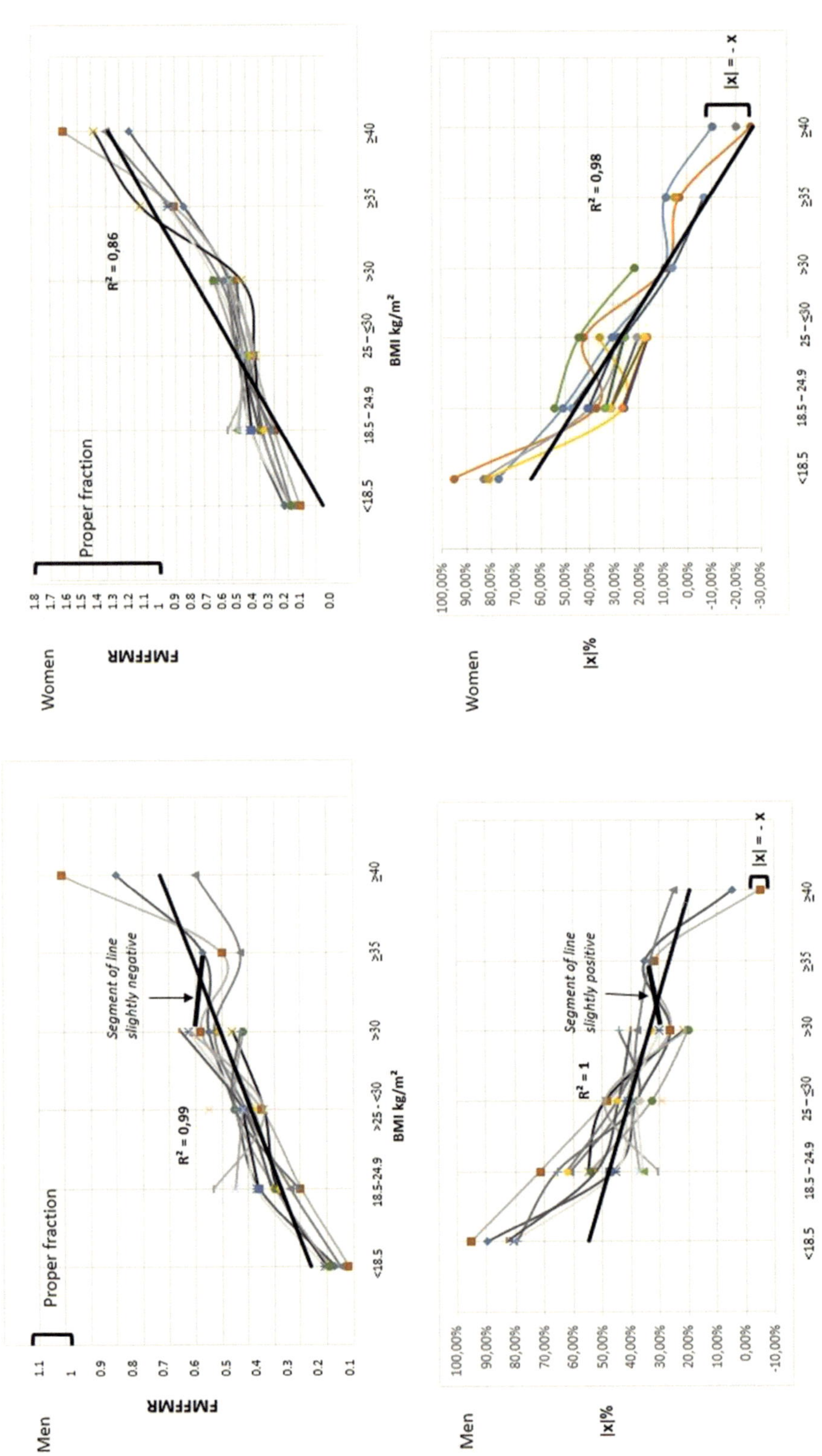

Figure 2.
*Scatterplots showing relationships between FMFFMR and |x|% with BMI across the entire risk spectrum and differentiating by sex. BMI: body mass index; FFM: fat-free mass; FM: fat mass; FMFFMR: fat mass-to-fat-free mass ratio; |x|: absolute difference between mean FM and FFM percentages. * All total mean values for FMFFMR and |x|% were significantly different between all risk categories (p < 0.001). ** Values for mean FM and FFM percentage within each risk category were significantly different sex by sex (p < 0.001). a. Values for FMFFMR between class I and II obesity in men determined a gap in the trend line. The "m" slope in this segment of line was negative and positive for FMFFMR and |x|%, respectively.*

DOI: http://dx.doi.org/10.5772/intechopen.1014539

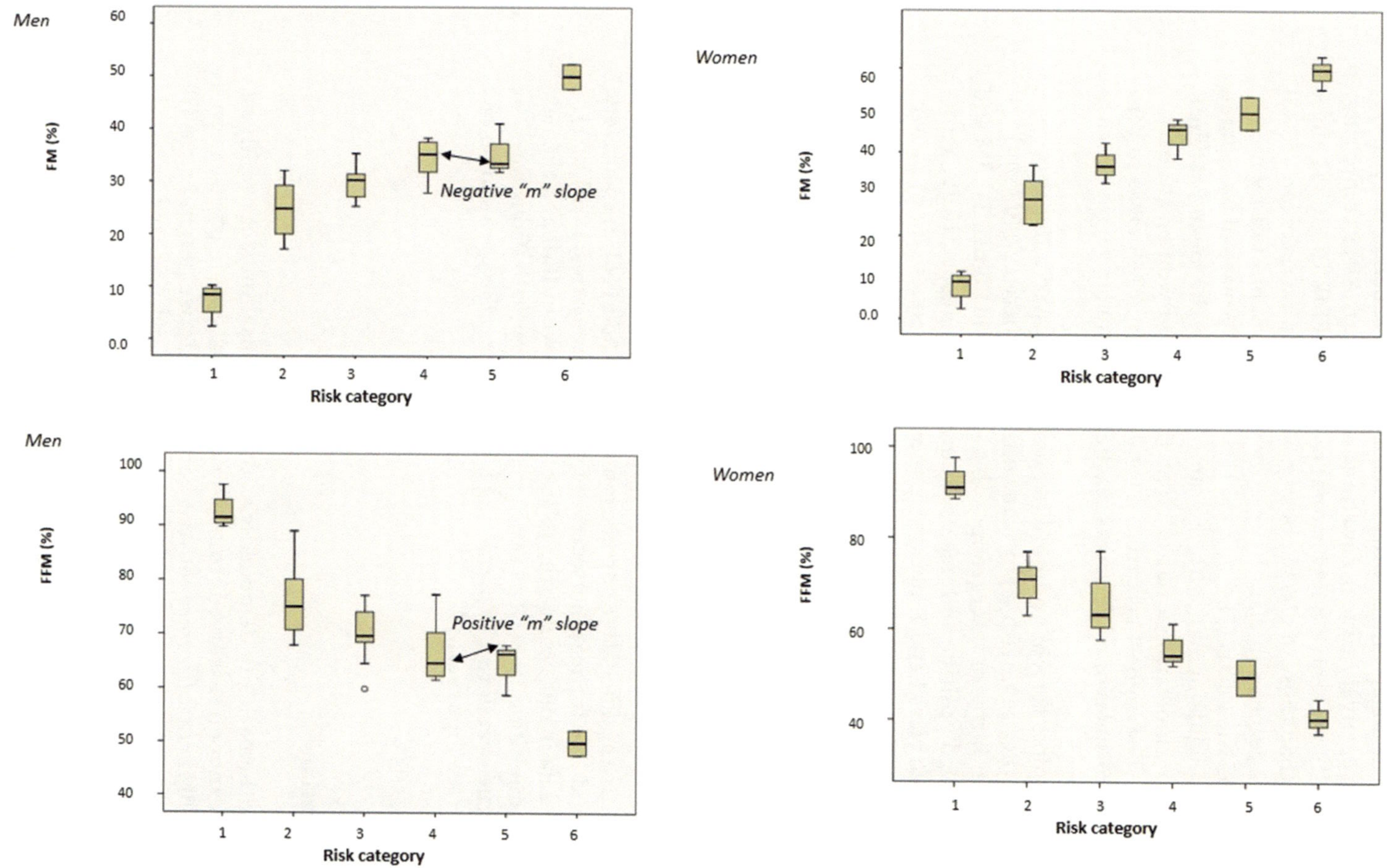

Figure 3.

Stem-and-leaf plots showing relationships between FM% and FFM% with BMI across the entire risk spectrum and differentiating by sex. *BMI: body mass index; FM: fat mass; FFM: fat-free mass. #The risk spectrum from BMI was divided into six categories: 1: BMI < 18.5 kg/m^2; 2: BMI ≥ 18.5–24.9; 3: BMI ≥ 25 to < 30; 4: ≥ 30 to < 35; 5: ≥ 35 – < 40; 6: ≥ 40. ##The scale on the y-axes may vary because men and women usually had significant differences between the fatty and non-fatty body components when comparing by sex. Only in underweight range, the body components for men and women were found similar (significance level was not measured). *All total mean values for FM% and FFM% were significantly different between all risk categories ($p < 0.001$). **Values for the total mean FM% and FFM% within each risk category were significantly different sex by sex ($p < 0.001$). ***Values between categories 4 (class I obesity) and 5 (class II obesity) in men showed a gap in the total linearity mostly due to a lower FM% in category 5 than in category 4, and subsequently, FFM% being higher in class II than in class I obesity. Accordingly, in men, the "m" slope in this segment of line was negative ("m" < 0) and positive ("m" > 0) for FM and FFM, respectively. Thus, in this range and sex, as BMI increased, FM and FFM decreased and increased, respectively. ****The maximum risk exposure level was located in category 6 in women with class III obesity, who presented a total mean FM% higher than that of FFM% (FM% > FFM%; |x|% = −x; $p < 0.001$). In men, category 6 showed a total mean FFM% > FM% and |x|% being equal to + x; $p < 0.001$.*

while that of $|x|\%$ moving in the opposite direction showed a strong negative correlation (see **Figure 2**). Regarding the partial trend, between class I and II obesity in men, there was a gap due to a negative and positive slope "m" for FMFFMR and $|x|\%$, respectively (linear equations not shown). After comparing, men with class II obesity presented a lower total mean FMFFMR ($p < 0.05$) and higher $|x|\%$ ($p = 0.08$) than those of class I obesity. The maximum risk from a total mean FMFFMR > 1 was reached in class III obesity by women, but not by men. A mean FMFFMR = 1 on the y-axis ("m" slope = 1) was already reached by women before class III obesity, while in men with the same category, the mean FMFFMR was lower than the unit, indicating a flatter slope than that of women (linear equations not shown). The highest risk from a total mean FMFFMR close to zero and total mean $|x| > 80\%$ in favor of FFM was reached in the underweight range in either sex ($p < 0.001$).

The stem-and-leaf plots for FM and FFM percentages showed a linear dose–response analysis in either sex, with significant differences between FM and FFM components either intra- or intergroups (all $p < 0.001$; see **Figure 3**). FM and FFM percentages showed positive and negative correlations, respectively, across all BMI ranges. Between class I and II obesity in men (linear equation not shown) FM and FFM showed a negative and positive slope "m", respectively, for indicating that class II obesity reached a lower mean FM% than that of class I obesity ($p = 0.05$), while for FFM% occurring vice versa ($p = 0.07$). In women with class III obesity an equivalent risk between FM% and BMI was reached (total mean FM% > 50%; $|x| = -x$; $p < 0.001$). In men with class III obesity, the total mean FM% was < 50% ($p < 0.001$). An equivalent risk between FFM% and BMI was reached in underweight range in either sex (total mean FFM% > 90%; $|x| = -x$; $p < 0.001$). Relationships for FMI and FFMI in each category and sex (not shown) were equal to those of FM and FFM, respectively, as expected (linear dose–response; positive and negative correlation for FMI and FFMI, respectively, and a gap in the trend line for men between the 4 and 5 categories; $p < 0.001$).

From real-world data in our results, the relationships between BMI and the new variables of body composition, as well as mathematical conceptualizations for understanding the true overall risk in predicting all-cause mortality, are shown on a graphical abstract (see **Figure 4**).

6. Discussion

6.1 General observation

This research mathematically demonstrates that the causal impact of BMI on all-cause mortality cannot be assumed from association measures in observational studies because all BMI cut-offs were located between underweight and class III obesity, and FM and FFM consistently showed inequality and non-risk equivalence with BMI in all epidemiological studies. Since weight is the sum of FM and FFM, it is impossible to ensure a causal risk from any BMI cut-off without demonstrating equality between both factors (i.e., difference in means = 0; FMFFMR = 1; "m" slope between FMFFMR and BMI = 1); and thus, only FM and FFM mathematically having the same risk consideration [18, 19, 32, 33]. If FM and FFM showed significant differences in favor of FFM within a total mean BMI, any BMI-associated risk may be biased. This is mainly due to a protective

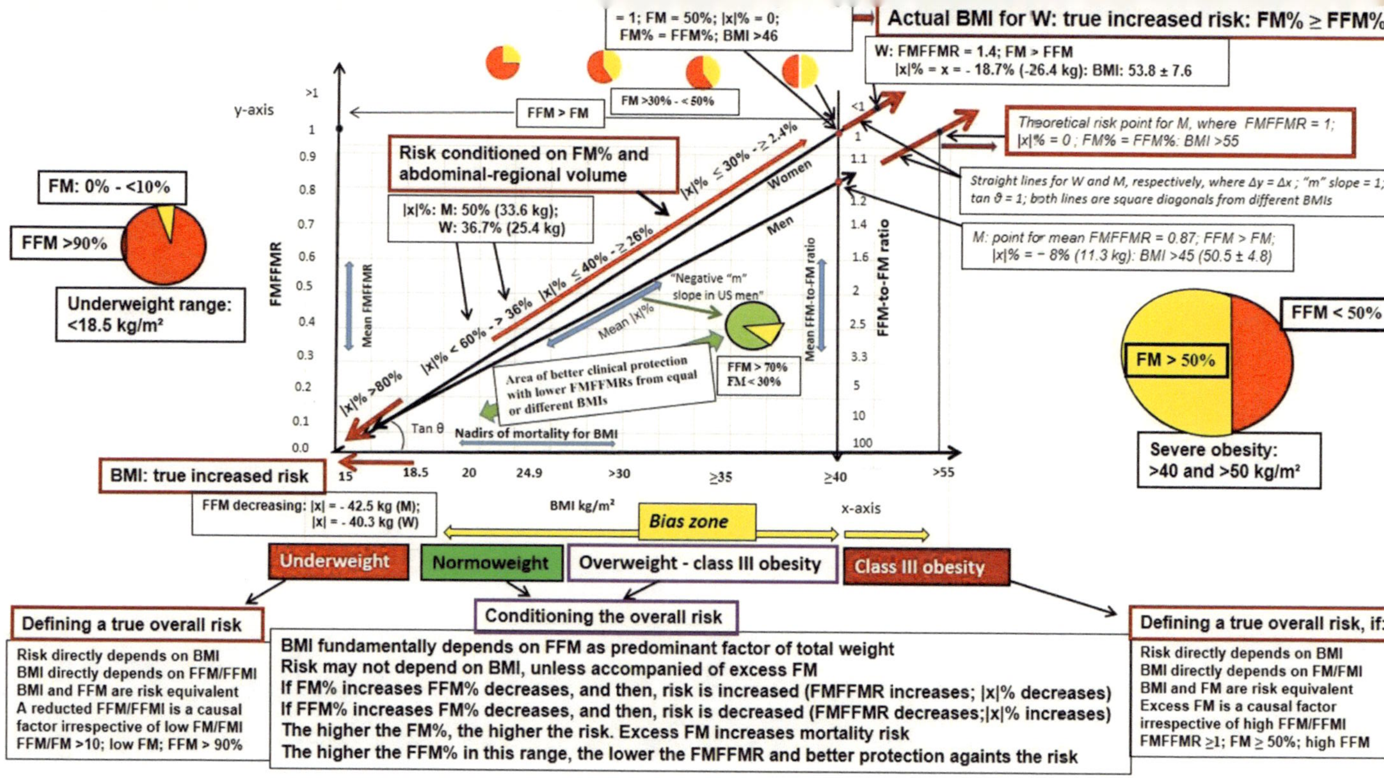

Figure 4.

Real relationships between BMI and new mathematical variables from associating body composition measures with all-cause mortality worldwide. Conceptualizations for understanding the true overall risk. BMI: body mass index in kg/m^2; FFM: fat-free mass in kg or %; FFMI: fat-free mass index in kg/m^2; FM: fat mass in kg or %; FMI: fat mass index in kg/m^2; FMFFMR: fat mass to fat-free mass ratio; M: men; "m": slope of a straight line between two Cartesian points ($\delta y / \delta x = \tan\theta$); W: women; |x|: absolute difference between FFM and FM, which may mathematically be + x or −x (±x), either in kg or in %.

** All values are means (standard deviation) from a pooled dataset, where FM and FFM were significantly different across all BMI categories ($p < 0.001$).*

a. Only in women with class III obesity does BMI capture 100% of mortality risk, and FM and BMI having the same sensitivity. In the underweight range in either sex, causal risk of mortality is captured entirely by a reduced FFM and BMI. From normoweight to class III obesity, a bias zone for BMIs may be found due to equal–different BMIs corresponding to different–equal FMFFMR and |x| values. In men between class I and II obesity, the segment of the line showed a slightly negative slope "m" mainly due to US adults who presented a lower FMFFMR in class II than that of class I obesity.

b. In each square diagonal, FMFFMR and BMI present different risk equivalence: a unit of 0.1 increased for FMFFMR (y-axis) is approximately equivalent to increasing 3.3 and 4 kg/m^2 of BMI (x-axis) in women and men, respectively: each unit of 0.1 between 0 and 1 for FMFFMR is equivalent to the proportional part of BMI between around 15 and severe and morbid obesity for women and men, respectively: when FMFFMR = 1, BMI is actually ≥46 in women and theoretically >55 in men.

c. Zero in the y-axis for FMFFMR is mathematically possible, although epidemiologically not compatible with full life. In contrast, the anthropological observation that one can have low or almost zero percentage of FM is not incompatible with the reality that one can be too lean (e.g., subcategories of normoweight individuals trained in endurance or athletes in overweight-obesity ranges or body builders) and having better clinical protection with lower FMFFMRs than those of other square diagonals, where risk equivalence between FMFFMR and BMIs from the same category are different.

overestimate of FFM with respect to FM when, in all BMI cut-offs referenced [2–19, 22–33, 36–38] FM was always significantly lower than FFM, and therefore, the risk value of the first is underestimated over the second. From a biological viewpoint, only a higher BMI variability, in accordance with a significantly increased central obesity and FM percentage, might be an accurate risk marker for CVD and cardiovascular mortality [18, 19, 29, 35, 38–43]. In this line, it is essential to understand that the biological risk may run in two opposing directions over time [16–20, 22–30]. This is in consonance with a recent systematic review and meta-analysis [13], where subgroup analysis, including diabetic patients, showed a greater mortality risk in the highest BMI (>35 kg/m^2) range. Besides, among the elderly and diabetic patients, BMI values <20 kg/m^2 were also associated with the highest risk.

From our findings, in any type of mortality occurring from normoweight to class III obesity in women [2–19, 22–31, 34, 37, 44–46], it is mathematically possible to say that FFM always presented a protective overestimate over FM. This is because, outside both ends of the BMI ranges, FM and FFM never reached equality (i.e., all mean $|x|$ values were >0; all FMFFMRs <1 and all differences between FM and FFM percentages were >were 1% and <50% in favor of FFM), and therefore, BMI and FM never being risk equivalent for a same causal risk [16–19, 22–31, 34, 37, 45, 46]. Only women in class III obesity presented a total mean for $|x|$ percentage and for FMFFMR where mean FM was higher than that of FFM (mean $|x| = -x$ and FMFFMR >1, respectively), and therefore, BMI directly depends on FM. This is coherent with a linear equation for women, where if FMFFMR as the y variable = 1, the BMI value as the x variable is equivalent to FMFFMR, and the "m" slope = 1, with both variables and values having the same sensitivity and measuring the same risk. In reverse, in the underweight range, BMI directly depends on FFM, and with FFM percentage being close to 100% of weight in either sex, BMI captures the maximum risk with the same sensitivity as that of FFM.

6.2 What studies tell us about associating BMI and body composition measures with all-cause mortality

Evidence indicates that the relationship between the FM percentage, high cardiometabolic risk, and specific-cause mortality risk on the right branches of the U- or J-shaped curves is predominantly driven by its correlation with visceral adiposity [18, 19, 32, 33, 35, 40–43, 47–53]. Similarly, from studies on myocardial infarction, it is well known that BMI underestimates whole-body fat and abdominal obesity as measured by relative abdominal volume and the waist-to-height ratio [18, 19, 32–35, 40, 43, 47, 48]. Conversely, weight loss with a reduced FFM and low BMI broadly impacts health and specific-cause mortality differently compared to increasing the FM percentage and abdominal fat volume [16–19, 22–30, 47–52]. Specific-causes of death associated with low BMIs are located on the left branches of the curve patterns [2–18]. Hence, if the association of BMI with all-cause mortality has always presented different epidemiological cut-offs between normal weight and slightly overweight or even upto 30 kg/m^2 [2–18, 21–23, 29, 53], something is wrong when inferring causality from BMI alone. If BMI is in itself a strong predictor of all-cause mortality both above and below an optimal range, BMI per se may not be the same causal factor for all-cause mortality.

Among millions of participants, a nadir of mortality between normoweight and 30 kg/m^2 has been widely debated [2–18]. In many studies measuring body composition, the mean or median FM and FFM always appeared significantly different in all BMI categories and when dividing by percentiles, quartiles, quintiles, and other classification criteria [18, 22–31, 34, 37, 45, 46] (see **Table S1**). From the UK Biobank, after recalculating relative FM from waist circumference and height, a causal association bias of BMI in predicting myocardial infarction was already proven, while significant inequalities between mean FM and FFM were mathematically demonstrated [18, 19, 34, 47]. Based on the same technologically validated anthropometric equations [34], a cohort study in a general Italian population was conducted on the association between BMI, relative FM, and mortality [31]. Thus, the mean or median BMI in the Italian population was in the overweight range in both sexes, while FM and FFM percentages were also significantly different in favor of FFM (mean FMFFMR <1: nadir for FM: 27.4 and 39.7 in men and women, respectively, both in the second quartile). From these findings, only men and women with BMI >35 kg/m^2, and men in the fourth quartile of relative FM showed an independent association with mortality, while women showed no association [31]. However, inconsistency may exist since the underweight range is not represented, and men and women in the first quartile presented a normal (23.9 ± 2.1) and high (34.3 ± 2.7) FM percentage of <25% and >30%, respectively [31]. Thus, all women showed higher mean FM and lower mean $|x|$ values than those of men, but a causal association bias occurred in either sex due to a protective overestimate of FFM over FM. In another recent study about all-cause mortality from the UK Biobank data [29], technologically measured FM-associated risk was concluded as not superior to that of BMI, with the BMI cut-off also being in the overweight range in either sex. Among the findings, FM (mean of 21.8 ± 7.8 in men and 26.3 ± 9.6 kg in women) showed a positive log-linear association in either sex, while appendicular skeletal muscle mass showed a positive log-linear association for men and a curvilinear association for women. However, after analyzing new anthropometric variables from the dataset, an inequality between mean FM and recalculated FFM, as well as a mean $|x|$ value of > zero, could also be proven. In this mathematical situation, the same FMFFMR may correspond to different BMIs and different $|x|$ values. However, BMI-associated risk was established from a unique mean BMI [18, 19, 39], and therefore, FM and FFM never have equality and the same risk consideration. Likewise, when classifying FM and muscle mass in quintiles, from mean weight and height, it is mathematically possible to calculate FMI, FFM, and FFMI. Under this analysis, the underweight range is not represented, and the first quintile corresponds to normoweight in both sexes. Similarly, the lowest values for FM, FMI, FFMI, and appendicular muscle mass may be found in the same first quintile. From there, all values progressively increase to the fifth quintile, where the highest values appear. Under this reading, FM and the musculoskeletal component may be associated with CVD and mortality risk [18, 19], but FFM is never a causative factor. This is because FM, FMFFMR, FFMI, and appendicular muscle mass linearly increase, but the final $|x|$ value and total FFM percentage decrease without reaching equality between components.

From other studies, a technologically measured or anthropometrically validated low lean body mass and FFM have been inversely associated with an increased risk of mortality in the lowest BMI range, suggesting that different contributions of FFM and FM to BMI may explain the shape of the association between BMI and mortality, as well as the controversial issue of the obesity paradox [16–19, 21–30, 34, 37, 45, 46, 54]. Similarly, other studies in Denmark, Canada, the United States, and European cohorts found that technologically measured FM percentage was significantly associated with an increased risk of total mortality [22, 25–28]. In this approach, mean or median BMIs were always located in overweight ranges, whereas body composition provides important prognostic information on an individual's mortality risk not provided by BMI. Thus, when some studies compared the top quintiles of lean mass/FFM/FFMI and FM/FMI versus the lowest, they concluded that excess FM is related to increased mortality risk and FFM protects against the risk of mortality (i.e., FFM showing an inverse association with mortality) [22, 25–28, 31]. This statement only holds true after understanding that FMFFMR linearly increases toward its maximum risk as FFM percentage increases, describing a flatter mortality risk line and, therefore, a lower overall risk (i.e., a lower FMFFMR). In this situation, a mean FMFFMR value of 1 (with a slope "m" slope = 1) could only be reached in very high BMIs and severe obesity. Of note, from the new variables analyzed in a representative sample of US adult men showing that lean mass was inversely associated with mortality [27], it is possible to demonstrate that in the fifth quintile (representing class II obesity), FM and FMI were higher than in the third quintile of overweight (as reference); however, the final FM percentage was lower in the top quintile (28.7%) than in the third (31.2%). Similarly, the final FFM percentage was higher in the fifth quintile (71.3%) than in the third quintile (68.8%). This demonstrates a higher mean $|x|$ (42.6%) and lower FMFFMR (0.40) in class II obesity than those of overweight, with 37.6% and 0.45 for mean $|x|$ and FMFFMR, respectively (see **Table S1**). Thus, when comparing European men [29, 31] with US participants [27], new findings may reveal new variables. Effectively, all presented a nadir of mortality at a mean BMI in the overweight range (between 26.9 and 27.4 kg/m^2); however, mean FMFFMR was similar in European men (0.34 and 0.38 for English and Italian men, respectively), but different from that of US men (mean FMFFMR = 0.45). Similarly, in the top quintiles or quartiles, BMI was around class II obesity (between 33 and 36.9 kg/m^2) in all; however, FMFFMR was 0.40 in US men and 0.48 and 0.50 in English and Italian men, respectively. This means that US men with BMIs similar to those of European men presented different FMFFMRs and $|x|$ values, justifying a lower mortality risk from the same high BMIs. Obviously, the US study [27] shows a higher mean FFM and lower FM than those of European studies [29, 31]. In this issue, the segment of the risk line that goes between overweight and class II obesity toward FMFFMR = 1 would be flatter than that of European men, with a lower slope justifying a protective effect of lean mass in that specific range of BMI. In contrast, those studies showing higher mean FMFFMR and lower $|x|$ percentage between any nadir of mortality and a mean FMFFMR = 1 presented greater risk because total FM percentage increased and mathematically related FFM percentage decreased, irrespective of FFMI or relative muscle mass increasing from the lowest to the highest quartiles or quintiles, as seen in European studies [29, 31]. So, when appendicular muscle mass or other relative musculoskeletal components directly appeared associated with CVD and mortality [29], they were never causative factors but rather a result of a spurious risk association [18, 19, 32, 33, 35, 43]. In the Melbourne Collaborative Cohort study [23], BMI and bioimpedance-assessed FM for men in the first and fifth quintiles were associated with mortality, while FM in women were not associated when comparing the top quintile with the second quintile. However, when analyzing the new variables, BMI in the 50th percentile showed an overweight range in either sex, and FM and FFM percentages showed inequality and significant differences in the same percentile for both sexes. Additionally, FM and FFM were significantly different in all percentiles ($|x| > 0$ in all), with FM showing a U-shaped association with all-cause mortality, while a risk equivalence between FM and BMI was demonstrated only in class III obesity in either sex. Thus, the linear positive association for the waist-to-hip ratio and waist circumference with mortality that was found in this study for both sexes may only derive from an enlarged waist circumference and high FM percentage and abdominal volume [18, 19, 23, 32, 33, 35, 36, 43, 48].

On the contrary, whole-body FM, visceral adiposity measured from different indices, and whole-body FFM have been associated with mortality, CVD, and different types of cancers, including pre- and postmenopausal breast cancer risk and colorectal cancer risk in men [29, 47–51, 55–68]. Similarly, a mean BMI in overweight/class I obesity, while FM and FFM take high mean values, has epidemiologically been correlated in many at-risk individuals [16–19, 21–35, 37–43, 45, 47, 60–68]. Based on these anthropometric profiles of high cardiometabolic risk, it is easy to establish a somatotype of high musculoskeletal and fatty components, simultaneously showing a high positive correlation with parameters of visceral fat accumulation and abdominal volume, especially measured by technology or indirectly by the waist-to-height ratio [18, 19, 29, 32, 33, 35, 42, 43, 47–51, 56–68]. Thus, if FFM and some muscle mass indices have inversely been associated with mortality [16–18, 21–30, 34, 37, 38], the musculoskeletal component, whether muscle mass, FFM/FFMI, appendicular muscle mass index, or mesomorphy, may artificially be associated with CVD, type II diabetes, and cancer, and besides, keep a high correlation with BMI, visceral adiposity, and mortality risk [18, 19, 29, 32, 33, 35, 38, 43, 47–53, 56, 59–61]. However, in these situations, a high BMI below class III obesity would capture an implausible part of the causal risk because the musculoskeletal component would constitute the largest proportion of BMI. Interestingly, from a study in Korean adults using validated anthropometric prediction models, the association of BMI and mortality was adjusted for the FFMI [45]. In this Asian population study, when participants were classified into four body composition types in agreement with tertile distributions for FMI and FFMI, FM and FFM showed a direct and inverse association with all-cause mortality, respectively. This is in consonance with the Shanghai Health Study, where the waist-to-hip ratio was linearly associated with all-cause and CVD mortality in either sex [46], although this index may also show a causal association bias with respect to waist circumference, overall when the mean waist-to-hip ratio has a value of < 1 [18, 19, 32, 33, 35, 46]. In addition, waist circumference has shown a positive linearity with mortality due to its high biological correlation with FM percentage [18, 19, 23, 26, 27, 29–33, 36, 41, 48]. In contrast, some studies using direct body composition measures in older women have associated both low and high adiposity with mortality from a mean BMI in the overweight range [54, 55]. From the Health ABC Cohort Study, which directly measured body components in older adults in the overweight range, total lean mass was not associated with mortality in either sex, while mid-thigh muscle area was significantly associated (in an inverse relationship) [37]. Nevertheless, lean mass and FM were also significantly unequal in either sex. This means that excluding a part of FFM, between-group lean mass may not be significantly different from a mean BMI in the normoweight/overweight range, but when accounting for total FFM, this component might or might not appear to be associated. So, from similar BMI cut-offs in the normoweight/overweight range, other studies have shown that low FFM and lean mass, as well as low arm muscle circumference, were associated with mortality in men [16, 17, 22, 26, 27, 69].

6.3 Rationale

From wide reviews and studies, whether showing or not showing an association of body components with greater mortality risk [29, 34, 48, 54–56], a difference in means between FM and FFM may always be proven for demonstrating a causal inconsistency from any BMI-associated risk, either by the sample size or by excluding high-risk body compositions at both ends of the range of BMI. The same holds true when either a low FM (with low BMI) or high FFM/lean mass (with high BMI) appears to be associated with greater CVD, cancer, and mortality risk [29, 45–51, 57–68, 70], while mean FM and FFM always show significant differences in favor of FFM. In fact, inconsistency for causality in large studies occurred not due to the sample size, but due to unbalancing opposite components (mean FMFFMR < 1: mean $|x| > 0 = +x$ in all) and omitting whether variations in total FM and FFM percentages were increased or decreased from baseline to the final values [18, 19]. As we demonstrate here, a low FM close to zero percent may not be biologically responsible for greater mortality risk unless accompanied by a high FFM percentage in the lower range of BMI (i.e., the highest mean for $|x|$ percentage and for FFM-to-FM ratio). Similarly, a high FFM may never be responsible for excess rates of total mortality unless accompanied by a high FM percentage and high BMI (i.e., the lowest mean for $|x|$ percentage [close to zero] and the highest for FMFFMR [close to 1], or even both means being negative [$|x| = -x$] and > 1, respectively, in favor of FM). In our results, a linear dose–response analysis from the relationships between FM and FFM components may be demonstrated in associating excess rates of total mortality at both ends of the range of BMI, and after accounting for thousands of subjects in underweight and in class III obesity [22, 23, 27, 31, 71, 72]. In fact, linearity occurs after verifying a higher FM percentage, higher FMFFMR, lower FFM-to-FM ratio, and a lower $|x|$ percentage as FFM percentage decreased from underweight toward class III obesity in either sex. In our findings, a gap between class I and II obesity in men was found, mainly due to the US population who in class II obesity presented a higher musculoskeletal component and lower FMFFMR [27] than those of other populations, and thus, a negative slope "m" in that segment of the line was demonstrated. In addition, from all studies in men with class III obesity, the total mean FFM was always higher than that of FM, indicating the predominance of the first and a different risk consideration for both components, while FM and BMI never reached the same sensitivity. In general, the differences between the two components always appeared significantly different in all BMI categories or when comparing by different distributions of percentiles, tertiles, quartiles, or quintiles. This means that from the body composition, all BMI categories consistently differed. Thus, a mean BMI hardly represents the true risk of any population. Possible reasons for a given inconsistency of BMI in many associations include the lack of mutual adjustment for FM and FFM and the inability to determine the body composition and mortality relation across the entire risk spectrum, essentially due to small numbers of participants and deaths at both ends of the range of BMI or if they were excluded.

To our knowledge, obesity has direct adverse effects on cardiac structure and function and leads to CVD development independent of other cardiovascular risk factors, such as type II diabetes mellitus, dyslipidaemia, hypertension, and sleep disorders [1, 73, 74]. Thus, class II/III obesity has appeared to be an important predictor of overall mortality and different BMI-related diseases [22, 23, 27, 31, 71, 72]. However, any BMI cut-off located outside of severe obesity may never be equivalent in mortality burden to those of high BMI levels, with excess FM being an independent factor [18, 19]. Likewise, weight loss and FFM mathematically decreasing with a negative sign could never be comparable to the anthropometric risk profile of subjects with high FFMIs, especially when accompanied by the aforementioned cardiovascular risk factors. In any cause-specific mortality associated with weight loss and being in the lower range of BMI, it is possible to encounter a pathogenesis differing from that of weight gain, increasing FM, visceral adiposity/abdominal volume, or living years with obesity [16–19, 32, 33, 35, 41, 51, 53, 55–72]. In reality, epidemiologically, any BMI cut-off located from high normoweight to class III obesity is usually due to an increasing FM percentage, FMI, and visceral/central adiposity, and therefore, CVD, type II diabetes, and cancer risk increase [2–19, 21–30, 32, 33, 35, 41–43, 47–51, 57–72, 75–78]. Conversely, decreased energy reserves and low protein deposits coinciding with a reduced FFM (i.e., mathematically having a negative sign) due to undernutrition, severe sarcopenia, neurological disorders, or other clinical conditions [2–19, 21–30] lead to a biological risk, where " $\pm x$" values, FMFFMRs, FFM-to-FM ratios, FMIs, FFMIs, and BMIs in underweight ranges differ from those of high BMIs and higher cardiometabolic risk.

Since real-world data in non-experimental studies were not randomized, two different risk dimensions were epidemiologically overlapping. In this approach, the U- or J-shaped curve for the association of BMI and all-cause mortality [2–18, 40, 44, 52, 53] remains disentangled, and the "obesity paradox" controversy may be largely explained. This is because FM and FFM may demonstrate opposing causal effects on mortality while being independent predictors [16–19, 22–31, 44–46]. Moreover, from normoweight to up ≥40 kg/m^2 in women, BMI always depended on both FM and FFM, whereas a significant inequality and different risk considerations may be demonstrated. Regarding this issue, if, after using a mean BMI located in a healthy body composition, one ignores the mean of the individual differences between FM and FFM, one omits a confounding factor that distorts any causal inference from the BMI association [18, 19]. This is because if the percentages of both FM and FFM are different in two groups of comparison, the difference in means may never be equal to zero, and any mean $|x|$ value in the total sample will be > 0, demonstrating an unbalanced distribution and between-group comparisons for different high-risk body compositions. For the same reason, any mortality risk prediction in men compared with women always appeared with a higher bias error due to differences in body composition, and mean $|x|$ values were always higher in men than in women [16–19, 22–30, 34, 37] (see **Table 2**). This explains why women reached class III obesity with a mean FM > FFM (mean $|x| > 0 = -x$), while in men from the same category, FFM continued to be the predominant factor (mean FFM >

FM: $|x| > 0 = +x$). Otherwise, from a mean FMFFMR, men and women would present different "m" slopes until reaching a value of 1, where BMI and FM have the same sensitivity. Thus, a flatter slope in men implies that from underweight until an FMFFMR of 1, a similar BMI in either sex indicates a different body composition and mortality risk. Thus, after analyzing global results, the gender difference can only be attenuated in individuals with underweight and beyond class III obesity. In fact, only at both ends of the entire risk spectrum (in category 1 and beyond category 6) may the highest-risk body compositions in either sex be defined (i.e., when FFM percentage is higher than 90% in underweight and FM percentage is around 50% or higher beyond class III obesity).

Since association does not equate to causation, for the first time, it is possible to demonstrate that within the underweight range, FM may be associated with mortality risk but is never the causal factor because BMI is independent of FM. Similarly, between underweight and class III obesity, the lower the $|x|$ positive value, the higher the risk, mainly due to excess FM and the smaller difference between the final FM and FFM percentages. In this situation, while FFM is the largest contributor to BMI, no musculoskeletal component can ever be the causal factor. This role corresponds to a higher FM percentage resulting from a smaller difference with respect to FFM. Obviously, if a range of BMI increases due to an increasing FFM percentage (e.g., in muscled persons), FM percentage and overall risk decrease, despite BMI variation increasing toward a higher risk category. In this case, the final FMFFMR value becomes lower than the initial value, and the line segment flattens its slope, or even a negative slope results in a downward-trending line that describes a non-paradoxical protective area of better clinical prognosis (see **Figures 1** and **4**).

Although BMI may measure opposite high-risk exposure levels, no mean BMI in normoweight or from overweight to class III obesity would anthropometrically be valid for discriminating the same overall risk in all individuals. Regarding sex, age, and ethnicity, weight management in health assessment remains a misleading factor if one does not consider other crucial anthropometric indicators (i.e., mathematical relationships between FM and FFM as well as the relative abdominal fat volume as geometrically measured from the waist-to-height ratio or using weight, waist, and height to estimate whole-body fat) [18, 19, 26, 27, 31–33, 35, 36, 43, 48]. In this context, when BMI and musculoskeletal components within BMI appeared to be universally associated with mortality risk, accepting a causal overall risk from mean FMFFMRs of <1 was a false premise. This was because any BMI-associated risk where mean FMFFMR and $|x|$ were <1 and >0 ($|x| = +x$), respectively, may not represent the overall risk as a whole in mathematical terms. Only in situations of a low range of BMI, where the mean FFM exceeds 90% of weight, and mean FM is closer to zero, would a mean BMI (with a FMFFMR <1 and $|x| > 0$: $|x| = -x$) meet risk criteria for capturing 100% of risk, and only then, FFM and BMI being inversely associated with mortality. Similarly, high-risk exposure levels and different types of causality may be found in women with class III obesity, where FM exceeding 50% of weight may justify a high BMI of maximum risk, whereas FM keeps risk equivalence with the final BMI. By deduction, only if moderate-high BMIs with FFM exceeding 50% of weight were conditional (e.g., with propensity score methods) on high FM percentage and abdominal volumes (e.g., above their own risk cut-offs) would it be possible to accept a causal risk from BMI in high-normoweight, overweight, or obesity ranges. However, in those anthropometric situations, neither FFM nor musculoskeletal components (e.g., lean and appendicular skeletal muscle masses or mesomorphy, etc.) necessarily affect cause-specific mortality, CVD, or cancer, as might be suggested from high BMIs in different studies [2–15, 29, 47, 55, 56]. When pharmacologic interventions, without differentiating by body composition and sex, are clinically used to treat overweight or class I and II obesity to reduce the risk of disease and complications for a few years [79–81], it does not guarantee an improvement in the mathematical relationships between FM and FFM, and thus ensure healthier ratios for a long time, at least from a high initial BMI to up normoweight. This is because weight loss, with the proportions of FM and FFM lost in either sex, may be unbalanced in favor of lean mass, thus losing much of its value and protective function.

Since an obesity paradox in evaluating mortality risk has been repeatedly described [2–17, 81], for the first time, we demonstrate that class II obesity may involve a lower mortality risk than that of overweight/class I obesity, without it meaning a paradoxical effect. This is mostly due to class II obesity showing a lower and higher FMFFMR and $|x|$ percentage, respectively, than those of class I. In this approach, any mean BMI demonstrating an FMFFMR < 1 (far from 1) and $|x| > 0 = +x$ (far from zero) will always present an unbalanced distribution between FM and FFM, with BMI being a misleading indicator. That way, it is not possible to accept an "obesity paradox" when describing a U- or J-shaped curve pattern for the association between BMI and mortality. In reality, a linear relationship between opposite associations for FM and FFM with mortality may indicate BMI ranges without a true causal risk, while describing protective areas of overlapping, which were always hidden when ignoring the mathematical relationships between components. Thus, in the analysis of the body of the literature and after revising many studies, this research mathematically demonstrates that between any epidemiological BMI risk cut-off and a mean $|x|$ equal to zero in either sex (mean FMFFMR = 1; "m" slope = 1 and FM and BMI being risk equivalent), a bias zone exists where FFM shows a protective overestimate with respect to FM. Certainly, neither normoweight, overweight, nor BMI-defined class I-II obesity are accurate ranges for assessing overall mortality and health risks, at least while hiding anthropometric confounding factors and BMI never describing a linear pattern for the association with mortality and causal risk.

7. Strengths and limitations

Our research has several strengths. First, this research included BMI- and body composition-related anthropometric variables to demonstrate that associations may mathematically capture a spurious risk. Second, this research reviewed many study types with millions of participants and thousands of deaths worldwide, analyzing the relationships between BMI and new variables derived from body composition. Third, this research used manually measured weights, heights, and waist circumferences, as well as technological methods from all studies, to reproduce BMIs, FMs, FFMs, $|x|$ values, and FMIs and FFMIs. This enabled population homogeneity and increased the reliability of our results. Finally, this research revealed mathematical misconceptions to demonstrate that BMI presents a different–equal risk assignment between individuals with equal–different shapes and high-risk body compositions. Furthermore, the findings in this research are innovative and pioneering and have no mathematical limitations, although values and anthropometric measurement biases might remain. Similarly, although anthropometrically and technologically measured body components may vary in their concrete values, this does not alter the mathematical principles developed here. The findings determine good generalizability to other population studies. To mathematically demonstrate that BMI appeared biased in most studies, no further studies are needed. This research was a mathematical demonstration, which can be applied to any study where it is feasible to use the necessary body components.

8. Conclusions

This research mathematically demonstrates that a causal association bias occurred in most epidemiological studies worldwide when associating BMI and body composition measures with all-cause mortality. From two metabolically opposite body components – such as FM and FFM – other mathematically defined newer variables may demonstrate BMI-related biases, fundamentally by verifying that mathematical relationships between FM and FFM components were confounding factors omitted in most studies. Differences between FM and FFM are non-causative confounding factors that appeared to be associated with mortality risk, while demonstrating a significant inequality in all BMI categories and distributions compared. The high-risk body compositions and risk exposure levels detected in the cut-offs of BMI and body composition measures for associating mortality risk consistently differed between groups, never comparing the same overall risk in mathematical terms, and thus confounding clinical practice.

The impact of excess FM on mortality essentially derives from a highly accumulated abdominal fat volume, which alters the differences between the final FM and FFM percentages, generating biases and clinical misinformation from underweight to class III obesity in women. Only in women with class III obesity does BMI capture 100% of the mortality risk. On the contrary, weight loss and a reduced FFM in the underweight range produce a causal risk captured 100% by BMI and FFM, where neither FM nor abdominal fat volume may be independent causative factors in either sex. All BMI cut-offs > 18.5–20 and < 40 kg/m^2 impact all-cause mortality with causal association biases, because in that wide range BMI never captures 100% of the overall risk. Mathematically, between underweight and class III obesity, it is always possible to find individuals with similar BMIs and significant differences between FM and FFM percentages, assuming that different–equal variations for FM and FFM at baseline may correspond to equal–different final percentages. As demonstrated here, excess FM and a reduced FFM were never risk equivalent with BMI, except in women with class III obesity and in either sex, respectively; therefore, the true overall risk of mortality and other clinical processes consistently appeared biased in most studies owing to a protective overestimation of FFM over FM.

Universally, BMI directly impacts mortality and health due to a high-risk body composition defined at both ends of the entire risk spectrum (i.e., a low FM–very high FFM percentage in underweight individuals and a high FFM–very high FM percentage beyond class III obesity). From underweight to class III obesity, a body composition of risk should be conditioned on a mathematically defined linear function from two variables: the ratio between FM and FFM, and BMI. Really, it is the body composition that determines global health risks through a linear dose–response relationship from the ratios between FM and FFM percentages or from their absolute differences. That way, the overall risk is defined by a linear function, whose "m" slope depends on variations of FM and FFM percentages within BMI over time (i.e., controlling for ratios or $|x|$ on the y-axis and BMIs on the x-axis [$\Delta y/\Delta x$]).

9. Recommendations

It is time to shift the historical paradigm about BMI and health risks. Since BMI does not discriminate the body composition of risk or measure a risk volume per unit of height, any BMI-associated risk outside of the extremes of the risk spectrum may appear biased from a causal inference, mainly due to a protective overestimate of FFM over FM. When handling health and measuring weight or BMI alone, it is impossible to ensure control of the causal risk if FM and FFM are uncontrolled factors, whether gaining or losing weight. In modern clinical practice, it is essential to know the two body components of total weight.

Conflict of Interest

The author declares no conflict of interest.

Appendix: Supplementary material

Original association findings										Novel findings	
Reference, Country, publish ed	Study (*N*), sex, age	Follow-up	Deat hs (*N*)	BC	FM/FMI or VAT or other anthropo metrics	FFM/FF MI/LM/ SM/aSM M/ASMI ALM	BMIs	UW/ ≥ IIO (*N* or %)	FM/FMI versus FFM/FFMI or FM versus LBM	FMFFMR	|x|
Heitman et al. [21] Sweden (2000)	*N* = 787 Men age 60 y	1973–1995 22 y	460	T.B.P.	FM: linearly increasing A	FFM: linearly decreasing A	q3: 25.4; q1: 21.3; q2: 23.8; q4: OW: 27.1; q5: 30.2	No/No	FM vs. FFM: q3:23.4 vs. 53.7 q1: 17 vs. 48.1; q5: 33.1 vs. 59.3	q3: 0.43; q1: 0.34 q5: 0.54 <1 in all	29.6 % $\|x\| > 0 = +x$ $\|x\| > 0$ *
Bigard et al. [22] Denmark (2004)	*N* =57,053 Both Age:50–64 y	1993–2001 Median 5.8 y	1,851	BIA	FMI: J-shaped A Below 20th P inverse A, Above 20th P direct A	FFMI: reversed J – shaped A Below 60th P: inverse A Above 60th P: NA	P50: M: 26.2; W:24.8 P0 (UW): M: 15.4; W: 14.2 P100 (IIIO); M: 52.7. W: 58.6	Yes: 0.76%/-	FMI vs. FFMI: P50: M: 6.8 vs. 19.4; W: 8.6 vs. 16.3. P0: M: 0.8 vs. 14.6; W: 0.6 vs. 12. P100: M: 25.2 vs. 27.5; W: 32.4 vs. 26.2.	P50: M:0.35; W: 0.52 P0: M: 0.05; W: 0.05 P100: M: 0.91; W: 1.23 <1 in all excepting P100 in W: > 1	P50: M: 48%; W: 32% P0: M: -89%; W: -92% ($\|x\| = -x$)* P100: M: 4.4%; W: -10.5% ($\|x\| = -x$)*
Simpson et al. [23] Australia (2007)	*N* = 41,313 Both Age 27–75 y	1990–2003 Median 11 y	2,822	BIA WC WHR	M: FM: U-shaped A (Q1 vs. Q5) WC, WHR: linear positive A W: FM: NA (Q2 vs. Q5) WC, WHR: linear positive A	NA	P50 (OW): M: 26.9; W: 25.9 P0 (UW): M: 15.6; W: 14 P100 (IIIO); M: 54; W: 54.8	0.02% (M) and 0.9% (W) were underweight. 19% (M) and 22% (W) were obese	FM vs. FFM: P50: M: 23 (29%) vs. 56.3 (71%) W: 26.5 (40.2%) vs 39.4 (59.8%) P0: M: 1.9 (2.4%) vs. 77.2 (97.6%) W: 4.4 (8.1%) vs. 50 (91.9%) P100: M: 79 (52.5%) vs. 71.5 (47.5%) W: 94.2 (63%) vs. 55.3 (37%)	P50: M: 0.41; W: 0.67 P0: M: 0.02; W: 0.08 P100 (IIIO): M: 1.1; W: 1.7 <1 in all excepting P100 in both sexes	P50: M: (42%); W: 19.6%: $\|x\| = +x$ P0: M: -95%; W: -83%: $\|x\| = -x$ P100: M: +5%; W: -26% ($\|x\| = -x$) $\|x\| > 0$ in all*

Original association findings										Novel findings	
Reference, Country, publish ed	**Study (*N*), sex, age**	**Follow-up**	**Deat hs (*N*)**	**BC**	**FM/FMI or VAT or other anthropo metrics**	**FFM/FF MI/LM/ SM/aSM M/ASMI ALM**	**BMIs**	**UW/ ≥ IIO (*N* or %)**	**FM/FMI versus FFM/FFMI or FM versus LBM**	**FMFFMR**	**$\|x\|$**
Zong et al. [24] US (2016)	N = 9,471 Both Age ≥ 20 y	1999–2010 Mean 8.8 y	682	DXA	FM%: q1, q3,q4 and q4 vs. q2: direct A	FFM%: NA	q1: M: 19.5; W: 21.5. q2: M: 25.5; W: 24.9 q3: M: 28.2; W: 28.8 q4: M: 32; W: 34.6	No/No	q2: M: 25.5% vs. 74.5%; W: 37.1% vs. 62.9% q1: M: 19.5% vs. 80.5%; W: 30.1% vs. 69.9% q4 (IO): M: 34.4% vs. 65.6%; W: 47.2% vs. 52.8%	q2: M: 0.34; W: 0.58 q1: M: 0.24; W: 0.43 q3: M: 0.40; W: 0.70 q4: M: 0.52; W: 0.89 <1 in all	q2:M: 49%; W: 25.8% q1: M: 61%; W: 39% q3: M: 42%: W: 17% q4: 31.2%; W: 5.6% $\|x\| > 0 = +x$ in all*
Padwall et al. [25]. Canada (2016)	*N* = 54,420 Both ≥40 y	1999–2013 Med: 6.7/ 4.5 y	M: 984 W: 4,965	DXA	FM%: M: Q4, Q5: direct A W: Q1,Q2,Q3, Q5: direct A	FFMI/BMI: Q1,Q2: inverse A in either sex	Mean (OW): M: 27.4; W: 27	-/-	Mean: M: 29.5% vs. .70.1% W: 32.1% vs 67.9%	M: 0.42; W: 0.47 <1 in all	M: 40.6%: $\|x\|$ >0* W: 35.8%: $\|x\|$ >0*
Lee et al. [26] US (2018)	*N* = 38,006 Men Age ≥ 40 y	1987–2012 Mean 21.4 y	M: 12,356	APE	Predicted FM: mono-tonic posi-tive A	Predicted LBM: inverse A	Mean: OW: 25.4	0.3% / 0.5%	FM vs. FFM: UW: 13.3 vs. 47.5; NW: 14.5 vs. 49.6 OW: 27.2 vs. 59 9; IIO: 41.2 vs. 77	UW: 0.27; NW: 0.29 IIO: 0.53 <1 in all	UW: 56.4%: $\|x\| > 0$ * NW: 54.8%: $\|x\| > 0$ * IIO: 30%: $\|x\|$ >0 *

					Original association findings					Novel findings	
Reference, Country, publish ed	**Study (N), sex, age**	**Follow-up**	**Deat hs (N)**	**BC**	**FM/FMI or VAT or other anthropo metrics**	**FFM/FF MI/LM/ SM/aSM M/ASMI ALM**	**BMIs**	**UW/ ≥ IIO (N or %)**	**FM/FMI versus FFM/FFMI or FM versus LBM**	**FMFFMR**	**$\lvert x \rvert$**
Liu et al. [27] US (2022)	N = 55,818 Both Mean age 45 y	1988–2014 Median 9.7 y	10,408	APE	Predicte FM: U-shaped A Q1, Q2, Q5 vs. Q3: direct A	Predicted LBM: L-shaped A Q1, Q2 vs. Q3: Inverse A	OW: Q3: M: 26.9-27.0; W: 26.1 NW: Q1: M: 21.3; W:22.6 IIO: Q5: M: 36.9; W: 35.4	Excluded / 30%	FM vs. FFM: Q3: M: 24.1 (FMI: 8.4) Vs. 59.3 (FFMI:18.5): 31.2% vs. 68.8% W: 29.9 (41.7%) vs. 41.7 (58.2%) Q1: M: < 16.2 (FMI: <5.8) vs. ≥ 31 (FFMI ≥15.5): 27.2% vs. 72.8%. W: < 21 (37%) vs. < 35.7 (63%) Q5: M: ≥ 31 (FMI: >10.6) vs. ≥ 65.4 (FFMI: 26.3): 28.7% vs. 71.3% Q5:W: ≥ 39.6 (45.6%) vs. ≥47.2 (54.4%)	OW: Q3: M: 0.45; W: > 0.71 NW: Q1: M: 0.37 W: 0.58 OW (Q3): M: 0.45 W: 0.71 IIO(Q5): M: 0.40 W: 0.83 <1 in all	OW: Q3: M: 37.6%; W: 16.5% NW: Q1, M: 45.6%; W: 26% OW: M: 37.6%; W: 16.5% IIO: Q5 M: 42.6%; W: 8.8% $\lvert x \rvert > 0 = +x$ in all*
Sedlmei er et al. [28]	N = 16,155	1994–2000	1,347	BIA	FMI: J-shaped A. BMI: 25.3 ± 2.2	FFMI: Q1 (16.1) vs. Q2	OW: q2: 25.4 ± 2.3	No/Low	OW: q2: 7.3 (28.8%) vs. 18 (71.2%)	OW: q2: 0.40 (<1)	q2: 42.4%: $\lvert x \rvert$ >0 *
EU and US (2021)	Both Mean age 45 y	Median 14.3 y			Q2 (7.3) vs. Q4 (13): direct A	(21.9): inverse A. BMI: 25.5 ± 2.4	NW: q1: 22.8 OW: q3: 28 IO: q4: 33.3 ± 4.2		NW: q1: 5.2 (22.9%) vs. 17.5 (77%) OW: q3: 9.2 (32.8%) vs. 18.2 (67.2%) IO: q4: 13 (38.7%) vs. 20.5 (61%)	NW: q1: 0.29 (<1) OW: q3: 0.48 (<1) IO: q4: 0.63 (<1)	q1: 54.1%: $\lvert x \rvert$ >0 * q3: 34.4%: $\lvert x \rvert$ > 0 * q4: 22.3%: $\lvert x \rvert$ >0 *

					Original association findings					Novel findings	
Reference, Country, publish ed	**Study (N), sex, age**	**Follow-up**	**Deat hs (N)**	**BC**	**FM/FMI or VAT or other anthropo metrics**	**FFM/FF MI/LM/ SM/aSM M/ASMI ALM**	**BMIs**	**UW/ ≥ IIO (N or %)**	**FM/FMI versus FFM/FFMI or FM versus LBM**	**FMFFMR**	**$\|x\|$**
Knowle s et al. [29] UK (2021)	N = 356,590 Both age 40–69 y	2006–2010 Median 10.5 y	15,844	BIA	FM: J-shaped A: positive log-linear A	aSMM: J-shaped A: M: positive log-linear A W: cur-vilinear A	OW: Mean: M: 27.6 ± 4; W: 26.7 ± 4.9 NW: Q1: M: 23.3; W: 21.6 IO: Q5: M: 33.1; W: 33.9	No/No	FM vs. FFM: M: 21.8 (25.4%) vs. 64 (74.6%); W: 26.3 (36.8%) vs. 45.1 (63.2%) FMI vs. FFMI: Q1: M: 4 vs. 19.3; W: 5.7 vs. 15.9 Q3: M: 7.1 vs. 20.5; W: 9.8 vs. 16.9 Q5: M: 10.8 vs. 22.3; W: 15.5 vs. 18.4	Q3: M: 0.34; W: 0.58 Q1: M: 0.20; W: 0.35 Q5: M: 0.48; W: 0.84 <1 in all	OW: M: 49.2%; W: 26.4%. NW: Q1: M: 65.7%; W: 47.3%. IO: Q5: M: 34.7%; W: 8.5% $\|x\| > 0 = +x$ in all*
Jung et al. [30] Germany (2024)	N = 23,725 Both age 40–75 y	2014–2019 (median 4.7 y)	–	MRI	Mean VAT:3.3 dm^3 direct A	Mean SM: 12.6 ± 3.3 dm^3: inverse A Mean SMFF: direct A	Overall (OW): 27.7 ± 4.7	– / –	Mean SMFF (%): 15 ± 3.2: SM vs. FM: > 50% vs. <50%	FM > SM FMFFMR < 1	$\|x\| < 50\%$–>1% $\|x\| > 0 = +x^*$
Jung et al. [30] UK (2024)	N = 36,317 Both age 45–84 y	2006–2010 (median 4.7 y)	634	MRI	Mean VAT: 3.5 dm^3: direct A	Mean SM: 11.4 ± 3 dm^3: inverse A Mean SMFF: direct A	Overall (OW): 25.9 ± 4.3	– / –	Mean SMFF (%): 18 ±3.2: SM vs. FM: > 50% vs. <50%	FM > SM FMFFMR < 1	$\|x\| < 50\%$–>1% $\|x\| > 0 = +x^*$

			Original association findings						Novel findings		
Reference, Country, publish ed	**Study (*N*), sex, age**	**Follow-up**	**Deat hs (*N*)**	**BC**	**FM/FMI or VAT or other anthropo metrics**	**FFM/FF MI/LM/ SM/aSM M/ASMI ALM**	**BMIs**	**UW/ ≥ IIO (*N* or %)**	**FM/FMI versus FFM/FFMI or FM versus LBM**	**FMFFMR**	**$\|x\|$**
Ghulam et al. [31] Italy (2023)	*N* = 20,587 Both mean age: 54 ± 11y	2005–2010 Median 11.2 y	M: 751 W: 458	APE	RFM: M: U-shaped A: nadir: 27.4; W: NA: nadir: 39.7 q4: M: direct A (RFM: 33.4 ± 1.8)	BMI > 35: direct A in both sexes	Mean (OW): M: 27.4 ± 1.4; W: 27.6 ± 0.7 NW: q1: M: 23.4 ± 2.8; W: 22.6 ± 1.6 IO: q3: M: 31.9 ± 1.4; W: 32.1 ± 1.4 IIO: q4: M: 35.4 ± 2; W: 38.4 ± 3.3	No/5.6%	RFM (%) vs. FFM (%): q2: M: 27.6 vs. 72.4; W: 39.7 vs. 60.3. q1: M: 23.9 vs. 76.1; W: 36.6 vs. 63.4 q4: M: 33.4 vs. 66.6; W: 48 vs. 52. FMI: M: q1: 5.8; q2: 7.3; q3: 8.6; q4:11; W: q1: 7.8; q2: 10.2; q3: 12.3; q4:16 FFMI: M: q1:18.5; q2:19.4; q3:20; q4: 22; W:q1: 15; q2:10.2; q3:16.2; q4: 17.5	q2: M: 0.38; W: 0.65 q1: M: 0.31; W: 0.57 q3: M: 0.43; W: 0.76 q4: M: 0.50; W: 0.90 <1 in all	q2: M: 44.8%; W: 20.6% q1: M: 52.2%; W: 26.8% q3: M: 40%; W: 13.4% q4: M: 33.2%; W: 5% $\|x\| > 0 = +x$ in all*
Farsijani et al. [37] US (2021)	*N* = 2,911 Both age 70–79 y	1996–1997 Average 12 y	1,873	CT DXA	FM (kg) by DXA: M: inverse A; W: inverse A	LBM: NA CT mid-thigh muscle area: inverse A in both	Mean (OW): M: 28.9; W: 27.4	No/No	LM: M: 55.5; W: 39.3. FM vs. FFM: M: 24.3 (29.7%) vs. 57.3 (70.3%); W: 29 (41.3%) vs. 41.2 (58.7%)	M: 0.42; W: 0.70 < 1 in all	M: 40.6%; W: 17.4% $\|x\| > 0 = +x$ in all*
Abramo vitz et al. [38] US (2018)	*N* = 11,687 Both age: 45.3 y	1999–2004 Median 9.3 y	1,819	DXA	Mean FM %: 33.05 (both sexes) FM: NA	Mean ASMI: 6.86 kg/m^2 Inverse A	Mean: 25.3 (both sexes); NW: 22.3; OW: 27; IO: 32.5	No/No	NW: FM (29.7%) vs. FFM (70.3%) OW: FM (36%) vs. FFM (64%) IO: FM (40%) vs. FFM (60%)	NW: 0.42; OW: 0.56; IO: 0.66 <1 in all	NW: 40.6%; OW: 28%; IO: 20% $\|x\| > 0 = +x$ in all*

				Original association findings						Novel findings	
Reference, Country, publish ed	**Study (*N*), sex, age**	**Follow-up**	**Deat hs (*N*)**	**BC**	**FM/FMI or VAT or other anthropo metrics**	**FFM/FF MI/LM/ SM/aSM M/ASMI ALM**	**BMIs**	**UW/ ≥ IIO (*N* or %)**	**FM/FMI versus FFM/FFMI or FM versus LBM**	**FMFFMR**	**|*x*|**
Jang et al. [45] Korean (2023)	*N* = 153,248 Both age ≥ 40 y	2004–2019 Median 18 y	6,061	APE	FMI: monotonic A WC: monotonic positive A	FFMI: inverse monotonic A	Nadir: 23–24.9: OW for Asian population Ref for FMI: 8.1 Ref for FFMI: 15.2 UW: 17.7; NW: 21.4; IO: 26.7; IIO: 31.8	1.7% / 3.1%	OW: high FFMI > low FMI NW: 18.5–22.9: low FFMI > low FMI UW: low FFMI > low FMI IO: 25–29.9:high FFMI > high FMI IIO: ≥ 30: low FFMI/high FMI Positive linearity for WC	0.53 in the nadir: FMI vs. FFMI: 8.1 (35%) vs. 15 (65%) <1 in all excepting cases of IIO and very increased WC, where FMI > FFMI	|*x*| > 0 = + *x* in all*
Rolland et al. [54] France (2023)	*N* = 4,574 W. Age ≥ 74 y	1992–2011 Median 17.7 y	2,876	DXA	FMI: reversed J-shaped A FM: inverse A	LBMI: NA ASMI: NA	OW: 25.2 ± 3.8	2.7% / 1.2%	OW: FMI: 9.3 ± 3.1 (37%) vs. FFMI: 15 9 ± 3 (63%)	OW: 0.58 <1	OW: 26% |*x*| > 0 = + *x**
Bea et al. [55] US (2015)	*N* = 10,525 W	1993–1998 Median 13.6 y	1,762	DXA	FM (Q3): 32.6; Q1: 19.4; Q5: 48.5; mean FM: 43.8%	LM (Q3):37.6; Q1: 36;	Q2: 25.6; Q3: 28.2; Q1: 22.5; Q5: 35.2	65/192	Q2: FM (40.3%) vs. FFM (59.7%) Q3 FM (44.3%) vs. FFM (55.7%)	Q2: 0.67; Q3: 0.79; Q1: 0.49; Q5: 1.14	OW: Q2: 19,4% OW: Q3: 11.4%
	Age 50–70 y				50–59 y: linear +; >70 y: linear –	Q5:40; FFM: 56%. < 60 y: linear –; > 70 y: linear +	≥ 35: increased risk: + A		Q1: FM (33.2%) vs. FFM (66.8%) Q5: FM (53.4%) vs. FFM (46.6%)	< 1 in all	Q1: 33.6%; Q5: 6.8% |*x*| > 0 = + *x* in all*

				Original association findings						Novel findings	
Reference, Country, publish ed	**Study (*N*), sex, age**	**Follow-up**	**Deat hs (*N*)**	**BC**	**FM/FMI or VAT or other anthropo metrics**	**FFM/FF MI/LM/ SM/aSM M/ASMI ALM**	**BMIs**	**UW/ ≥ IIO (*N* or %)**	**FM/FMI versus FFM/FFMI or FM versus LBM**	**FMFFMR**	**|*x*|**
Lee et al. [56] China (2012)	*N* = 3,978 Both. < 65 y	2001–2003 Median 74.4 m	383	DXA	FM%: M: negative A; W: NA	NA	M: 23.2: low OW; W: 23.9: low OW	No/No	M: FM: 24% (5.2) vs. FFM: 86% W: FM: 34.2% (6.1) vs. FFM: 65.8%	M: 0.27; W: 0.51 <1 in both: far from 1	M: 62%; W: 31.6% |*x*| > 0 = + *x**
Wanna methee [69] UK (2007)	*N* = 4,017 Men age 60–79 y	1978–2005 Mean 6 y	713	BIA	FMI: NA	FFMI: NA MAMC: inverse A	Mean: OW: q2: 25–27.4 UW men were excluded. q1: NW q3: 27.5–30. q4 ≥ 30	0.6% (excluded)/ –	FMI vs. FFMI: q1: < 7.6 vs. < 16; q2: 7.6–9.4 vs. 16–17.1; q3: 9.4–11.5 vs. 17.1–18.4; q4: ≥ 11.5 to ≥ 18.4 FM vs. FFM: q1: < 32.1% vs. > 67.9%; q2: –35.4% vs. –64.6%; q3: –38.4% vs. –61.6%; Q4: ≥ 38.4% vs. ≤ 61.6%	q1: NW: < 0.47 q2: 0.47 to < 0.54 q3: 0.54 to < 0.62 q4: ≥ 0.62 < 1 in all	q1: NW: > 35.8% q2: 35.8 to > 29.2% q3: 29.2% to > 23.2% q4: > 0 to < 23.2% |*x*| > 0 = + *x* in all*
Kitahara et al. [71] US (2023)	*N* = 280,611 Both	1976–2009 Median 10 y	16,769 (999 in class III)	WC APE	Class IIIO: direct A	High FFMI (FFMI > FMI) in both sexes	NW (ref) vs. class IIIO IIIO: > 45 (median)	No/9,215 in class IIIO	FM vs. FFM in class IIIO: M: 37.5% vs 62.5%; W: 59.8% vs. 40.2% FMI vs. FFMI in class IIIO: M: 16.8 vs. 28.2; W: 26.9 Vs. 28.1	M: 0.6 (<1) W: 1.48 (>1)	M: 25%: |*x*| >0 = + *x* W: –19.6%: |*x*| = –*x* |*x*| > 0 *
Batsis et al. [82] US (2017)	*N* = 4,984 Both Age ≥ 60	1999–2004 Median 102 m	2,002	DXA	FM ≥ 25%: M: A FM ≥ 35%: W: NA	ALM: M: A; W: NA ALM + obesity: M: A; W: NA	Mean BMI: M: 28.2 ± 0.1 W: 28.3 ± 0.1	No/No	M: FM: 30.9% (0.2) vs. FFM: 69% W: 42% (0.13) vs. FFM: 58%	M: 0.44 W: 0.72 < 1 in both	M: 38.2%; W: 16% |*x*| = + *x* in both |*x*| > 0 *

Original association findings										Novel findings	
Reference, Country, publish ed	**Study (*N*), sex, age**	**Follow-up**	**Deat hs (*N*)**	**BC**	**FM/FMI or VAT or other anthropo metrics**	**FFM/FF MI/LM/ SM/aSM M/ASMI ALM**	**BMIs**	**UW/ ≥ IIO (*N* or %)**	**FM/FMI versus FFM/FFMI or FM versus LBM**	**FMFFMR**	**|*x*|**
Graft el al. [83] Switzrerland (2015)	N = 3,181 Both Age > 65 y	1990–2011 -	1,777	BIA	FMI: NA	FFMI: M: negative A W: NA	Mean BMI: M: 24.6 (4.8); W: 24.6 (6.1) q1: M: 20.9; W: 20.3 q4: M: 27.6; W: 28	10%/4%	M: FMI: 6.7 vs. FFMI: 18 FM: 26.2% vs. FFM: 73.8%. W: FMI: 9.4 vs. FFMI: 15.3. FM: 36.8% vs. FFM: 63.2%. q1: FMI: M: < 4.7; W: < 6.8 FFMI: M: < 16.2; W: < 13.5 q4: FMI: M: > 8.2; W: > 11.4 FFMI: M: > 19.4; W: > 16.6	NW: M: 0.35; W: 0.58 Low NW: q1: M: 0.28; W: 0.50 OW: q4: M: 0.42; W: 0.68 <1 in all	NW: M: 47.6%; W: 26.4% q1: M: 55.2%; W: 33.2% q4: M: 40.6%; W: 18.6% |*x*| > 0 = + *x* in all*
Chang et al. [84] Taiwan (2022)	N = 1,199 Both	2009–2018 Median 5.8 py	103	BIA	FM: NA FMI and VFAI: + A in W	FFMI and SMMI: – A in both sexes	Mean: 24.2 (3.5)	–/–	FM: 31.4% (8.2) vs. FFM: 68.6% FMI: 7.8 (2.9); Mean FFMI: 16.3 (2) SMMI: 8.8 (1.25) VFAI: 49.4 (12.8)	NW: 0.45: < 1	NW: 37.2% |*x*| > 0 = + *x* *
Howell et al. [85] US-residing Mexican – Americans (2018)	N = 10,329 Both	1988–2010 Mean 10 y	1,423	BIA	FM%, LM, FM: NA Ref value for FM: M: 22.5%; W: 35.8% WC, WHtR: M: NA; W: + A	LM: NA Ref value for BMI: 25	Mean: 28.1 (5.6)	–/–	FM: 31.5% vs. FFM: 68.5% (both sexes) FM (kg): 23.9 vs. FFM: 51.9 (both sexes) FM for NA: M: 22.5% vs. FFM: 77.5%; W: 35.8% vs. FFM: 64.2%	OW: 0.45 Mean for NA: M: 0.29 (NW); W: 0.55 (low OW) <1 in all	OW: 37% Mean for NA: M: 55%; W: 28% (low OW): |*x*| >0 = + *x* in all*

					Original association findings					Novel findings	
Reference, Country, publish ed	**Study (*N*), sex, age**	**Follow-up**	**Deat hs (*N*)**	**BC**	**FM/FMI or VAT or other anthropo metrics**	**FFM/FF MI/LM/ SM/aSM M/ASMI ALM**	**BMIs**	**UW/ ≥ IIO (*N* or %)**	**FM/FMI versus FFM/FFMI or FM versus LBM**	**FMFFMR**	**|*x*|**
Lee JS et al. [79] Hong Kong (2012)	*N* = 3,978 Both	2001–2003 Median 74.4 m	361	DXA	FM, RAF: M: reverse A W: NA Mean BF%: M: 24.05 (5.1); W: 34.2 (6.1)	FFM%: – Mean FFM %: M: 76 W: 65.8	M: 22,7 (3); W: 24 (4) Q1: M: 20.2 (2.6) Q3: M: 23.9 (2.4) Q5: 25.7 (2.8)	-/-	Quintiles of RFA in men: Q1 (ref): FM%: 18.9 vs. FFM%: 80.1 Q3: FM%: 25.4 (3.6) vs. FFM%: 74.6 Q5: FM%: 27.3 (3.7) vs. FFM%: 72.7	M: Q1 (ref): 0.23; Q3: 0.34; Q5: 0.37 W: mean: 0.51 <1 in all	M: Q1 (ref): 61.2% Q3: 49%; Q5: 45.4% W: mean: 31.6% |*x*| > 0 = +*x* in all*
Kimberl y et al. [86] United States (2025)	*N* = 1,291 Both	2009–2021 Median 3.9 y	111	BIA	Mean BF%: M: 25.8 (7.4): NA W: 36.4 (8.9): NA	Mean LBM: M: 61.9 (9.5): NA; W: 43.5 (7.5): – A	Mean: M: 27.4 (6.1); W: 27.3 (6.0)	-/-	Quintiles of BF %: Q1 (ref): M: < 19.7; W: <28.2 Q3: M: 25.8 (7.4); W: 36.4 (8.9)	Q1: M: < 0.25; W: < 0.39 Q3: M: 0.34; W: 0.57 <1 in all	M: Q1: 60%; Q3: 48% W: Q1: 44%; Q3: 27% |*x*| > 0 = +*x* in all*

A: association; APE: anthropometric prediction equations; aSMM: appendicular skeletal muscle mass (kg); ASMI: appendicular skeletal muscle mass index; ALM: appendicular lean mass (kg); BC: body composition; BIA: bioimpedance analysis; BF: body fat; BMI: body mass index (kg/m2); CT: computed tomography; DXA: dual-energy X-ray absorptiometry; FFM: fat-free mass (kg or %); FFMI: fat-free mass index (kg/m2); FM: fat mass (kg or %); FMI: fat mass index (kg/m2); LBM: lean body mass (kg or %); LM: lean mass (kg); M: men; MAMC: midarm muscle circumference (cm); MRI: magnetic resonance imaging; NA: no association; NW: normal weight; OI: class I obesity; OII: class II obesity; OIII: class III obesity; OW: overweight; P: percentile; q: quartile; Q: quintile; RFM: relative fat mass (%); RAF: relative abdominal fat; SMMI: skeletal muscle mass index; VAT: visceral adipose tissue; VFAI: visceral fat area index; W: women; WC: waist circumference; WHR: waist-to-hip ratio; WHtR: waist-to-height ratio; UW: underweight; |x|, modulus "x" as the absolute difference between FFM and FM (may be in kg or %, |x| may be + x or −x).

**Significance level: p <0.05, |x| > 0.5 kg or |x| exceeding 1% of weight in favor of FFM or FM as appropriate.*

***Data are means (standard error), medians, or representative means. Sums of percentages may not equal 100% due to rounding.*

****Body composition studies include those studies that assessed measurements of FFM, FFMI, LBM, aSMM, ASMI, muscle areas, and/or FM, FMI, VAT from techniques such as bioimpedance analysis, CT, MRI, total body potassium, DXA, and APE that, among other anthropometrics, included WC and height. Specific studies of sarcopenia, muscle quality, and mortality are not included because they are not applicable. Studies of BMI alone or body fat distribution indices, without accounting for body composition measures, are not included.*

Table S1.
Relevant studies in the literature review of associations between body composition measures and mortality (previously omitted variables derived from datasets or recalculations are included to support novel association findings).

Author details

Angel Martin Castellanos
Spanish Society of Sports Medicine, Cáceres, Spain

*Address all correspondence to: angelmartincastellanos@gmail.com

References

[1] ESC Scientific Document Group, Koskinas KC, Van Craenenbroeck EM, Antoniades C, Blüher M, Gorter TM, Hanssen H, et al. Obesity and cardiovascular disease: An ESC clinical consensus statement. European Heart Journal. 2024;ehae508. DOI: 10.1093/eurheartj/ehae508

[2] GBD Obesity Collaborators. Health effects of overweight and obesity in 195 countries over 25 years. New England Journal of Medicine. 2017;**377**:13–27

[3] Dramé M, Godaert L. The obesity paradox and mortality in older adults: A systematic review. Nutrients. 2023;**15**(7):1780. DOI: 10.3390/nu15071780

[4] Flegal KM, Kit BK, Orpana H, Graubard BI. Association of all-cause mortality with overweight and obesity using standard body mass index categories: A systematic review and meta-analysis. JAMA. 2013;**309**(1):71–82. DOI: 10.1001/jama.2012.113905

[5] Aune D, Sen A, Prasad M, et al. BMI and all cause mortality: Systematic review and non-linear dose-response meta-analysis of 230 cohort studies with 3.74 million deaths among 30.3 million participants. BMJ. 2016;**353**:i2156

[6] Joshy G, Korda RJ, Bauman A, Van Der Ploeg HP, Chey T, Banks E. Investigation of Methodological Factors Potentially Underlying the Apparently Paradoxical Findings on Body Mass Index and All-Cause Mortality. PLoS ONE. 2014;**9**(2):e88641. DOI: 10.1371/journal.pone.0088641

[7] Bhaskaran K, Dos-Santos-Silva I, Leon DA, Douglas IJ, Smeeth L. Association of BMI with overall and cause-specific mortality: A population-based cohort study of 3·6 million adults in the UK. The Lancet Diabetes & Endocrinology. 2018;**6**(12):944–953. DOI: 10.1016/S2213-8587(18)30288-2

[8] Duarsa AB, Widiyanto A, Putri SI, Anulus A, Atmojo JT, Fajriah AS. The association between body mass index and all-cause mortality: A meta-analysis. International Journal of Health Sciences. 2022;**6**(S4):367–383. DOI: 10.53730/ijhs.v6nS4.5521

[9] Mehran L, Amouzegar A, Fanaei SM, Masoumi S, Azizi F. Anthropometric measures and risk of all-cause and cardiovascular mortality: An 18 years follow-up. Obesity Research & Clinical Practice. 2022;**16**(1):63–71. DOI: 10.1016/j.orcp.2021.12.004

[10] Prospective Studies Collaboration. Body-mass index and cause-specific mortality in 900 000 adults: Collaborative analyses of 57 prospective studies. The Lancet. 2009;**373**(9669):1083–1096. DOI: 10.1016/S0140-6736(09)60318-4

[11] Lu C-Y, Chen -H-H, Chi K-H, Chen P-C. Obesity indices and the risk of total and cardiovascular mortality among people with diabetes: A long-term follow-up study in Taiwan. Cardiovascular Diabetology. 2023;**22**(1):345. DOI: 10.1186/s12933-023-02072-3

[12] Consortium GCR, Magnussen C, Ojeda FM, Leong DP, Alegre-Diaz J, Amouyel P, Aviles-Santa L, et al. Global Effect of Modifiable Risk Factors on Cardiovascular Disease and Mortality. New England Journal of Medicine. 2023;**389**(14):1273–1285. DOI: 10.1056/NJMoa2206916

[13] Nowak MM, Niemczyk M, Gołębiewski S, Pączek L. Impact of Body Mass Index on All-Cause Mortality in Adults: A Systematic Review and Meta-Analysis. Journal of Clinical Medicine. 2024;**13**(8):2305. DOI: 10.3390/jcm13082305

[14] Taha MB, Javed Z, Nwana N, Acquah I, Satish P, Sharma G, et al. Body Mass Index and All-Cause and Cardiovascular Mortality in United States Adults With and Without Atherosclerotic Cardiovascular Disease: Findings from the National Health Interview Survey. Population Health Management. 2023;**26**(4):254–267. DOI: 10.1089/pop.2022.0280

[15] Visaria A, Setoguchi S. Body mass index and all-cause mortality in a 21st century U.S. population: A National Health Interview Survey analysis. PLoS One. 2023;**18**(7):e0287218. DOI: 10.1371/journal.pone.0287218

[16] Baumgartner RN, Heymsfield SB, Roche AF. Human body composition and the epidemiology of chronic disease. Obesity Research. 1995;**3**:73–95

[17] Allison DB, Faith MS, Heo M, Kotler DP. Hypothesis concerning the U-shaped relation between body mass index and mortality. American Journal of Epidemiology. 1997;**146**(4):339–349. DOI: 10.1093/oxfordjournals.aje.a009275

[18] Martin-Castellanos A. Why predicting health risks from either body mass index or waist-to-hip ratio presents causal association biases worldwide: A mathematical demonstration. Acta Scientific Medical Sciences. 2023;**7**(7):112–120. DOI: 10.31080/ASMS.2023.07.1605

[19] Castellanos AM. Association of body mass index and abdominal obesity with myocardial infarction: We reveal confounding factors that historically distorted causal inferences. Medical Research Archives. 2024;**12**(3). DOI: 10.18103/mra.v12i3.5102

[20] Wang ZM, Pierson Jr RN, Heymsfield SB. The five-level model: A new approach to organizing body-composition research. The American Journal of Clinical Nutrition. 1992;**56**(1):19–28. DOI: 10.1093/ajcn/56.1.19

[21] Heitmann BL, Erikson H, Ellsinger B-M, Mikkelsen KL, Larsson B. Mortality associated with body fat, fat-free mass and body mass index among 60-year-old Swedish men—a 22-year follow-up. The study of men born in 1913. International Journal of Obesity. 2000;**24**(1):33–37. DOI: 10.1038/sj.ijo.0801082

[22] Bigaard J, Frederiksen K, Tjønneland A, Thomsen BL, Overvad K, Heitmann BL, Sørensen TI. Body fat and fat-free mass and all-cause mortality. Obesity Research. 2004;**12**(7):1042–1049. DOI: 10.1038/oby.2004.131

[23] Simpson JA, MacInnis RJ, Peeters A, Hopper JL, Giles GG, English DR. A comparison of adiposity measures as predictors of all-cause mortality: The Melbourne Collaborative Cohort Study. Obesity (Silver Spring). 2007;**15**:994–100

[24] Zong G, Zhang Z, Yang Q, Wu H, Hu FB, Sun Q. Total and regional adiposity measured by dual-energy X-ray absorptiometry and mortality in NHANES 1999-2006. Obesity. 2016;**24**:2414–2421

[25] Padwall R, Leslie WD, Lix LM, Majumdar SR. Relationship Among Body Fat Percentage, Body Mass Index, and All-Cause Mortality: A Cohort

Study. Annals of Internal Medicine. 2016;**164**(8):532–541. DOI: 10.7326/M15-1181

[26] Lee DH, Keum N, Hu FB, Orav EJ, Rimm EB, Willett WC, et al. Predicted lean body mass, fat mass, and all cause and cause specific mortality in men: Prospective US cohort study. BMJ (Clinical Research Ed.). 2018;**362**(2575). DOI: 10.1136/bmj.k2575

[27] Liu M, Zhang Z, Zhou C, Ye Z, He P, Zhang Y, Li H, Liu C, Qin X. Predicted fat mass and lean mass in relation to all-cause and cause-specific mortality. Journal of Cachexia, Sarcopenia and Muscle. 2022;**13**(2):1064–1075. DOI: 10.1002/jcsm.12921

[28] Sedlmeier AM, Baumeister SE, Weber A, Fischer B, Thorand B, Ittermann T, et al. Relation of body fat mass and fat-free mass to total mortality: Results from 7 prospective cohort studies. The American Journal of Clinical Nutrition. 2021;**113**(3):639–646. DOI: 10.1093/ajcn/nqaa339

[29] Knowles R, Carter J, Jebb S, Bennet D, Lewington S, Piernas C. Associations of Skeletal Muscle Mass and Fat Mass With Incident Cardiovascular Disease and All-Cause Mortality: A Prospective Cohort Study of UK Biobank Participants. Journal of the American Heart Association. 2021;10e019337. DOI: 10.1161/JAHA.120.019337

[30] Jung M, Raghu VK, Reisert M, Rieder H, Rospleszcz S, Pischon T, et al. Deep learning-based body composition analysis from whole-body magnetic resonance imaging to predict all-cause mortality in a large western population. EBioMedicine. 2024;**110**:105467

[31] Ghulam A, Gianfagna F, Bonaccio M, Costanzo S, Di Castelnuovo A, De Curtis A, et al. Association between BMI, RFM and mortality and potential mediators: Prospective findings from the Moli-sani study. International Journal of Obesity. 2023;**47**(8):697–708. DOI: 10.1038/s41366-5

[32] Martin Castellanos A. Anthropometrics in Predicting Cardiovascular Disease Risk: Our Research Work Mathematically Demonstrates that Cardiovascular Sciences Were Always Confused for a Long Time [Internet]. Novel Pathogenesis and Treatments for Cardiovascular Disease. IntechOpen. 2023;333–359. DOI: 10.5772/intechopen.105098

[33] Castellanos AM. Anthropometrics and Myocardial Infarction Risk: A Misleading Evidence Was Accepted by Cardiovascular Sciences When Errors of Bias Were Overlooked Worldwide. When Should We End Discussion about the Optimal Metric? Medical Research Archives. 2022;**10**(7):2–16. DOI: 10.18103/mra.v10i7.2917

[34] Castellanos AM. Waist-to-Height Ratio is an Optimal Metric in Predicting Myocardial Infarction Risk. Other Anthropometrics Widely used by Cardiology to Promote Cardiovascular Health Present Association Biases. MRA. 2023;**10**(12):1–16. DOI: 10.18103/mra.v10i12.3463

[35] Castellanos AM. Anthropometric measures in predicting myocardial infarction risk. Do we know what we are measuring? Bias in research occurred worldwide when the true unhealthy body composition was not well compared. Medical Research Archives. 2021;**9**(6):1–19

[36] Woolcott OO, Bergman RN. Relative fat mass (RFM) as a new

estimator of whole-body fat percentage — A cross-sectional study in American adult individuals. Scientific Reports. 2018;**8**:1):10980. DOI: 10.1038/s41598-018-29362-1

[37] Farsijani S, Xue L, Boudreau RM, Santanasto AJ, Kritchevsky SB, Newman AB. Body Composition by Computed Tomography vs Dual-Energy X-ray Absorptiometry: Long-Term Prediction of All-Cause Mortality in the Health ABC Cohort. The Journals of Gerontology. Series A, Biological Sciences and Medical Sciences. 2021;**76** (12):2256–2264. DOI: 10.1093/gerona/glab105

[38] Abramowitz MK, Hall CB, Amodu A, Sharma D, Androga L, Hawkins M. Muscle mass, BMI, and mortality among adults in the United States: A population-based cohort study. PLoS One. 2018;**13**:e0194697. DOI: 10.1371/journal.pone.0194697

[39] Almuwaqqat Z, Hui Q, Liu C, Zhou JJ, Voight BF, Ho YL, et al. Long-Term Body Mass Index Variability and Adverse Cardiovascular Outcomes. JAMA Network Open. 2024;7(3): e243062. DOI: 10.1001/jamanetworkopen.2024.3062

[40] Li S, Fu Z, Zhang W. Association of anthropometric measures with all-cause and cause-specific mortality in US adults: Revisiting the obesity paradox. BMC Public Health. 2024;**24**(1):929. DOI: 10.1186/s12889-024-18418-9

[41] Feng Q, Beśević J, Conroy M, Omiyale W, Woodward M, Lacey B, et al. Waist-to-height ratio and body fat percentage as risk factors for ischemic cardiovascular disease: A prospective cohort study from UK Biobank. The American Journal of Clinical Nutrition. 2024;**119**(6):1386–1396. DOI: 10.1016/j.ajcnut.2024.03.018

[42] Georgoulis M, Damigou E, Chrysohoou C, Barkas F, Kravvariti E, Tsioufis C, et al. Increased body weight and central adiposity markers are positively associated with the 20-year incidence of cardiovascular disease: The ATTICA epidemiological study (2002–2022). Nutrition Research. 2024;**121**:1–15

[43] Martín-Castellanos A, Cabañas MD, Martín-castellanos P, Barca Durán FJ. The body composition and risk prediction in myocardial infarction men. Revealing biological and statistical error bias for both general obesity and waist-to-Hip ratio. Cardiovascular Research Medicine. 2018;**2**:13–20

[44] Mboya IB, Fritz J, da Silva M, Sun M, Wahlström J, Magnusson PKE, et al. Time trends of the association of body mass index with mortality in 3.5 million young Swedish adults. Annals of Epidemiology. 2024;**97**:23–32

[45] Jang H, Kim R, Lee J-T, Lee DH, Giovannucci EL, Oh H. Overall and abdominal obesity and risks of all-cause and cause-specific mortality in Korean adults: A pooled analysis of three population-based prospective cohorts. International Journal of Epidemiology. 2023;**52**(4):1060–1073. DOI: 10.1093/ije/dyac242

[46] Warren Andersen S, Shu XO, Gao YT, Zhang X, Cai H, Yang G, et al. Prospective Cohort Study of Central Adiposity and Risk of Death in Middle Aged and Elderly Chinese. PLoS One. 2015;**10**(9):e0138429. DOI: 10.1371/journal.pone.0138429

[47] Peters SAE, Bots SH, Woodward M. Sex Differences in the Association Between Measures of General and Central Adiposity and the Risk of Myocardial Infarction: Results From the UK Biobank. Journal of the

American Heart Association. 2018;7(5): e008507. DOI: 10.1161/ JAHA.117.008507

[48] Lee DH, Giovannucci EL. Body composition and mortality in the general population: A review of epidemiologic studies. Experimental Biology and Medicine. 2018;**243** (17-18):1275–1285. DOI: 10.1177/ 1535370218818161

[49] Abdi Dezfouli R, Mohammadian Khonsari N, Hosseinpour A, Asadi S, Ejtahed H-S, Qorbani M. Waist to height ratio as a simple tool for predicting mortality: A systematic review and meta-analysis. International Journal of Obesity. 2023;**47**:1286–1301. DOI: 10.10 38/s41366-023-01388-0

[50] Tewari A, Kumar G, Maheshwari A, Tewari V, Tewari J. Comparative Evaluation of Waist-to-Height Ratio and BMI in Predicting Adverse Cardiovascular Outcome in People With Diabetes: A Systematic Review. Cureus. 2023;**15**(5):e38801. DOI: 10.7759/cureus.38801

[51] Chan V, Lo K. People with normal waist circumference but with elevated waist-to-height ratio: An overlooked population with increased cardiometabolic risk? the American Journal of Clinical Nutrition. 2024;**119** (6):1379–1380. DOI: 10.1016/j. ajcnut.2024.04.013

[52] Afzal S, Tybjærg-Hansen A, Jensen GB, Nordestgaard BG. Change in Body Mass Index Associated With Lowest Mortality in Denmark, 1976-2013. JAMA. 2016;**315**(18):1989–1996. DOI: 10.1001/jama.2016.4666

[53] Nalini M, Sharafkhah M, Poustchi H, Sepanlou SG, Pourshams A, Radmard AR, et al. Comparing Anthropometric Indicators of Visceral and General Adiposity as Determinants of Overall and Cardiovascular Mortality. Archives of Iranian Medicine 2019;**22**:301–309

[54] Rolland Y, Gallini A, Cristini C, Schott AM, Blain H, Beauchet O, et al. Body-composition predictors of mortality in women aged ≥75 y: Data from a large population-based cohort study with a 17-y follow-up. The American Journal of Clinical Nutrition. 2014;**100**(5):1352–1360. DOI: 10.3945/ ajcn.114.086728

[55] Bea JW, Thomson CA, Wertheim BC, Nicholas JS, Ernst KC, Hu C, et al. Risk of mortality according to body mass index and body composition among postmenopausal women. American Journal of Epidemiology. 2015;**182**:585–596

[56] Lee JS, Auyeung TW, Kwok T, Li M, Leung J, Woo J. Survival benefit of abdominal adiposity: A 6-year follow-up study with Dual X-ray absorptiometry in 3,978 older adults. Age (Dordr). 2012;**34**(3):597–608. DOI: 10.1007/s113 57-011-9272-y

[57] Parra-Soto S, Boonpor J, Lynskey N, Araya C, Ho F, Pell JP, et al. Association between visceral adiposity index and cancer risk in the UK Biobank cohort. Cancer. 2025;**131**. DOI: 10.1002/ cncr.35576

[58] Zhang X, Ma N, Lin Q, Chen K, Zheng F, Wu J, et al. Body Roundness Index and All-Cause Mortality Among US Adults. JAMA Network Open. 2024;7(6):e2415051. DOI: 10.1001/ jamanetworkopen.2024.15051

[59] NY K, JC K. A new body shape index predicts mortality hazard independently of body mass index.

PLoS One. 2012;7e39504. DOI: 10.1371/journal.pone.0039504

[60] Aoki KC, Mayrovitz HN. Utility of a Body Shape Index Parameter in Predicting Cardiovascular Disease Risks. Cureus. 2022;**14**(4):e23886. DOI: 10.7759/cureus.23886

[61] Tang L, Zeng L. Comparative efficacy of anthropometric indices in predicting 10-year ASCVD risk: Insights from NHANES data. Frontiers in Cardiovascular Medicine. 2024;**11**:1341476. DOI: 10.3389/fcvm.2024.1341476

[62] Medina Inojosa BJ, Somers VK, Lara-Breitinger K, Johnson LA, Medina-Inojosa JR, Lopez-Jimenez F. Prediction of presence and severity of metabolic syndrome using regional body volumes measured by a multisensor white-light 3D scanner and validation using a mobile technology. European Heart Journal - Digital Health. 2024;ztae059. DOI: 10.1093/ehjdh/ztae059

[63] Frija-Masson J, Mullaert J, Vidal-Petiot E, Pons-Kerjean N, Flamant M, d'Ortho M-P. Accuracy of smart scales on weight and body composition: Observational study. JMIR mHealth and uHealth. 2021;**9**:e22487. DOI: 10.2196/22487

[64] Lv Y, Zhang Y, Li X, Gao X, Ren Y, Deng L, et al. Body mass index, waist circumference, and mortality in subjects older than 80 years: A Mendelian randomization study. European Heart Journal. 2024;**45**(24):2145–2154. DOI: 10.1093/eurheartj/ehae206

[65] Guasch-Ferré M, Bulló M, Martínez-González MA, Corella D, Estruch R, Covas MI, et al. Waist-to-height ratio and cardiovascular risk factors in elderly individuals at high cardiovascular risk. PLoS One. 2012;7(8):e43275. DOI: 10.1371/journal.pone.0043275

[66] Cai Z, Chen G, Zhao W, Wei Z, Wang X, Huang Z, et al. Increased Risk of Cardiometabolic Disease in Ideal Weight Adults With History of Overweight/Obesity in China: A Prospective Cohort Study. Journal of the American Heart Association. 2024;**13**(9):e033610. DOI: 10.1161/JAHA.123.033610

[67] World Cancer Research Fund/American Institute for Cancer Research. Continuous Update Project Expert Report 2018. Body fatness and weight gain and the risk of cancer. Available from: dietandcancerreport.org; https://www.wcff.org/wp-content/uploads/2024/10/Body-fatness-and-weight-gain_0.pdf

[68] Reges O, Test T, Dicker D, Karpati T. Association of Waist Circumference and Body Mass Index Deciles Ratio with All-Cause Mortality: Findings from the National Health and Nutrition Examination Survey. Nutrients. 2024;**16**(7):961. DOI: 10.3390/nu16070961

[69] Wannamethee SG, Shaper AG, Lennon L, Whincup PH. Decreased muscle mass and increased central adiposity are independently related to mortality in older men. The American Journal of Clinical Nutrition. 2007;**86**:1339–1346. DOI: 10.1093/ajcn/86.5.1339

[70] Sanchez-Lastra MA, Ding D, Dalene KE, Del Pozo Cruz B, Ekelund U, Tarp J. Body composition and mortality from middle to old age: A prospective cohort study from the UK Biobank. International Journal of Obesity. 2023;**47**(8):709–716. DOI: 10.1038/s41366-023-01314-4

[71] Kitahara CM, Flint AJ, Berrington de Gonzalez A, Bernstein L, Brotzman M, MacInnis RJ, et al. Association between Class III Obesity (BMI of 40–59 kg/m2) and Mortality: A Pooled Analysis of 20 Prospective Studies. PLoS Medicine. 2014;**11**(7):e1001673. DOI: 10.1371/journal.pmed.1001673

[72] Group of Vascular Diseases from Albacete, Ponce-Garcia I, Simarro-Rueda M, Carbayo-Herencia JA, Divisón-Garrote JA, Artigao-Ródenas LM, Botella-Romero F, et al. Prognostic value of obesity on both overall mortality and cardiovascular disease in the general population. PLoS One. 2015;**10**(5)e0127369. DOI: 10.1371/journal.pone.0127369

[73] Tanamas SK, Ng WL, Backholer K, Hodge A, Zimmet PZ, Peeters A. Quantifying the proportion of deaths due to body mass index- and waist circumference-defined obesity. Obesity (Silver Spring). 2016;**24**(3):735–742. DOI: 10.1002/oby.21386

[74] Abdullah A, Wolfe R, Stoelwinder JU, de Courten M, Stevenson C, Walls HL, et al. The number of years lived with obesity and the risk of all-cause and cause-specific mortality. International Journal of Epidemiology. 2011;**40**(4):985–996. DOI: 10.1093/ije/dyr018

[75] Farchan A, Helda H, Qonita Nur S, Rahma H, Ramadhani R, Ramadlani I, et al. Surrogate Biomarker to Identify Obesity and Predict Cardiovascular Disease Risk: A Systematic Review. Journal Health Sains. 2024;(5/7):410–428. DOI: 10.46799/jhs.v5i7.1302

[76] Bioletto F, Ponzo V, Goitre I, Stella B, Rahimi F, Parasiliti-Caprino M, et al. Complementary Role of BMI and EOSS in Predicting All-Cause and Cause-Specific Mortality in People with Overweight and Obesity. Nutrients. 2024;**16**(20):3433. DOI: 10.3390/nu16203433

[77] Tuccinardi D, Watanabe M, Masi D, Monte L, Meffe LB, Cavallari I, et al. Rethinking weight loss treatments as cardiovascular medicine in obesity, a comprehensive review. European Journal of Preventive Cardiology. 2024;**31**(10):1260–1273. DOI: 10.1093/eurjpc/zwae171

[78] Batsis JA, Mackenzie TA, Emeny RT, Lopez-Jimenez F, Bartels SJ. Low lean mass with and without obesity, and mortality: Results from the 1999–2004 National Health and Nutrition Examination Survey. The Journals of Gerontology. Series A, Biological Sciences and Medical Sciences. 2017;**72**:1445–1451. DOI: 10.1093/gerona/glx002

[79] Lincoff AM, Brown-Frandsen K, Colhoun HM, Deanfield J, Emerson SS, Esbjerg S, et al. Semaglutide and cardiovascular outcomes in obesity without diabetes. New England Journal of Medicine. 2023;**389**:2221–2232

[80] Ma C, Avenell A, Bolland M, Hudson J, Stewart F, Robertson C, et al. Effects of weight loss interventions for adults who are obese on mortality, cardiovascular disease, and cancer: Systematic review and meta-analysis. BMJ. 2017;**359**:j4849–j4849

[81] Donini LM, Pinto A, Giusti AM, Lenzi A, Poggiogalle E. Obesity or BMI Paradox? Beneath the Tip of the Iceberg. Frontiers in Nutrition. 2020;7:53. DOI: 10.3389/fnut.2020.00053

[82] Graf CE, Karsegard VL, Spoerri A, Makhlouf AM, Ho S, Herrmann FR, et al. Body composition and all-cause

mortality in subjects older than 65 y. The American Journal of Clinical Nutrition. 2015;**101**:760–767

[83] Chang CS, Liu IT, Liang FW, Li CC, Sun ZJ, Chang YF, et al. Effects of age and gender on body composition indices as predictors of mortality in middle-aged and old people. Scientific Reports. 2022;**12**(1):7912. DOI: 10.1038/s41598-022-12048-0

[84] Howell CR, Mehta T, Ejima K, Ness KK, Cherrington A, Fontaine KR. Body Composition and Mortality in Mexican American Adults: Results from the National Health and Nutrition Examination Survey. Results from the National Health and Nutrition Examination Survey. Obesity (Silver Spring). 2018;**26**(8):1372–1380. DOI: 10.1002/oby.22251

[85] Lee JS, Auyeung TW, Kwok T, Li M, Leung J, Woo J. Survival benefit of abdominal adiposity: A 6-year follow-up study with Dual X-ray absorptiometry in 3,978 older adults. Age (Dordr). 2012;**34**(3):597–608. DOI: 10.1007/s11357-011-9272-y

[86] Ogbonnaya C, Kindred M, Lavie CJ, Hannah O, Shin M-J, Sui X, et al. Association Between Trunk Fat Mass Index and Diabetes in a Multinational Population. Mayo Clinic Proceedings: Innovations, Quality & Outcomes. 2025;**9**(5):100658. DOI: 10.1016/j.mayocpiqo.2025.100658

Section 2

BMI in Pediatric and Adolescent Populations: Alternative Risk Stratification Strategies

Chapter 3

Beyond BMI in Childhood and Adolescence: Limitations and Alternatives

Ken Kiyono and Madhur Mangalam

Abstract

Accurate assessment of body size in growing children is a central challenge in pediatrics, with implications for both clinical care and public health. The body mass index (BMI), though widely used, was developed for adults, where body weight scales approximately with the square of height. In adults, this scaling reflects stable skeletal proportions after growth, allowing BMI to function as a height-adjusted indicator. In children, however, the weight–height relationship shifts systematically with age, sex, and maturation. Thus, the conventional definition of a *height-adjusted* index – minimizing correlation with height – fails to remove growth-related bias. Even if the BMI exponent p in weight/height^p is tuned to eliminate correlation, misclassification of thinness or obesity may still occur. We analyzed 7.86 million Japanese schoolchildren aged 5–17 years using an allometric framework and identified two distinct regimes. In the *uni-scaling* regime, observed after skeletal maturity (≥ 16 years in males, ≥ 14 in females), all weight-for-height centile curves share a common exponent ($p \approx 2$), producing BMI distributions invariant to height. In the *multi-scaling* regime, characteristic of younger children, exponents differ across centiles, causing BMI to overestimate obesity in taller children and underestimate it in shorter ones. To address this, we introduce *population-statistical objectivity* – requiring not only independence of the mean or median, but invariance of the entire distribution across heights – as the criterion for valid adjustment. For multi-scaling ages, centile-specific methods or direct use of weight centiles by sex, age, and height may offer a more accurate and interpretable basis for pediatric assessment.

Keywords: pediatrics, body mass index (BMI), anthropometry, weight-for-height centile analysis, growth and development, skeletal maturity, allometry, scaling laws, obesity and thinness

1. Introduction: Purpose and scope

Despite its widespread clinical use, no fully validated, height-adjusted metric exists for accurately assessing body mass in growing children. This persistent gap represents a critical opportunity for re-evaluation in pediatric medicine. Assessing body size during growth is a central task with far-reaching implications for both

 IntechOpen

clinical decision-making and public health policy. The body mass index (BMI) – originally developed for adults – remains the predominant tool for evaluating childhood nutritional status, even amid long-standing debate over its validity in developing populations [1–4]. Its theoretical basis lies in the empirical observation that, in the general adult population, typical body weight increases in proportion to height squared, rendering BMI largely independent of height. This property, grounded in the physiology of fully matured skeletal structures, has made BMI a practical and widely adopted screening tool for adults. However, applying a metric conceived for adults directly to children – without rigorous validation across the dynamic stages of growth – raises fundamental questions for evidence-based pediatric practice.

In this chapter, we revisit the scientific rationale and historical development of BMI – its conceptual foundations, successes, and limitations – to explore whether a genuinely height-adjusted body size index for children can be derived from routinely measured anthropometrics. Our goal is not to dismiss BMI by cataloging its weaknesses, but to clarify what BMI is – and what it is not – as a height-adjusted measure, thereby identifying principles for constructing a practical screening tool for childhood thinness and obesity using only height and weight.

Experience from adult practice offers important lessons. Firstly, two simple, inexpensive, and universally obtainable measurements – height and weight – can together form the basis of a large-scale screening metric for detecting both underweight and obesity. Secondly, the scalability of these measurements enables reduced statistical uncertainty and reproducible decision thresholds. Thirdly, although imperfect, BMI exhibits meaningful associations with body fatness and the prevalence of weight-related health conditions, supporting its role as an initial screening metric.

However, why these adult lessons fail to translate directly to children has been largely overlooked. Traditionally, a *height-adjusted* index has been defined as one showing minimal correlation with height. For growing children, this criterion is fundamentally flawed: The weight–height relationship shifts systematically with age, sex, and maturation, and eliminating statistical correlation does not eliminate growth-related bias. Indeed, in pediatric populations, even when BMI-type indices of the form weight/height^p are constructed using an exponent p estimated to remove correlation with height, such an adjustment does not necessarily yield the expected improvement in assessment accuracy. Our central argument is that BMI's practical role is not to achieve zero correlation with height, but rather to approximate a child's weight ranking within a same-height reference group – effectively, its weight centile position. This reinterpretation, detailed in the sections that follow, reveals why adult-derived indices underperform in pediatric contexts and suggests a more appropriate framework for childhood body size assessment.

The question is not whether simple anthropometric indices are inherently inadequate in pediatrics, but rather what form of height adjustment is appropriate during development. By making explicit the assumptions that support BMI's use in adults and identifying which ones break down in children, we argue that a principled, height-adjusted body size index for children is achievable. Such an index must be grounded in empirically observed weight–height scaling patterns throughout growth, rather than imported wholesale from adult models.

In this article, we (i) address the long-standing lack of systematic examination of the scientific rationale for constructing BMI in children, clarifying its conceptual and methodological gaps; (ii) define the conditions under which a height-adjusted index can be made approximately independent of height during development; and (iii) propose a methodology for constructing and validating such an index from large-scale height–weight datasets, with the aim of improving screening for both thinness and obesity in children.

In this review, we present findings from our analysis of the largest pediatric anthropometric dataset to date – comprising 7.86 million Japanese children aged 5–17 years and examine height–weight distributions in detail by sex and age. This review is based on three recent publications from our group [5–7]. Our analysis reveals the height dependence of BMI-type indices, weight/height^p, and changes markedly between the post-skeletal maturity period and the growth phase. At ages corresponding to skeletal maturity, the conditional distribution of BMI given height is essentially height-invariant, making BMI comparisons within a sex–age group effectively equivalent to comparing weight centile positions within the same height group (**Figure 1**). By contrast, during growth, BMI distributions vary strongly with height, so that BMI ceases to function as a truly height-adjusted index – rendering its comparisons difficult to interpret and of limited practical value.

We seek to give readers an intuitive understanding of the contrast between two biological states: skeletal maturity and skeletal immaturity. To classify and distinguish these differences more rigorously, we introduce a minimal but sufficient set of mathematical concepts. Specifically, we distinguish between uni-scaling – corresponding to the conventional notion of allometric scaling, in which a single exponent fully characterizes the weight-for-height relationship and multi-scaling, in which the relationship is described by a range of scaling exponents, reflecting variation in scaling behavior across the centile curves of the weight-for-height distribution.

2. Historical foundation of BMI

To explore where gaps in understanding have persisted within the conceptual foundations of BMI, we first briefly review the historical development of BMI for adults and the subsequent attempts to adapt it for use in children.

In his 1832 work and subsequently in the major 1835 treatise *Sur l'Homme et le Développement de ses Facultés, ou Essai de Physique Sociale* (Chapter II, Section 2 in [8]), the Belgian-French astronomer, mathematician, statistician, and sociologist Adolphe Quetelet presented a detailed statistical analysis of the relationship between human height and weight. Quetelet reasoned that if humans grew geometrically in all dimensions, body weight would be proportional to the cube of height ($\propto$ height^3). However, his empirical observations indicated otherwise: excluding the growth period, "the weight of the average man – an ideal type toward which nature tends – varies approximately in proportion to the square of the height" [8]. This suggested that, for adults, the ratio of weight to height squared remains nearly constant, making it a useful index for comparing body size between individuals. Quetelet himself did not name this ratio. Later researchers honored his contribution by calling it the Quetelet Index (now known as BMI). He further noted that during the growth period, weight increases approximately in proportion to the 2.5th power of height – a scaling relationship distinct from that observed in fully developed adults. This early recognition of the distinct scaling laws for children and adults is noteworthy, as it

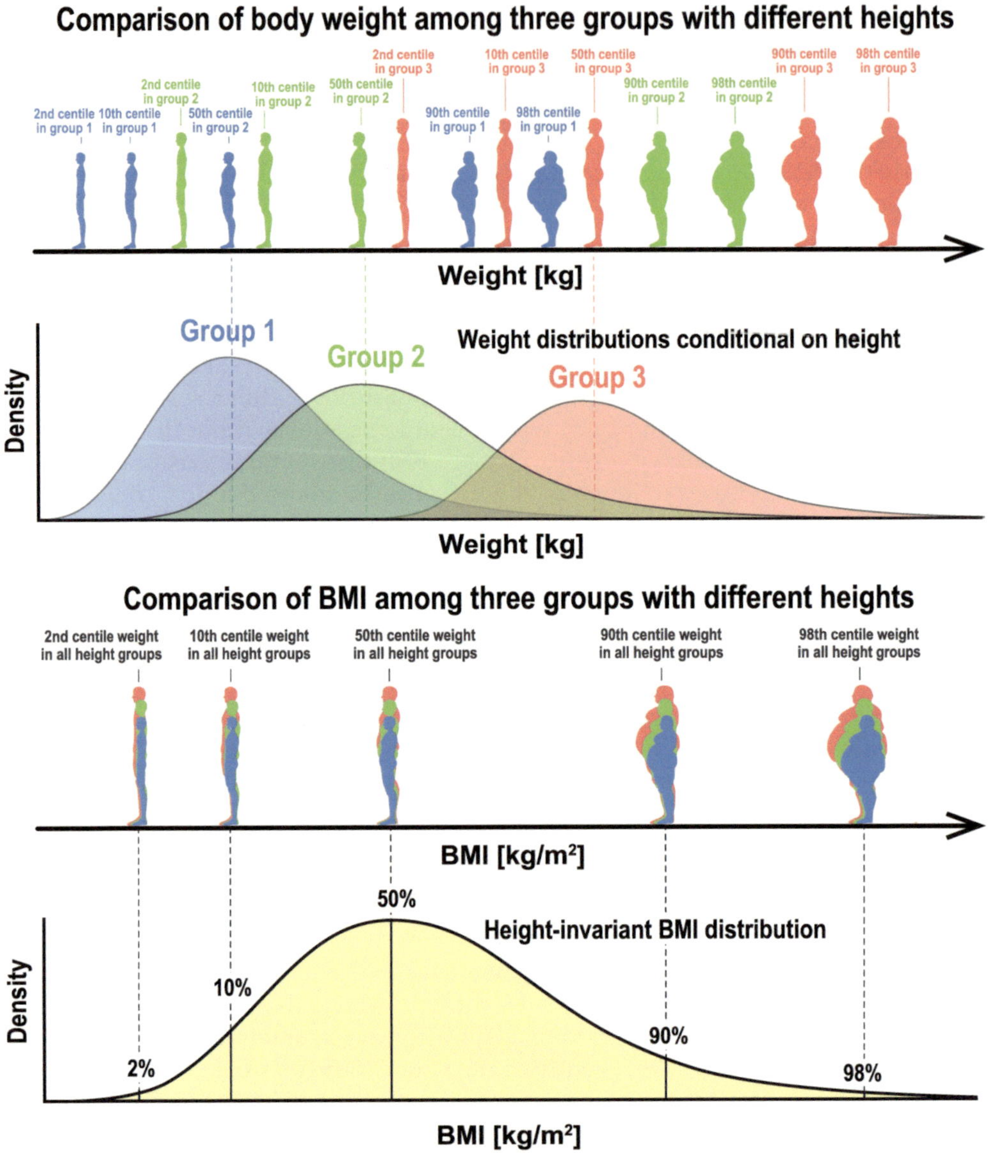

Figure 1.
An appropriately chosen BMI removes the influence of height, enabling comparison based on conditional weight distribution centiles. Top: Body weight in three height groups, with silhouettes indicating the 2nd, 10th, 50th, 90th, and 98th centiles. Because weight distributions shift with height, weight alone cannot objectively compare obesity or thinness across groups. Bottom: appropriately chosen BMI in the same three height groups, where centile positions now align across heights and distributions overlap – illustrating the height-adjusting property of BMI in late adolescents after skeletal maturity.

anticipates later developments in the quantitative understanding of growth and body mass indices. In light of modern research on pediatric BMI, which emphasizes the need to account for age-dependent changes in the weight–height relationship when assessing adiposity in children, Quetelet's observation can be regarded as a prescient contribution that foreshadowed current debates on the validity and adjustment of BMI for growing populations.

In addition to his contributions to anthropometry, Quetelet's introduction of the concepts of *l'homme moyen* (the average man) and social physics marked a profound shift in understanding both individuals and society through quantitative means. By demonstrating that human characteristics – whether physical traits or social behaviors – cluster around a statistical mean and follow predictable patterns, he laid foundational groundwork for applying mathematical principles not only to social phenomena but also to understanding human nature itself. These ideas underpin many modern statistical and social science methods, earning him recognition as one of the founding figures of modern statistics and social science.

The empirical observation that adult body weight is proportional to the square of height can also be derived from fundamental physiological principles [7, 9, 10]. According to Kleiber's law, proposed by the Swiss physiologist Max Kleiber in the 1930s, the basal metabolic rate B of warm-blooded animals scales with body mass M [11]:

$$B \propto M^{3/4}. \tag{1}$$

This scaling law, observed across a wide range of mammals and birds, is thought to arise from a combination of factors, including body surface area, hierarchical vascular networks, and energy transport efficiency [11, 12]. In endothermic animals, the heat generated by basal metabolism must balance the heat lost through the body surface to maintain thermal equilibrium. Because heat loss is proportional to surface area, and because the body can be reasonably approximated as a series of cylindrical segments, it follows from geometric considerations that adult body weight should scale approximately with the square of height. The proportionality between weight and height squared in adult warm-blooded animals is therefore not merely a statistical artifact but is grounded in metabolic scaling and thermoregulatory demands. The study of such scaling relationships between body size and biological function is known as *allometry*. In simple terms, allometry is the study of how the shape, physiology, or behavior of organisms changes with size. It examines how different biological traits scale with body size, often revealing consistent patterns across species or developmental stages [13].

Recent work by Ogata *et al.* [7] has extended this allometric approach, demonstrating that the characteristics of growing individuals cannot be fully captured by a single power-law scaling with a fixed exponent. In late adolescents, after skeletal maturity, body weight relative to height follows a single allometric scaling law, and deviations from this relationship can be used to assess obesity or thinness. In this context, weight-for-height centile curves share a common exponent – a pattern referred to as *allometric uni-scaling* (or *single-exponent allometric scaling*). By contrast, during the period of rapid skeletal growth in childhood, weight-for-height centile curves display varying exponents across centiles, a phenomenon termed *allometric multi-scaling* (or *multiple-exponent allometric scaling*), which likely reflects the complex physiological and body-composition changes occurring throughout growth.

2.1 Emergence of BMI as a height-adjusted index

In human anthropometry, the relationship between height and weight in what Quetelet termed the "average man" – an ideal type toward which nature tends – provides a conceptual foundation for constructing body size indices. In the modern history of BMI, the index was selected as the height-adjusted measure showing the weakest correlation with height [14–17]. This criterion of *height uncorrelatedness* ensures that the expected value (mean or median) of the index, conditional on a given height, does not depend on height.

In the 1970s, Ancel Keys, using anthropometric data, demonstrated that BMI (weight/height^2) was superior to the body build index (weight/height) and ponderal index (also known as the corpulence index, defined as weight/height^3) for population-level epidemiological studies, primarily because of its weaker correlation with height [14]. Keys also noted, however, that BMI could not reliably distinguish between muscle and fat mass and should not be used as a sole diagnostic metric for individual health without considering other relevant physiological factors. Following Keys' work, the height-uncorrelated criterion became widely recognized as a key justification for height-adjusted body mass assessment.

Tim Cole later conducted systematic investigations to determine, for children, the optimal exponent p in the relationship between weight and height^p that would eliminate correlation with height [18]. He demonstrated that this exponent varies with age, suggesting that an age-dependent p could, in principle, yield a more accurate height adjustment for pediatric populations. This work represents a detailed, quantitative extension of an idea already noted by Quetelet, who had observed nearly two centuries ago that the scaling exponent between weight and height changes systematically during growth. Although *extended BMI* formulations incorporating age-specific exponents have been proposed, current evidence does not indicate that they outperform the standard BMI in predicting fat mass or health risk [19, 20], although some studies have reported improvements in certain age groups or populations [20–22].

The continued use of BMI (with $p = 2$) for children is supported by several empirical findings:

- **Correlation with fat mass**: BMI shows a strong correlation with total body fat measured by direct methods (e.g., DXA), with coefficients typically around $r \approx 0.8 - 0.9$ and particularly strong discriminatory power at the upper end of the distribution [23–25].

- **Sensitivity and specificity**: BMI-for-age ≥ 85th percentile yields sensitivity and specificity in the 0.7–0.9 range for identifying children with elevated adiposity, as measured by DXA or comparable standards; this pattern has been demonstrated consistently across cohorts and summarized in multiple reviews [26, 27].

- **Epidemiological application**: BMI with $p = 2$ remains a practical and robust approximation, even though the height exponent minimizing residual association with stature may increase to $p \approx 2.5 - 3.0$ during puberty [21, 28]. It is widely used in national and international epidemiological surveillance to estimate and compare obesity and thinness prevalence in large populations over time [29].

Although these findings support the continued utility of BMI in pediatric populations, several important caveats and limitations remain. A strong correlation with fat mass does not eliminate systematic height-related bias: BMI tends to overestimate adiposity in taller children and underestimate it in shorter ones, particularly during puberty [21]. Sensitivity and specificity are method- and sample-dependent, and they vary across race/ethnicity [27, 30–32]. Finally, the persistence of $p = 2$ in epidemiological applications is driven largely by convention and cross-study comparability rather than by physiological optimality, which may obscure meaningful differences in growth patterns across developmental stages.

These observations highlight important methodological challenges and point to fundamental limitations in constructing body size indicators solely from the weight–height relationship. Historically, a widely accepted approach to constructing height-adjusted body size indices has been to derive a formula describing the relationship between average weight and height, then use this formula to set a reference value for each height or to create an index uncorrelated with height. The conventional BMI follows this principle: It has served both as a population-level indicator for identifying degrees of thinness or obesity that are rare in the general population and as a simple screening tool to flag individuals who may require further evaluation.

However, this approach does not translate well to children. In practice, indices of weight and height^p that demonstrably achieve uncorrelatedness with height are often not used; instead, the conventional BMI with the exponent $p = 2$ continues to be applied, despite its weak theoretical basis. As noted earlier, BMI cutoff values derive from statistical centiles, which reflect the probability of a given body size within a reference population. In pediatric populations, the weight–height relationship is intrinsically shaped by both age and stage of maturation, and clear, universally accepted principles for defining valid cutoffs remain lacking. This uncertainty highlights the need to reconsider how body size assessment criteria are developed for growing individuals. Expecting a single index – based solely on a formula relating height and weight – to capture health risks associated with underlying body fat across diverse ages and maturational stages is likely unrealistic and extends well beyond the intended scope of a simple screening metric for monitoring trends in obesity or thinness.

In conclusion, the criterion of height uncorrelatedness is inadequate for developing robust and meaningful height-adjusted indices for assessing thinness and obesity. As illustrated in **Figure 1**, we argue that the rarity of certain body shapes in the general population – that is, their low probability of occurrence – should serve as the primary reference point for defining *abnormal* body size. This reframing offers a more conceptually sound and empirically grounded basis for evaluation, particularly in growing individuals. While we recognize that further refinement and validation are needed, we put forward this approach as a necessary and timely departure from conventional assumptions, providing a foundation for critical reassessment and more accurate future practice. Historically, degrees of obesity or thinness have been interpreted in terms of statistical rarity within the population – body shapes that are infrequent and thus warrant attention. Indeed, major organizations such as the WHO [33], CDC [34], and IOTF [35, 36] have relied on BMI centiles or z-scores to define cutoffs for overweight and thinness, rather than direct assessments of body fat or health outcomes, implicitly reinforcing this probabilistic interpretation.

3. Current evidence on the validity and limitations of BMI-type indices

Efforts to determine the optimal exponent in weight/height^p-type indices for children have repeatedly failed to yield a satisfactory solution. We argue that developing a truly appropriate body size index for pediatric use first requires understanding why these attempts have fallen short. The answer, we contend, lies in fundamental differences between the body size distributions of adults and those of children – a distinction that must be clearly recognized, as it calls for a thorough rethinking of how body size in children is assessed.

In this section, we clarify the conditions that an appropriate height-adjusted body size index should satisfy. As a starting point, we empirically examine data from late adolescence – a period when skeletal growth has largely matured – to illustrate in what sense BMI serves as a well-calibrated and objectively meaningful body size index. Remarkably, our findings suggest that adult BMI reflects a coherent biological design, revealing an internal consistency that is both unexpected and scientifically compelling. Using these conditions as criteria, we show that BMI and other weight/height^p-type indices used to date do not qualify as height-adjusted indices in the context of growth and development. Based on the findings reported in [5–7], we present results from our analysis of a large-scale national dataset containing age, sex, height, and weight measurements for 7,863,520 Japanese schoolchildren aged 5–17 years. These data were collected between 2008 and 2019 through the Ministry of Education, Culture, Sports, Science, and Technology's annual School Health Statistics Research, which uses stratified random sampling to ensure nationwide representativeness [5, 7].

As shown in **Figure 2**, in 17-year-old late adolescents of both sexes – after skeletal maturity – BMI proves to be, perhaps surprisingly, an effective metric for evaluating the rarity (i.e., the probability of occurrence) of a given body shape [7]. In this age group, the estimated BMI distributions across different height strata (*right panels* of **Figure 2**) exhibit nearly identical shapes. The curves align closely at both tails of the distribution, whereas the corresponding weight distributions differ markedly in both location and overall form. In the BMI plots, the 2nd centiles (*circles*) cluster very tightly at nearly a single point across all height strata, and the 98th centiles (*diamonds*) likewise show only minimal variation. This striking consistency underscores BMI's utility as an objective, population-level parameter for assessing thinness and obesity, since the centiles of the conditional weight distribution given height remain stable and reproducible regardless of stature.

Because males typically reach adult height by about age 16 and females by about age 14, BMI-type indices ($\approx$ weight/height^2) in individuals above these ages can be considered a valid height-adjusted body size measure – uncorrelated with height in the population-statistical sense. For further interpretation, see the explanation accompanying **Figure 1**. While we used the conventional BMI with $p = 2$ in this analysis, it is also possible to estimate statistically the optimal exponent p that best aligns BMI distributions across different height strata. In **Figure 2**, however, the estimated optimal p is very close to 2, the conventional value, reinforcing the appropriateness of the conventional BMI formulation in late adolescence.

Although the BMI formulation appears valid in late adolescents, its validity breaks down during periods of rapid skeletal growth. In these developmental stages, the criterion of height uncorrelatedness loses relevance for evaluating low-probability body shapes – specifically, the distributional extremes associated with thinness and obesity. To examine this paradox, we next present examples of index distributions during the growth period. In growing children, the condition we refer to as *population-statistical objectivity* – the alignment of weight centiles independent of height – no longer holds. As shown, the BMI distribution shifts systematically with

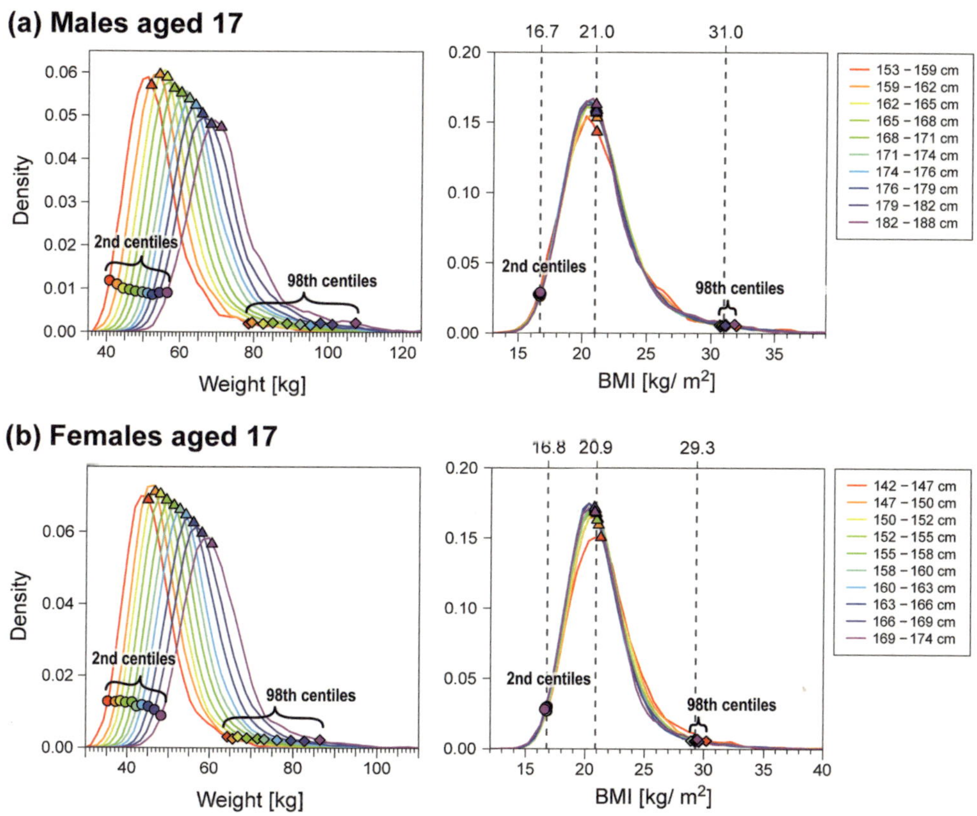

Figure 2.
At skeletal maturity, BMI is an appropriate height-adjusted index. (a) 17-year-old males (n = 238,851). (b) 17-year-old females (n = 240,958). Left panels: Weight distributions across height strata, showing clear height-dependent patterns. Right panels: BMI distributions across height strata, showing nearly identical patterns across heights. In all panels, circles indicate the 2nd centile points of weight (underweight side), triangles indicate the median 50th centile points, and diamonds indicate the 98th centile points (obese side). The objectivity of BMI is ensured by the fact that, given height, the probability of having a high weight (obesity) or a low weight (underweight) depends little on stature. Accordingly, in the right panels, the 2nd centiles (circles), the 50th centiles (triangles), and the 98th centiles (diamonds) all cluster at nearly identical positions across height strata, demonstrating independence from height.

height during growth, thereby undermining its usefulness for comparing weight centiles across height strata.

As illustrated in **Figure 3**, using the example of 11-year-old males, skeletally immature children do not exhibit height-invariant distributions for any weight/height^p-type index, regardless of the value of p, the exponent. With the conventional BMI ($p = 2$; **Figure 3b**), all centile positions vary systematically across height strata: the 2nd centile on the underweight side (*circles*), the median 50th centile (*triangles*), and the 98th centile on the obese side (*diamonds*). When p is optimized to align the median of the index distribution (**Figure 3c**) – rather than to satisfy the height-uncorrelated criterion – the 50th centile (*triangles*) becomes approximately aligned across height strata. However, the 2nd centiles (*circles*) and 98th centiles (*diamonds*) still display a clear and consistent height dependence. Interestingly, adjusting the

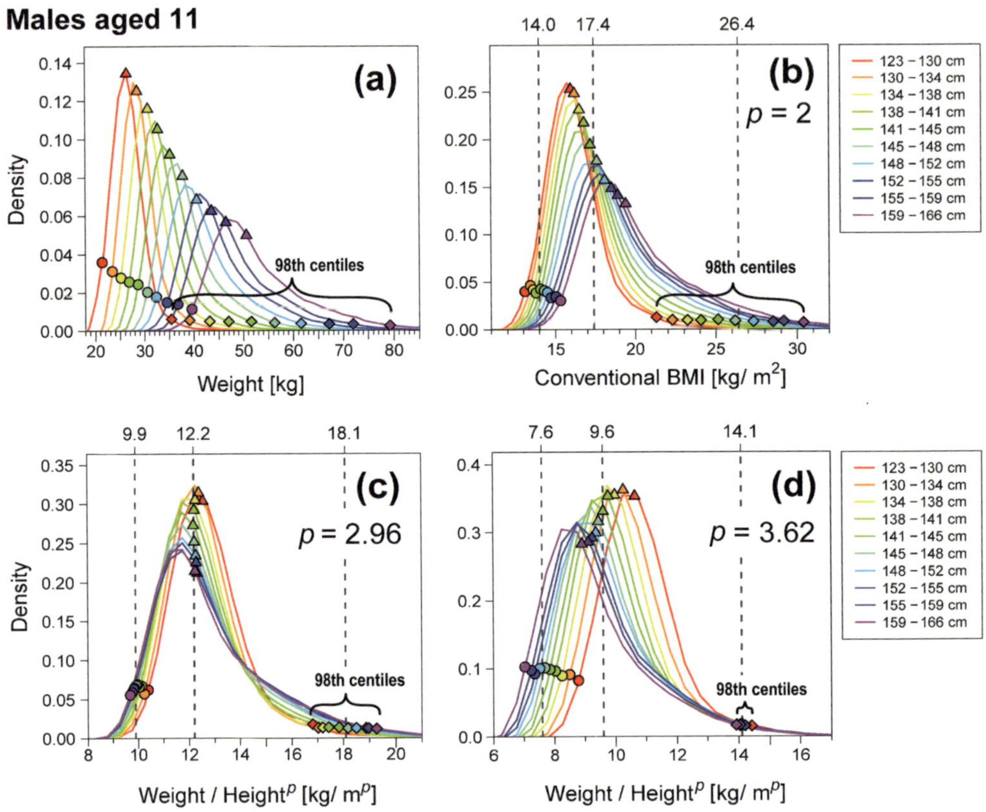

Figure 3.
In skeletally immature children, an index based on the height-independent condition is not truly height-adjusted, exemplified using data for 11-year-old males (n = 262,405). (a) Weight distributions across height strata. (b) Conventional BMI (p = 2) distributions across height strata. (c) Distributions of weight/height^p with p = 2.96 across height strata. (d) Distributions of weight/height^p with p = 3.62 across height strata. For weight/height^p-type indices, no distribution invariant to height exists. However, adjusting the exponent p can approximately align a particular centile. In (d), for example, p was selected so that the 98th centile (diamonds) is as independent of height as possible. In all panels, circles indicate the 2nd centile points of weight (underweight side), triangles indicate the median 50th centile points, and diamonds indicate the 98th centile points (obese side). This illustrates that although centile-specific alignment can be forced by tuning p, no single exponent removes the overall height dependence, demonstrating the lack of population-statistical objectivity in skeletally immature children.

exponent allows alignment of any chosen centile across height groups; for example, in **Figure 3d**, p is selected to align the 98th centile across height strata.

In Ogata *et al*. [7], the values of p (denoted as α in that study) required to align the 2nd, 10th, 90th, and 98th centiles – together with the corresponding cutoff values – are reported. (*Note:* Throughout this chapter, we use p to denote a fixed BMI-type exponent (as in weight/height^p), and $\alpha(q)$ to denote centile-specific exponents estimated via quantile regression.) This centile-specific adjustment offers a potential approach to achieving population-statistical objectivity, defined here as the alignment of weight centiles across height strata using a weight/height^p-type index. The optimal exponent p was estimated by fitting a power-law model, $w_q(h) = C_q h^{\alpha(q)}$, to the qth centile curve of the weight-for-height distribution using quantile regression, which estimates the conditional quantile (centile) by minimizing a weighted sum of absolute residuals. For additional methodological details, see [7].

As illustrated in **Figure 4**, a valid height-adjusted body size index must satisfy more than the simple *height-uncorrelated* criterion. Historically, the absence of correlation between BMI and height has been treated as a key feature. However, the essential property lies not in uncorrelatedness itself, but in what it signifies – namely that the distribution of the index remains nearly invariant across height strata. In this view, the height uncorrelatedness observed in adult BMI serves only as a proxy for a deeper and more meaningful condition: distributional invariance with respect to height.

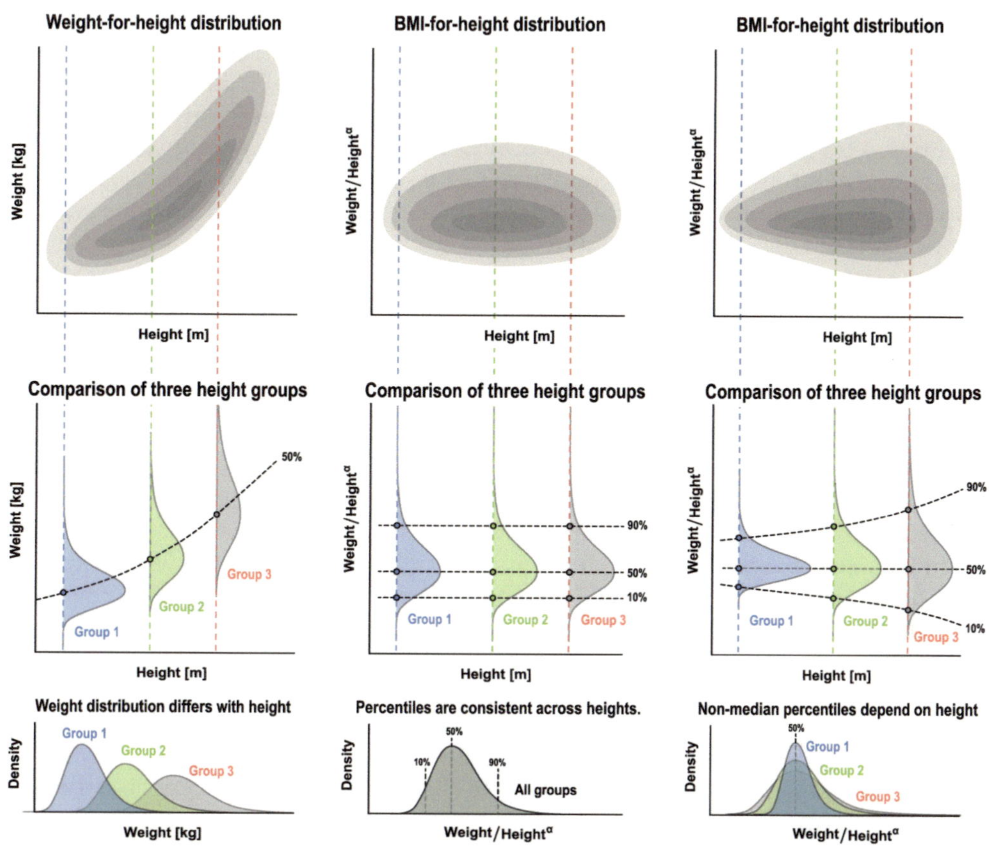

Figure 4.
The height-uncorrelated criterion is not sufficient for a height-adjusted body size index. The figure illustrates three scenarios for weight–height relationships and their corresponding weight/height^{p}-type index distributions. Left: Raw weight-for-height relationship showing how weight distributions vary systematically with height across three height groups (blue, green, red). Middle: An ideal height-adjusted index where the central tendency is uncorrelated with height and the distributional shape remains consistent across height groups, resulting in equivalent centile interpretations regardless of stature. Right: A problematic scenario where an index is uncorrelated with height in terms of central tendency but exhibits height-dependent distributional properties – the degree of obesity or thinness varies with height, rendering centile-based classifications unreliable. The top row shows bivariate density plots with color intensity representing probability density. The middle row compares the conditional distributions across the three height groups, with centile lines (10th, 50th, 90th) indicated in each panel. The bottom row displays the overlaid marginal distributions, demonstrating how distributional equivalence (middle) versus distributional dependence (right) affects the interpretation of body mass indices. This distinction reveals why the weight–height correlation minimization alone is insufficient for creating a valid height-adjusted body size index in pediatric populations.

It is therefore not sufficient for only the central tendency (e.g., the mean or median) to be independent of height; rather, the entire conditional distribution given height should retain essentially the same shape and spread across all height groups. In other words, the positions of lower centiles (such as the 2nd) and upper centiles (such as the 98th) must remain consistent and comparable regardless of stature.

We refer to this stronger requirement as the *population-statistical objectivity* condition. This condition ensures that each centile of the index corresponds to the same degree of thinness or obesity for individuals of different heights. From this perspective, thinness and obesity are assessed objectively in terms of statistical rarity – that is, according to their probability of occurrence within the general population (e.g., being among the thinnest or heaviest 1 in 10 or 1 in 50 individuals).

Importantly, we do not expect this statistical rarity to be strongly or consistently correlated with actual body fat percentage. Rather, we regard it as a broadly useful reference point for identifying individuals whose body size may warrant further attention – for instance, as a potential indicator of atypical growth or underlying health conditions. In this sense, population rarity functions not as a direct measure of adiposity but as a screening signal to prompt closer examination when body size lies in the extreme tails of the distribution.

If the population-statistical objectivity condition is not met, an index may appear height-uncorrelated in terms of average values, yet still exhibit systematic shifts in its distributional tails across height groups. This results in biased assessments — overestimating or underestimating thinness or obesity depending on stature. Such violations are particularly common in pediatric populations, where ongoing growth alters both body proportions and distributional shapes. This illustrates why minimizing correlation with height alone is insufficient. To construct a truly valid index for children, both the alignment of centile positions and the invariance of the index distribution shape across height strata must be verified.

In fact, our analysis revealed clear evidence of height-related bias when applying BMI-based criteria [5, 7]. The IOTF cutoffs for overweight, obesity, and thinness are age- and sex-specific BMI thresholds derived by statistically projecting childhood BMI centile curves so that they intersect the internationally recognized adult BMI cutoffs at age 18: 25 kg/m^2 for overweight, 30 kg/m^2 for obesity, and 18.5 kg/m^2 for Grade I thinness, with additional lower thresholds for Grades II and III thinness [35, 36]. As shown in **Figure 5**, applying these cutoffs revealed that among males aged 11–13 and females aged 10–11, those in the shortest quartile were classified as underweight up to five times more frequently than those in the tallest quartile. Conversely, among males aged 8–11 and females aged 7–10, those in the tallest quartile were classified as overweight or obese four to five times more often than their shortest peers.

These disparities arise because the BMI-for-age reference curves used by the IOTF do not fully account for the age and height-related changes in the weight-for-height distribution during growth. As a result, they systematically overestimate thinness in shorter children and obesity in taller ones. This finding indicates that similar height-related biases are very likely to occur when using other BMI-based standards, such as those developed by the WHO and CDC.

Notably, this height dependence becomes negligible once skeletal growth is largely complete – typically by about age 16 in males and age 14 in females (**Figure 5**). In late adolescence, BMI functions more reliably and consistently as a

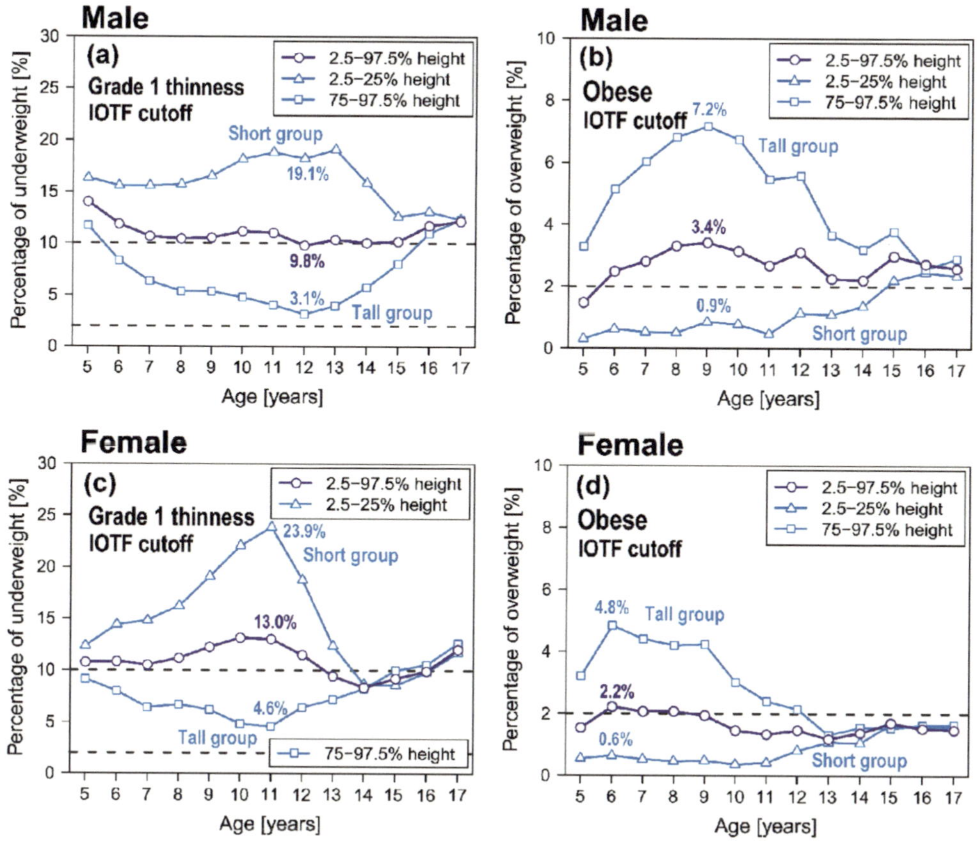

Figure 5.
Age- and height-related variation in the prevalence of underweight and overweight classifications among children and adolescents, based on anthropometric data from 2018. ***Top:*** *males;* ***Bottom:*** *females. (a, c) Prevalence of underweight using IOTF cutoffs for Grade I thinness. (b, d) Prevalence of overweight/obesity using IOTF cutoffs for obesity. These panels illustrate body size assessment with BMI, applying the age-specific IOTF reference cutoffs [35, 36]. Further methodological details are provided in [5].*

height-adjusted index, exhibiting minimal bias across stature. These results also offer indirect support for the validity of adult BMI, suggesting that the distributional stability observed in late adolescence can, with reasonable confidence, be extended to the adult population.

The key point is that the height-independent consistency observed in these late adolescents arises because the height dependence of each centile curve is nearly proportional to the square of height. This is illustrated in **Figure 6**, which compares the WHO centile-based BMI cutoffs (*dashed lines*) with the corresponding empirical weight centile curves (*solid lines*) across height strata. For adolescents at ages when skeletal growth is complete (approximately 16 years for males and 14 years for females), the WHO-defined BMI cutoff lines align closely with the observed weight centile curves, indicating strong concordance. Although WHO reference curves are shown here, applying the IOTF standards produces nearly identical results. This agreement supports the conclusion that our dataset is well aligned with established international reference distributions.

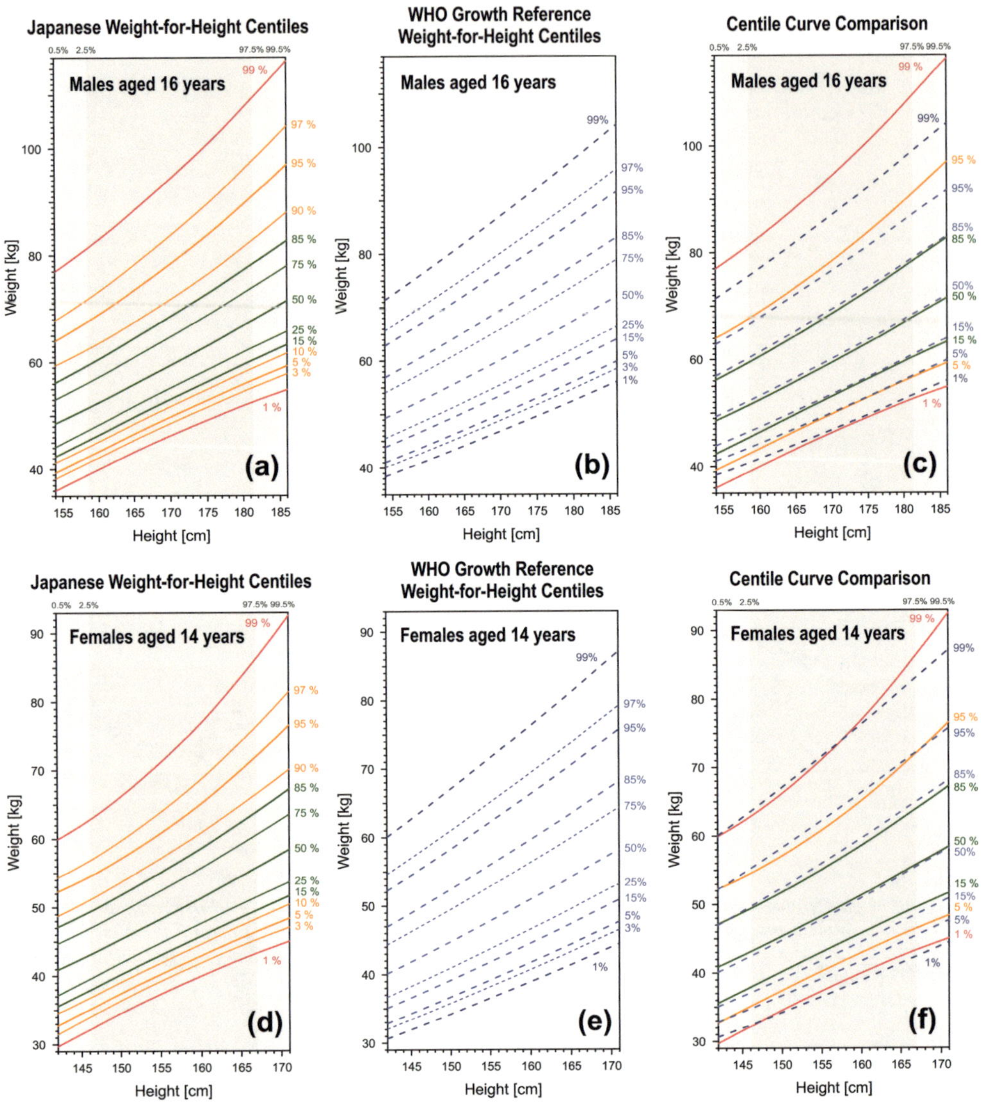

Figure 6.
At skeletal maturity, the centile curves of weight-for-height closely match those derived from BMI. Left: centile curves of weight-for-height estimated from a large Japanese dataset (for details on the estimation method, see [5]). ***Center:*** *WHO BMI growth reference plotted on a weight-for-height graph. Right: direct comparison of the two sets of curves. Top: males aged 16 years; bottom: females aged 14 years. For males aged 16 years and older and females aged 14 years and older, the weight-for-height centile curves (solid lines) and the BMI centile curves (dashed lines) are in close agreement. The horizontal axis for height extends from the 0.5th to the 99.5th centiles of the height distribution.*

In contrast, **Figure 7** presents the corresponding results for 9-year-old males and females, who are still in the growth phase. As shown in the *right panels* of **Figure 7**, the WHO BMI cutoff lines (*dashed*) intersect the actual weight centile curves (*solid*), thereby failing to satisfy the population-statistical objectivity condition and producing a pronounced height-related bias. If overweight is defined using the WHO 85th BMI centile cutoff, the regions where this cutoff overestimates compared with the actual 85th weight-for-height centile are shaded in pink, and the regions where it underestimates are shaded in light blue. This discrepancy illustrates how BMI-based thresholds, even when internationally standardized, can result in systematic misclassification during periods of active growth.

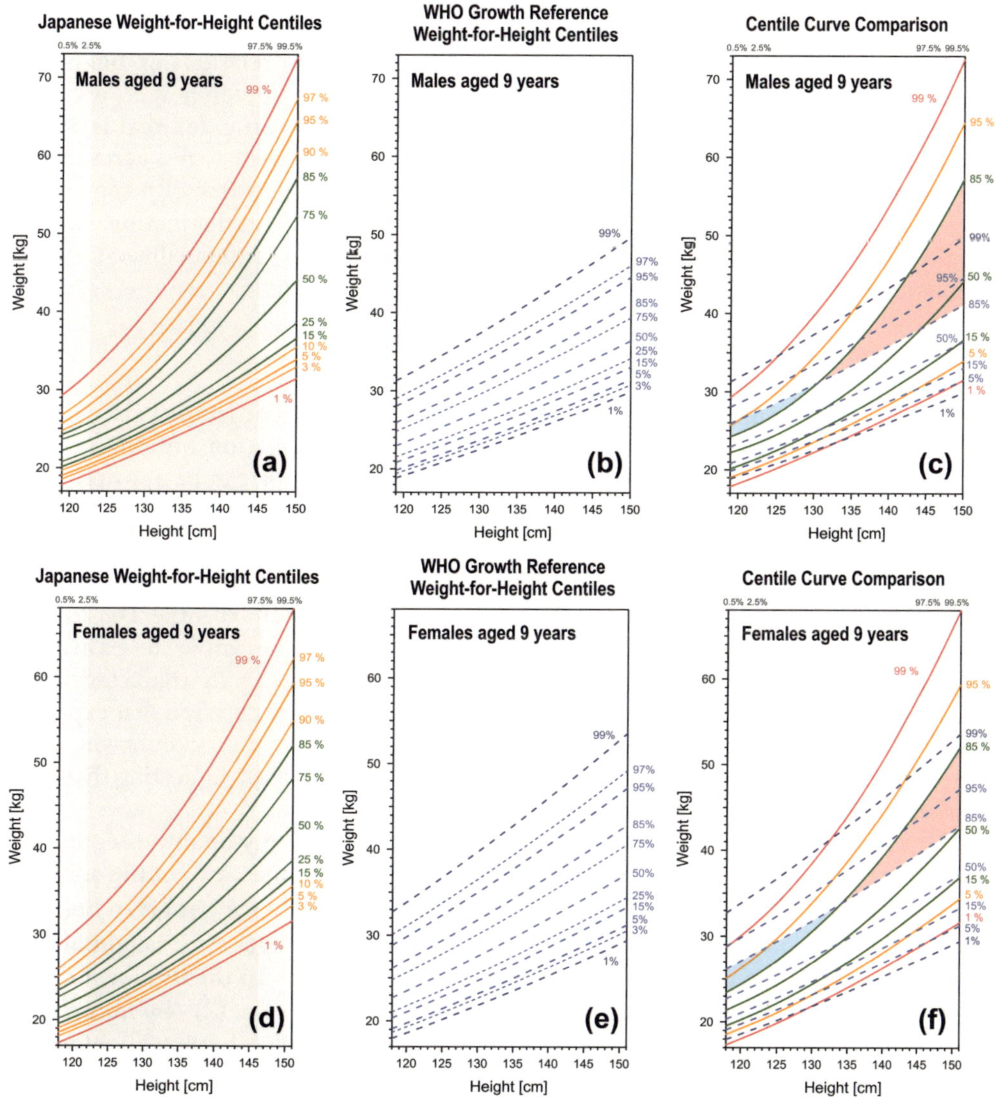

Figure 7.

During childhood growth, BMI shows a strong height-related bias. Plot analogous to ***Figure 6****. Top: males aged 9 years; bottom: females aged 9 years. In the right panels, the weight-for-height centile curves (solid lines) and the WHO BMI growth reference curves (dashed lines) intersect, resulting in height-dependent misclassification of obesity and underweight. If overweight is defined using the WHO 85th BMI centile cutoff, regions where it overestimates compared with the actual 85th weight-for-height centile are shaded in pink, and regions where it underestimates are shaded in light blue. For example, in tall 9-year-old males (upper right), the actual 50th weight centile aligns near the 95th BMI centile, while the WHO 50th BMI centile corresponds to approximately the 15th weight centile. Such mismatches between weight and BMI centiles highlight the risk of systematic misclassification in tall children during growth. This figure is adapted from* ***Figure 3*** *of Isoyama* et al. *[5] under the terms of the Creative Commons Attribution 4.0 International License (CC BY 4.0) and has been modified from the original.*

4. Multi-scaling allometric patterns observed in skeletally immature children

To clarify the conditions under which a weight/height^p-type index fails to function as a valid height-adjusted measure, it is useful to outline its mathematical basis. In allometric scaling, the relationship between body weight w and height h in a population can often be expressed as a power law, $w = Ch^\alpha$, where α is the scaling exponent, and C is a proportionality constant. If this scaling relationship holds uniformly across the entire set of weight centile curves for a given height, dividing weight by h^α will remove the height dependence, producing an index that is, in principle, height-adjusted. However, when the scaling exponent varies across the centile curves of the weight-for-height distribution, no single value of p can eliminate height dependence for all centiles simultaneously. This distinction – and its implications for the validity of weight/height^p-type indices – is formalized in the concepts of uni-scaling and multi-scaling described below.

4.1 Uni-scaling and multi-scaling

The concepts of *uni-scaling* and *multi-scaling* in the allometric framework describe fundamentally different patterns in the weight-for-height relationship. In our approach, we assume that the qth centile curve of weight $w_q(h)$can be approximated by the power-law function:

$$w_q(h) = C_q h^{\alpha(q)}, \tag{2}$$

where $\alpha(q)$ is the scaling exponent associated with that specific centile. *Uni-scaling* arises when $\alpha(q)$ is constant across all centiles, so the slopes of the centile curves in a log–log weight–height plot are parallel. In this case, a single exponent fully characterizes the scaling of the entire distribution, and dividing weight by height raised to that exponent yields a distribution independent of height. By contrast, *multi-scaling* occurs when $\alpha(q)$ varies with q centiles; here, the centile curves have different slopes, indicating that body size scales differently across distinct regions of the distribution.

To estimate the parameters C_q and $\alpha(q)$ in Eq. (2), we apply quantile regression [37] to the weight-for-height distribution stratified by sex, age, and centile q. In this framework, $w_q(h)$ denotes the conditional q^{th} centile of body weight given height, $\alpha(q)$ is the scaling exponent that quantifies how weight changes with height at that centile, and C_q is the proportionality constant corresponding to the intercept on the log–log scale. Quantile regression fits the power-law model –Eq. (2) –by minimizing a weighted sum of absolute residuals at the specified quantile, thereby allowing the slope $\alpha(q)$ to vary across centiles. This approach enables direct testing of the uni-scaling condition –where $\alpha(q)$ is constant for all q centiles – and the identification of multi-scaling behavior when depends on q. Once C_q and $\alpha(q)$ are estimated for a given centile, they can be used to construct centile-specific, height-adjusted indices and to derive corresponding cutoff values for assessing thinness and obesity.

4.2 Why uni-scaling matters

The distinction between uni-scaling and multi-scaling is critical for determining whether an index is a valid height-adjusted body size measure. Under uni-scaling, applying the appropriate exponent p produces weight/height^p index distributions whose centile positions align across height strata. Such alignment ensures that the meaning of a given centile–such as the 2nd or 98th – remains consistent for both short and tall individuals, thereby satisfying the condition of population-statistical objectivity. This condition requires more than independence of the central tendency from height; it also demands that the entire conditional distribution, given height, retains the same shape. When uni-scaling holds, indices such as BMI in skeletally mature adolescents and adults meet this requirement, enabling objective comparisons of thinness and obesity across stature.

In the presence of multi-scaling, no single exponent can fully eliminate height dependence across the entire distribution. Even if the median (50th centile) is rendered approximately independent of height, the lower and upper tails will still vary systematically with stature. This produces substantial height-dependent biases in centile-based classifications, such as overestimating thinness in shorter children and obesity in taller ones. Such violations of the population-statistical objectivity condition are particularly common during growth, when weight and height follow different developmental trajectories that yield distinct centile-specific scaling exponents. Recognizing whether a population follows a uni-scaling or multi-scaling regime is therefore essential for selecting or designing a truly valid and practically useful height-adjusted body size index.

To illustrate these concepts, **Figure 8a** presents an example of uni-scaling in 17-year-old males, where the double-logarithmic plot of weight versus height shows that the regression lines for the 2nd, 50th, and 98th centiles are nearly parallel, with estimated scaling exponents $\alpha(2) = 2.0$, $\alpha(50) = 1.9$, and $\alpha(98) = 2.1$. This close agreement across centiles indicates that a single exponent can adequately characterize the scaling relationship, thereby fulfilling the uni-scaling condition. In this case, as shown in **Figure 2**, applying $p \approx 2$ to construct a weight/height^p index yields distributions whose centile positions are essentially aligned across height strata, enabling height-invariant comparisons of thinness and obesity.

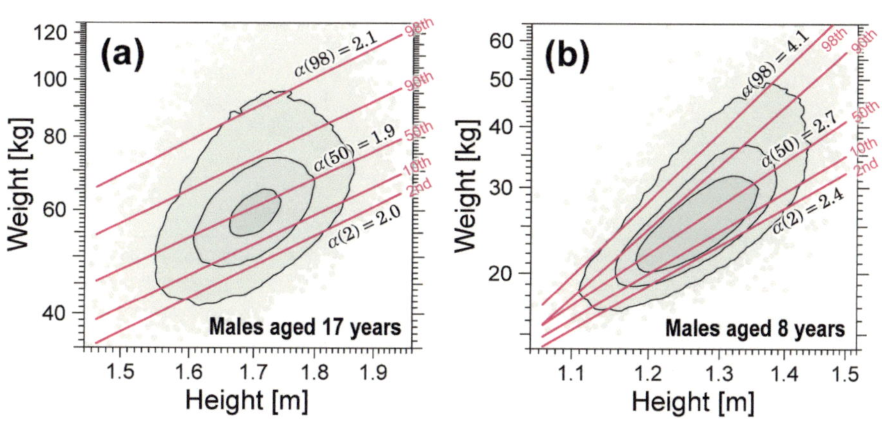

Figure 8.
*Extended allometric analysis results. (a) 17-year-old males. (b) 8-year-old males. Solid lines represent quantile regression fits for the 2nd, 10th, 50th, 90th and 98th centiles on a double-logarithmic scale. The estimated scaling exponents (slopes), such as α(2), α(50), and α(98), are shown in each panel. This figure is adapted from **Figure 8** of Ogata et al. [7] under the terms of the Creative Commons Attribution 4.0 International License (CC BY 4.0) and has been modified from the original.*

By contrast, **Figure 8b** illustrates a clear multi-scaling pattern in 8-year-old males. The slopes of the centile curves differ markedly: $\alpha(2) = 2.4$, $\alpha(50) = 2.7$, and $\alpha(98) = 4.1$. Higher-weight centiles exhibit much steeper exponents, suggesting that heavier children tend to gain body mass more readily than their lighter peers. This divergence in slopes implies that no single exponent p can align all centile positions simultaneously; even if the median is adjusted to be height-independent, the lower and upper tails will still shift with stature. As shown in **Figure 8**, such multi-scaling patterns are common in younger age groups but gradually converge toward uni-scaling as skeletal maturity is reached.

The age- and centile-dependent trends in the scaling exponent $\alpha(q)$ are summarized in **Figure 9**. In both males (**a**) and females (**b**), $\alpha(q)$ varies systematically with age and centile, particularly during the growth phase prior to skeletal maturity. The rainbow-colored lines represent 12 different centiles of the weight-for-height distribution: A large vertical spread indicates a multi-scaling pattern, whereas convergence of all lines toward a single value signifies a uni-scaling pattern. For males aged 5–14 years and females aged 5–11 years, high-weight centiles (e.g., 90th and 95th) exhibit much steeper exponents than the median or lower centiles, showing that heavier children gain weight disproportionately with height compared to their leaner peers. This divergence across the distribution is precisely the multi-scaling pattern described earlier.

As children approach adolescence, the $\alpha(q)$ curves for different centiles begin to converge noticeably. In males, this convergence typically occurs around age 14, and in females around age 12, with the scaling exponents becoming largely independent of centile position and gradually approaching a uni-scaling pattern. The uni-scaling exponent itself declines steadily from approximately 2.5 toward 2. These findings indicate that, for males aged 16 years and older and females aged 14 years

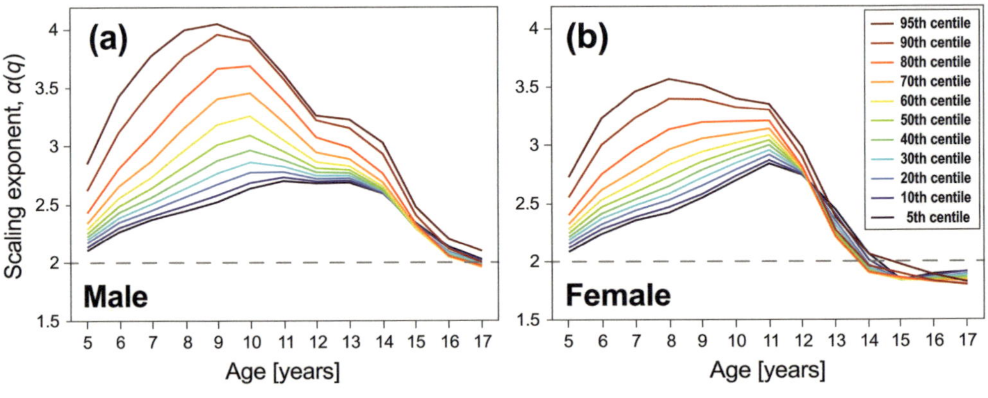

Figure 9.
Age- and centile-dependent scaling exponents in males and females aged 5–17 years. The scaling relationship between weight and height varies systematically with age and growth (height) centiles, using data from males (a) and females (b). Unlike the traditional BMI, which assumes a fixed exponent (weight/height^2), these plots demonstrate that the optimal scaling exponent $\alpha(q)$ changes across both age and centile. In early childhood, higher-weight centiles display much steeper exponents, indicating that standard BMI underestimates adiposity in heavier, shorter children. In contrast, for taller females—particularly during adolescence—the exponent often falls below 2, meaning that BMI overestimates adiposity in lean, tall females. Around ages 13–15 years, scaling patterns converge toward the standard BMI formula, but this convergence is temporary and differs by sex. These results underscore the need for age- and centile-adjusted indices to more accurately assess weight status and minimize misclassification in pediatric populations.

and older, the conventional BMI with $p = 2$ functions reliably as a valid height-adjusted index. This age-dependent transition from multi-scaling to uni-scaling generally coincides with the completion of the pubertal growth spurt, raising important physiological questions about the mechanisms underlying human growth and body composition changes. Collectively, these age- and centile-dependent patterns strongly highlight the need to account for both factors when constructing height-adjusted indices, since neglecting them can lead to systematic misclassification of thinness and obesity in pediatric populations.

4.3 Future directions

Looking ahead, the approach outlined here will be particularly valuable for future studies aiming to establish valid height-adjusted body size indices in populations beyond those analyzed in the present work. For instance, we have not examined data for children aged 0–5 years, nor have we analyzed datasets from countries outside Japan. Extending this framework to such populations would enable the development of indices that remain valid across a broader range of growth stages and demographic contexts. Importantly, the starting point should not be the traditional *height-uncorrelated* criterion, but rather a direct evaluation of weight-for-height centile curves in terms of their uni-scaling and multi-scaling patterns, as described in this review.

A further and equally important challenge remains: How to implement body size assessment for children in age groups that exhibit a clear multi-scaling pattern. In our recent work [7], we proposed a method that evaluates body size by combining the scaling exponent and cutoff value for each centile. While this approach is theoretically sound, it may be perceived as cumbersome in practical use. Implementing such calculations in a PC or smartphone application would remove this inconvenience. Moreover, if such an application were to be developed, it might be preferable to bypass BMI-type indices altogether and instead use the directly estimated weight centile value conditional on sex, age, and height as the index. This would yield a measure whose interpretation, as an evaluation of statistical rarity, is clearer. In any case, for assessing body size in children during the growth phase before skeletal maturity, it is necessary to return to first principles and reconstruct the evaluation method from the ground up.

5. Conclusion: Toward a fundamental reconstruction of pediatric anthropometric assessment

In this chapter, we have re-examined the conceptual and empirical foundations of BMI as a height-adjusted index, with a particular focus on its application to growing children. Drawing on an unprecedentedly large dataset of 7.86 million Japanese schoolchildren, we demonstrated that the scaling relationship between weight and height changes systematically with age, sex, and body size centile. The framework of allometry describes this scaling well, but its form differs fundamentally between skeletally mature adolescents and children in active growth.

Our analyses revealed two distinct regimes. In the uni-scaling regime – that is, observed after skeletal maturity – weight-for-height centile curves share a common scaling exponent ($p \approx 2$), yielding BMI distributions that are height-invariant in both central tendency and overall shape. Under these conditions, BMI operates as a statistically objective index, allowing meaningful comparisons of thinness and obesity across individuals of different stature. In contrast, the multi-scaling regime – characteristic of younger, skeletally immature children –shows that different centiles follow different scaling exponents. In this context, reliance on conventional BMI introduces systematic height-related biases, consistently overestimating obesity in taller children while underestimating it in shorter ones.

From this perspective, the traditional criterion of *height uncorrelatedness* is inadequate as the basis for a valid height-adjusted body size index. Instead, we have argued for the stronger requirement of population-statistical objectivity, in which the entire conditional distribution given height – not just its mean or median – remains invariant across height strata. This reframing shifts the focus from minimizing statistical correlation to aligning weight centile positions, thereby interpreting thinness and obesity explicitly in terms of rarity within the population distribution.

Our findings also have practical implications. For late adolescents (≥ 16 years in males, ≥ 14 years in females), conventional BMI with $p = 2$ is both theoretically and empirically justified, aligning closely with international reference centiles. For younger children, however, robust assessment requires approaches that explicitly account for multi-scaling. We have proposed one such method – centile-specific scaling exponent and cutoff estimation –which achieves height adjustment at chosen centiles but is computationally more demanding [7]. While software implementation could remove this barrier, an even more transparent approach may be to bypass BMI-type transformations altogether and directly use weight centile values conditional on sex, age, and height as the primary screening metric.

Ultimately, the assessment of body size in children before skeletal maturity demands a return to first principles. A valid index must be grounded in empirically observed scaling patterns throughout growth, rather than imported wholesale from adult models. By distinguishing uni-scaling from multi-scaling, and by introducing population-statistical objectivity as a guiding principle, this work lays the conceptual and methodological groundwork for developing height-adjusted indices that are both scientifically sound and practically useful. Extending this framework to younger age groups and to diverse international populations is a critical next step toward more accurate, equitable, and interpretable assessments of thinness and obesity in the pediatric population.

Author details

Ken Kiyono[1,2*†] and Madhur Mangalam[2†]

1 Graduate School of Engineering Science, University of Osaka, Toyonaka, Osaka, Japan

2 Department of Biomechanics, University of Nebraska at Omaha, Omaha, NE, USA

† These authors contributed equally.

*Address all correspondence to: kiyono.ken.es@osaka-u.ac.jp

References

[1] NC ADV, Pérez-Treviño P, Cepeda Lopez AC, Murillo-Torres RM, Castillo EC, Gutierrez-Cantu D, Tamez-Rivera O, Paez Flores M, Flores-Ayuzo I, Luévano-Martinez LA, et al. Beyond BMI: A comprehensive approach to pediatric obesity assessment. Frontiers in Pediatrics. 2025;**13**:1597309. DOI: 10.3389/fped.2025.1597309

[2] O'Connor LE, Lopez-Perez L, Martinez RX, Spill MK, Peña-Rosas JP, MacFarlane AJ. Report of a meeting: An expert consultation on body composition and adiposity for children and adolescents in all their diversity. Current Developments in Nutrition. 2025;**9**(7):107475. DOI: 10.1016/j.cdnut.2025.107475

[3] Rubino F, Cummings DE, Eckel RH, Cohen RV, Wilding JPH, Brown WA, Stanford FC, Batterham RL, Farooqi IS, Farpour-Lambert NJ, et al. Definition and diagnostic criteria of clinical obesity. The Lancet Diabetes & Endocrinology. 2025;**13**(3):221–262. DOI: 10.1016/s2213-8587(24)00316-4

[4] Wright CM, Cole TJ, Fewtrell M, Williams JE, Eaton S, Wells JC. Body composition data show that high BMI centiles overdiagnose obesity in children aged under 6 years. American Journal of Clinical Nutrition. 2022;**116**(1):122–131. DOI: 10.1093/ajcn/nqab421

[5] Isoyama Y, Nose-Ogura S, Ijitsu MJ, Kruse JGS, Nagai N, Kayaba M, Ogata H, Mangalam M, Kiyono K. Age- and height-dependent bias of underweight and overweight assessment standards for children and adolescents. Frontiers in Public Health. 2024;**12**:1379897. DOI: 10.3389/fpubh.2024.1379897

[6] Mangalam M, Isoyama Y, Ogata H, Nose-Ogura S, Kayaba M, Nagai N, Kiyono K. Multi-scaling allometry in human development, mammalian morphology, and tree growth. Scientific Reports. 2024;**14**:19957. DOI: 10.1038/s41598-024-69199-5

[7] Ogata H, Isoyama Y, Nose-Ogura S, Nagai N, Kayaba M, Kruse JGS, Seleznov I, Kaneko M, Shigematsu T, Kiyono K. Allometric multi-scaling of weight-for-height relation in children and adolescents: Revisiting the theoretical basis of body mass index of thinness and obesity assessment. PloS One. 2024;**19**(7):e0307238. DOI: 10.1371/journal.pone.0307238

[8] Quetelet A. A Treatise on Man and the Development of His Faculties. Translated by R. Knox, original work published in 1835. Edinburgh, Scotland: William and Robert Chambers; 1842

[9] Agrawal D. Metabolic rate M 0.75 in human beings. Physics Education. 2014;**49**(6):685. DOI: 10.1088/0031-9120/49/6/685

[10] Agrawal DC. Teaching Body mass index and Kleiber law. The Physics Educator. 2019;**1**(04):1920010. DOI: 10.1142/S2661339519200105

[11] Kleiber M. Body size and metabolism. Hilgardia. 1932;**6**(11):315–353. DOI: 10.3733/hilg.v06n11p315

[12] West GB, Brown JH, Enquist BJ. A general model for the origin of allometric scaling laws in biology.

Science. 1997;**276**(5309):122–126. DOI: 10.1126/science.276.5309.122

[13] Huxley JS. Problems of Relative Growth. London, England: Methuen & Co. Ltd; 1932

[14] Keys A, Fidanza F, Karvonen MJ, Kimura N, Taylor HL. Indices of relative weight and obesity. Journal of Chronic Diseases. 1972;**25**(6-7):329–343. DOI: 10.1016/0021-9681(72)90027-6

[15] Khosla T, Lowe CR. Indices of obesity derived from body weight and height. British Journal of Preventive & Social Medicine. 1967;**21**(3):122–128. DOI: 10.1136/jech.21.3.122

[16] Komaroff M. For researchers on obesity: Historical review of extra body weight definitions. Journal of Obesity. 2016;**2016**:2460285. DOI: 10.1155/2016/2460285

[17] Pray R, Riskin S. The history and faults of the body mass index and where to look next: A literature review. Cureus. 2023;**15**(11):e48230. DOI: 10.7759/cureus.48230

[18] Cole TJ. Weight/height^p compared to weight/height^2 for assessing adiposity in childhood: Influence of age and bone age on p during puberty. Annals of Human Biology. 1986;**13**(5):433–451. DOI: 10.1080/03014468600008621

[19] Frontini MG, Bao W, Elkasabany A, Srinivasan SR, Berenson G. Comparison of weight-for-height indices as a measure of adiposity and cardiovascular risk from childhood to young adulthood: The Bogalusa heart study. Journal of Clinical Epidemiology. 2001;**54**(8):817–822. DOI: 10.1016/S0895-4356(01)00343-2

[20] Sun J, Yang R, Zhao M, Bovet P, Xi B. Tri-ponderal mass index as a screening tool for identifying body fat and cardiovascular risk factors in children and adolescents: A systematic review. Frontiers in Endocrinology. 2021;**12**:694681. DOI: 10.3389/fendo.2021.694681

[21] Hudda MT, Aarestrup J, Owen CG, Baker JL, Whincup PH. Varying optimal power for height-standardisation of childhood weight, fat mass and fat-free mass across the obesity epidemic. International Journal of Obesity. 2025;**49**:84–92. DOI: 10.1038/s41366-024-01619-y

[22] Peterson CM, Su H, Thomas DM, Heo M, Golnabi AH, Pietrobelli A, Heymsfield SB. Tri-ponderal mass index vs body mass index in estimating body fat during adolescence. JAMA Pediatrics. 2017;**171**(7):629–636. DOI: 10.1001/jamapediatrics.2017.0460

[23] Boeke CE, Oken E, Kleinman KP, Rifas-Shiman SL, Taveras EM, Gillman MW. Correlations among adiposity measures in school-aged children. BMC Pediatrics. 2013;**13**:99. DOI: 10.1186/1471-2431-13-99

[24] Freedman DS, Wang J, Maynard LM, Thornton JC, Mei Z, Pierson RN, Dietz WH, Horlick M. Relation of BMI to fat and fat-free mass among children and adolescents. International Journal of Obesity. 2005;**29**:1–8. DOI: 10.1038/sj.ijo.0802735

[25] Pietrobelli A, Faith MS, Allison DB, Gallagher D, Chiumello G, Heymsfield SB. Body mass index as a measure of adiposity among children and adolescents: A validation study. Journal of Pediatrics. 1998;**132**(2):204–210. DOI: 10.1016/S0022-3476(98)70433-0

[26] Freedman DS, Sherry B. The validity of BMI as an indicator of body fatness and risk among children. Pediatrics. 2009;**124** (Supplement_1):S23–S34. DOI: 10.1542/peds.2008-3586E

[27] Mei Z, Grummer-Strawn LM, Pietrobelli A, Goulding A, Goran MI, Dietz WH. Validity of body mass index compared with other body-composition screening indexes for the assessment of body fatness in children and adolescents. American Journal of Clinical Nutrition. 2002;**75**(6):978–985

[28] Mackay NJ. Scaling of human body mass with height: The body mass index revisited. Journal of Biomechanics. 2010;**43**(4):764–766. DOI: 10.1016/j.jbiomech.2009.10.038

[29] Abarca-Gómez L, Abdeen ZA, ZA H, Abu-Rmeileh NM, Acosta-Cazares B, Acuin C, Adams RJ, Aekplakorn W, Afsana K, Aguilar-Salinas CA, et al. Worldwide trends in body-mass index, underweight, overweight, and obesity from 1975 to 2016: A pooled analysis of 2416 population-based measurement studies in 128.9 million children, adolescents, and adults. The Lancet. 2017;**390**(10113):2627–2642. DOI: 10.1016/S0140-6736(17)32129-3

[30] Freedman DS, Wang J, Thornton JC, Mei Z, Pierson RN, Dietz WH, Horlick M. Racial/ethnic differences in body fatness among children and adolescents. Obesity (Silver Spring). 2008;**16**(5):1105–1111

[31] Hudda MT, Nightingale CM, Donin AS, Fewtrell MS, Haroun D, Lum S, Williams JE, Owen CG, Rudnicka AR, Wells JCK, Cook DG, Whincup PH. Body mass index adjustments to increase the validity of body fatness assessment in UK Black African and South Asian children. International Journal of Obesity. 2017;**41**:1048–1055

[32] Nightingale CM, Rudnicka AR, Owen CG, Cook DG, Whincup PH. Patterns of body size and adiposity among UK children of South Asian, black African–Caribbean and white European origin: Child Heart And health Study in England (CHASE Study). International Journal of Epidemiology. 2011;**40**(1):33–44

[33] World Health Organization. Physical status: The use and interpretation of anthropometry. Report of a WHO expert committee. WHO Technical Report Series. 1995;854. World Health Organization, Geneva, Switzerland. Available from: https://www.who.int/publications/i/item/9241208546

[34] Kuczmarski RJ, Ogden CL, Grummer-Strawn LM, Flegal KM, Guo SS, Wei R, Mei Z, Curtin LR, Roche AF, Johnson CL. CDC Growth Charts: United States. Hyattsville, MD: National Center for Health Statistics; 2000

[35] Cole TJ, Bellizzi MC, Flegal KM, Dietz WH. Establishing a standard definition for child overweight and obesity worldwide: International survey. BMJ. 2000;**320**(7244):1240. DOI: 10.1136/bmj.320.7244.1240

[36] Cole TJ, Flegal KM, Nicholls D, Jackson AA. Body mass index cut offs to define thinness in children and adolescents: International survey. BMJ. 2007;**335**(7612):194. DOI: 10.1136/bmj.39238.399444.55

[37] Koenker R, Bassett G. Regression quantiles. Econometrica. 1978;**46** (1):33–50

Chapter 4

From BMI to Waist Circumference: Advancing Pediatric Risk Stratification for Obesity-Related Cardiometabolic Disease

Maria-Zinaida Dobre, Bogdana Virgolici, Andreea-Consuela Timnea-Florescu, Olivia Timnea and Daciana Costina Andrada Stefan

Abstract

Visceral adiposity drives atherosclerosis and ectopic fat deposition, including hepatic steatosis, and is a major determinant of cardiometabolic risk in pediatric obesity. In adolescents, both BMI and WC are linked to cardiometabolic comorbidities, though their predictive accuracy differs. BMI is widely used due to its simplicity, low cost, and standardized reference values, but it cannot distinguish fat from lean mass, provides no information on fat distribution, and may misclassify children during rapid growth or puberty. Its association with metabolic risk also varies by sex, ethnicity, and developmental stage, limiting its value as a standalone indicator. Measures of central adiposity, including WC and waist-to-height ratio (WHtR), have gained increasing attention because they better capture visceral fat burden and show stronger associations with early metabolic dysfunction. Both WC and BMI are positively associated with elevated blood pressure and triglyceride concentrations and inversely associated with high-density lipoprotein cholesterol. Evidence shows that WC correlates more strongly than BMI with atherogenic lipid profiles, insulin resistance, alanine aminotransferase, and serum uric acid levels. Despite these advantages, the routine use of WC in pediatric practice is limited by the lack of standardized measurement protocols and universally accepted reference charts. Emerging evidence indicates that combining BMI and WC improves risk stratification compared with BMI alone. A two-step approach—using BMI for initial screening followed by WC or WHtR to assess central adiposity—may better identify high-risk children. Future research should integrate anthropometry with advanced imaging, molecular biomarkers, and AI-based models to enhance precision in cardiometabolic risk prediction.

Keywords: waist circumference, body mass index, pediatric obesity, cardiometabolic risk, visceral adiposity, insulin resistance

1. Introduction

Pediatric obesity has become one of the most pressing global health crises of our time. According to the World Health Organization, by 2022, over 390 million children and adolescents aged 5–19 were identified as overweight, including about 160 million classified as obese [1]. This shift is not limited to high-income countries – low – and middle-income regions are experiencing rapidly rising rates as well [2, 3, 4]. Further, recent data show that the prevalence of obesity among children aged 5 to 19 has increased from about 1.9% in 1990 to around 8.2% in 2022 [1].

Alongside overall rising obesity rates, there is accumulating evidence that visceral adiposity – fat stored within the abdominal cavity around internal organs – is increasing and contributing disproportionately to the cardiometabolic burden. Visceral fat is more metabolically active than subcutaneous fat and is associated with insulin resistance, inflammation, and ectopic fat deposition (for example, in liver and muscle). Recent anthropometric and imaging studies indicate that waist-based measures are more closely aligned with visceral adiposity than global adiposity indices [5].

Traditional anthropometric indicators, particularly Body Mass Index (BMI), have formed the backbone of obesity screening and epidemiologic surveillance in children. BMI is simple, inexpensive, and well-standardized for age and sex. Nonetheless, it has major limitations: it does not discriminate between fat and lean mass; it provides no information on fat distribution; it may misclassify children during growth spurts or puberty; and its correlation with metabolic risk varies across sex, ethnicity, and developmental stage [6, 7].

In contrast, measures of central or abdominal adiposity – such as waist circumference (WC) and waist-to-height ratio (WHtR) – are gaining attention for their ability to better capture visceral fat burden and for their stronger associations with early metabolic dysfunction. Recent longitudinal analyses demonstrate that WHtR exhibits better agreement over time with dual-energy X-ray absorptiometry (DEXA) measured fat mass, both total and trunk fat, compared with BMI in children followed from age 9 into young adulthood [8]. Additionally, studies suggest combining WC with BMI may improve identification of adolescents at increased cardiometabolic risk beyond what either measure alone offers [9].

However, despite mounting evidence, WC and related indices are underused in many clinical settings, partly due to lack of standardized reference percentiles in different populations, differing measurement techniques, and uncertainty about cut-offs that best predict long-term risk. For example, a very recent study from Macao established new age – and sex-specific percentile curves for WC among 6 – to 20-year-olds, highlighting differences in growth patterns and cut-off trajectories compared to other populations [10].

1.1 Aim of this chapter

To critically compare waist circumference vs BMI as predictors of cardiometabolic risk in children and adolescents. This chapter will examine the epidemiology of pediatric obesity, the biological plausibility of visceral fat as a driver of metabolic disease, empirical evidence from recent pediatric studies, and the clinical and public health implications of adopting waist-based measures alongside or instead of BMI in routine screening.

2. Anthropometric assessment of pediatric adiposity

2.1 Body mass index (BMI): Strengths and limitations

2.1.1 Simplicity and widespread use

BMI, defined as weight in kilograms divided by height in meters squared, remains the most widely used index for assessing overweight and obesity in children and adolescents. Its appeal lies in its simplicity, low cost, and standardization by age and sex, which make it suitable for both surveillance and clinical screening[11]. Recent analyses confirm that elevated BMI in youth is significantly associated with higher total body fat, supporting its utility as a first-line screening too [12].

2.1.2 Poor reflection of fat distribution

Despite its utility, BMI does not differentiate between fat and lean mass and provides no information about fat distribution. Two adolescents with identical BMI values may differ substantially in visceral fat burden and cardiometabolic risk [11]. Cross-sectional pediatric studies demonstrate that BMI z-scores correlate well with total fat mass but less strongly with relative fat percentage, especially in children younger than 9 years [13]. Moreover, during puberty, changes in lean mass can obscure true adiposity when relying solely on BMI [14].

2.1.3 Influence of age, sex, puberty, ethnicity

Interpretation of BMI in pediatric populations requires adjustment for age, sex, and pubertal stage. A BMI percentile deemed "normal" for one child may correspond to a very different metabolic risk profile in another [11]. Ethnic differences further complicate this picture: Asian children, for example, may experience higher metabolic risk at lower BMI thresholds compared to peers of European descent [15].

In sum, BMI is a practical and valuable tool, but it should not be considered a definitive measure of adiposity or risk in children.

2.2 Waist circumference (WC) and waist-to-height ratio (WTHR)

2.2.1 Measurement methodology and feasibility

Waist circumference is measured using a calibrated, non-stretchable tape at a standardized anatomical site (often the midpoint between the lowest rib and iliac crest or at the umbilicus). The procedure is inexpensive, rapid, and minimally invasive. The waist-to-height ratio (WtHR) is derived by dividing WC by standing height, thereby adjusting for stature [15].

2.2.2 Advantages: Surrogate marker of visceral fat

WC and WtHR more closely reflect central adiposity and visceral fat, which are metabolically more detrimental than subcutaneous fat. A longitudinal cohort of over

7,200 participants followed from childhood into young adulthood demonstrated that WtHR was more strongly correlated with dual-energy X-ray absorptiometry (DEXA) measures of trunk and total fat than BMI, and better distinguished lean from fat mass [16]. Similarly, cross-sectional studies consistently show stronger associations of WC and WtHR with dyslipidemia, insulin resistance, and hypertension compared to BMI [17].

2.2.3 Proposed pediatric thresholds

A frequently cited cut-off for WtHR is **0.5**, summarized in the aphorism "keep your waist less than half your height." [18] While pragmatic, this threshold may not capture ethnic and sex-specific variations in risk, and meta-analyses suggest that optimal cut-offs may differ across populations [19]. Recently, new percentile curves for WC were generated for children and adolescents in Macao, underscoring the variability in normative values between populations and the need for regional reference data [10].

Overall, WC and WtHR provide practical and clinically meaningful improvements over BMI by better capturing visceral adiposity, although consensus on standardized pediatric cut-offs remains elusive.

2.3 Advanced body composition techniques (DXA, MRI, ADP, BIA)

2.3.1 Higher accuracy compared to anthropometrics

Imaging-based and advanced techniques provide direct and more accurate quantification of fat distribution. DEXA can differentiate fat and lean mass regionally and has been validated as a reference for body composition in children. For instance, Verduin et al. used DEXA to establish percentiles of visceral adipose tissue in 10–11-year-olds independent of BMI and WC [20]. MRI is a noninvasive research tool widely used to measure visceral and hepatic fat without ionizing radiation, offering precise quantification of intra-abdominal adiposity in children [21]. Air displacement plethysmography (ADP) is often considered a reference method in pediatric body composition, while bioelectrical impedance analysis (BIA) provides a more accessible, noninvasive alternative albeit with acknowledged limitations in precision [22, 23].

2.3.2 Limitations: Cost, accessibility, and radiation (for DXA)

Despite their precision, these methods are resource-intensive. DXA involves low-level radiation exposure and is not universally available; MRI is expensive and time-consuming; ADP requires specialized equipment; and BIA, while portable and inexpensive, is sensitive to hydration status and body geometry, limiting its reliability in obese children [22, 24].

2.3.3 Comparative insights

Advanced imaging offers excellent precision but is impractical for widespread pediatric screening; hence anthropometric measures – especially WC and WtHR –

are indispensable in public health and clinical practice, given continued validation against imaging techniques [25].

3. Visceral fat and cardiometabolic dysfunction in children

3.1 Mechanistic links

3.1.1 Free fatty acid overflow

Visceral adipocytes have a high lipolytic rate and release a significant flux of free fatty acids (FFAs) into the portal circulation. This overflow of FFAs to the liver impairs hepatic insulin signaling, enhances gluconeogenesis, and stimulates lipoprotein production (especially VLDL), thereby contributing to hypertriglyceridemia and systemic insulin resistance [26].

Furthermore, the accumulation of FFAs is a well-recognized driver of ectopic lipid deposition and lipotoxic stress in non-adipose tissues [27].

3.1.2 Adipokines: Leptin, adiponectin, resistin

Visceral fat behaves as an endocrine organ by secreting adipokines that modulate metabolism and inflammation. In children with central obesity, leptin levels tend to be elevated (reflecting leptin resistance), which disrupts energy homeostasis and appetite regulation [28]. In parallel, adiponectin – known for its insulin-sensitizing and anti-inflammatory roles – is consistently found at lower concentrations in youth with visceral adiposity; lower adiponectin levels correlate with dyslipidemia and insulin resistance [26]. Resistin, predominantly from visceral depots, may amplify inflammatory pathways and impair endothelial function, though data in pediatric populations remain less abundant [29].

3.1.3 Low-grade inflammation and oxidative stress

Visceral fat expansion evokes recruitment of immune cells (macrophages, T cells) and secretion of proinflammatory cytokines (TNF-α, IL-6), activating NF-κB and other inflammatory cascades; this chronic low-grade inflammation undermines insulin signaling and contributes to vascular injury and atherogenesis [30, 31].

Simultaneously, hypertrophied adipocytes generate reactive oxygen species (ROS), which exacerbate oxidative stress, damage mitochondrial function, and blunt insulin receptor pathways. The intersection of inflammation and oxidative stress is central to the pathophysiology linking visceral fat to metabolic dysfunction [26].

3.1.4 Endothelial dysfunction and prothrombotic milieu

Inflammation and oxidative stress from visceral adiposity reduce nitric oxide (NO) bioavailability, impairing endothelial vasodilatory function – a key early step toward atherosclerosis [32]. Moreover, visceral fat promotes a prothrombotic environment by increasing plasminogen activator inhibitor-1 (PAI-1) and fibrinogen levels, contributing to coagulation risk [33].

3.2 Ectopic fat deposition

3.2.1 Liver (NAFLD/MASLD)

Excess FFAs from visceral adiposity lead to triglyceride accumulation in hepatocytes and promote hepatic steatosis. In pediatric cohorts, the prevalence of non-alcoholic fatty liver disease (NAFLD) (or the newer term MASLD – Metabolic Dysfunction Associated Steatotic Liver Disease) is increasing, and central adiposity is among the main predictors of hepatic fat content and elevated ALT levels [28].

In a large cohort of 10-year-olds, liver fat quantified by MRI showed that even within the so-called "normal" range (<5%) is linearly associated with higher blood pressure, insulin resistance, triglycerides, and clustering of metabolic risk, independent of BMI [34].

3.2.2 Heart

Visceral adiposity may also manifest in or influence the heart via epicardial adipose tissue (EAT). In adolescents, increased EAT thickness measured by imaging correlates with insulin resistance and early indices of cardiac dysfunction [35].

EAT, being contiguous with the myocardium, may exert paracrine and mechanical effects, accelerating local inflammation and remodeling [36].

3.2.3 Kidney

Perirenal and renal sinus fat depots are emerging as potentially pathogenic ectopic fat tissues. In obese children, higher perirenal fat volume has been associated with elevated blood pressure and impaired renal hemodynamics, possibly through mechanical compression of renal structures and sodium handling alterations [37].

3.3 Clinical consequences

3.3.1 Anthropometric indices as predictors of MASLD in overweight and obese children in children

Metabolic Dysfunction Associated Steatotic Liver Disease (MASLD) is diagnosed by the presence of hepatic steatosis together with at least one cardiometabolic risk factor.: 1) BMI ≥ the 85th percentile for age/sex or waist circumference (WC) > the 95th percentile; 2) fasting plasma glucose (FPG) ≥5.6 mmol/L; 3) BP ≥ the 95th percentile33 or ≥130/80 mmHg for children aged <13 years and ≥130/85 mmHg for children aged ≥13 years; 4) serum triglyceride (TG) concentration ≥1.15 mmol/L for children <10 years-old and ≥1.70 mmol/L for children ≥10 years-old; 5) high-density lipoprotein cholesterol (HDL-C) concentration ≤1.0 mmol/L [38].

MASLD is increasingly prevalent in pediatrics and, if untreated, contributes to greater metabolic disease burden in adulthood. Adiposity and weight gain worsen MASLD, while weight reduction improves outcomes. Hepatic steatosis may also result from other illnesses, alcohol use, genetic disorders, nutritional deficiencies, medications, gut microbiota changes, or endocrine disorders, so these causes must be ruled out rather than assuming obesity alone is responsible [39].

The North American Society for Pediatric Gastroenterology, Hepatology and Nutrition (NASPGHAN) guidelines recommend screening for MASLD in children aged 9–11 with obesity or in overweight children with additional risk factors, while the European Society for Pediatric Gastroenterology, Hepatology and Nutrition (ESPGHAN) advises the use of ultrasound alongside ALT for diagnosis [40]. MASLD is the most common liver disease in adolescents with obesity. In a study of 758 adolescents with severe obesity (BMI z-score >2), researchers evaluated which indicators best reflected the prevalence and severity of MASLD. Waist-to-height ratio was the most sensitive measure, the hepatic steatosis index showed the strongest association, and the liver enzymes alanine aminotransferase and aspartate aminotransferase were most closely linked to the presence and severity of the disease [41].

It was demonstrated that adolescents, males, Mexican Americans, and those with high waist circumference and BMI greater than 85th percentile are more likely to have MASLD [42].

In adults, waist circumference and metabolic indices serve as early markers of MASLD, where timely diagnosis can prompt lifestyle changes to prevent progression [43]. Also, in a review of studies up to 2014, the authors evaluated in adults, both body mass index (a measure of general obesity) and waist circumference (a measure of central obesity) in relation to the risk of nonalcoholic fatty liver disease, adjusting for body mass index. While both measures were independently associated with the disease, only central obesity showed a statistically significant association [44].

In children, as in adults, waist circumference, body mass index, and abdominal subcutaneous fat thickness are predictive of severe non-alcoholic fatty liver disease. Ultrasonography was used to assess fatty liver and its severity in 110 children aged 6.2–17.9 years who were overweight or obese, with waist circumference showing the highest predictive accuracy. Among the parameters, waist circumference and abdominal subcutaneous fat thickness were predictive in specific age groups [45].

Weng et al. analyzed data from 1,559 U.S. children and adolescents in the 2017–2020 NHANES survey and found that larger arm circumference (AC) was positively associated with NAFLD risk and greater liver steatosis severity. They also observed a non-linear relationship with an inflection point at 34.5 cm. The study suggests AC may serve as a useful marker for childhood NAFLD [46].

The latest American Association for the Study of Liver Diseases guidelines recommend ALT as the primary screening tool for MASLD in children aged 10 years, or earlier in those with cardiometabolic risk factors, family history, or severe obesity, with ultrasound considered as an initial imaging modality to support diagnosis [39].

In a study of 322 children (median age 13 years), higher ALT levels were associated with increased age, BMI, and waist circumference, with a male predominance. ALT was an effective initial screening tool for detecting increased liver stiffness, suggestive of significant fibrosis, in children with obesity or overweight and additional risk factors [47].

A study of 219 children with obesity (79 with MASLD and 140 without) assessed demographic, anthropometric, body composition, and biochemical variables. Multivariable logistic regression, stratified analyses, machine learning methods (Random Forest, LASSO regression), mediation analysis, and a nomogram were employed. This model integrating weight, waist circumference, body fat mass, and alanine aminotransferase (ALT) predicted metabolic dysfunction-associated steatotic liver disease with an AUC of 0.861, surpassing single-parameter approaches. These factors act synergistically to increase disease risk, with ALT mediating approximately one-third of the adiposity–MASLD relationship while maintaining an independent role. The validated nomogram offers individualized risk assessment, emphasizing the value of early ALT monitoring and adiposity management, particularly in children with obesity lasting more than three years [48].

In addition, a study published in The Lancet Regional Health, that employed machine learning methods demonstrated that the waist-to-height ratio (WHtR) represents a simple and practical tool for predicting pediatric MASLD. A cutoff of WHtR ≥0.48 may support early detection and management, particularly in populations with an obesity prevalence of ≥12.0%. For individual screening, the combination of WHtR ≥0.48 and lipid accumulation product (LAP) ≥668.22 cm × mg/dL is recommended. When integrated with regional obesity prevalence, these indices not only enable estimation of MASLD burden but also highlight the potential benefits of targeted screening strategies across populations with different levels of obesity risk [49].

The first prospective study on the natural history of pediatric NAFLD, using per-protocol timed liver biopsies in children from the placebo arms of two large multicenter clinical trials, was published in 2020. Participants received only standard lifestyle counseling consistent with routine primary care for children with overweight or obesity. Progression to definite NASH and fibrosis was associated with adolescent age, elevated transaminases, higher waist circumference, higher LDL cholesterol, and worsening liver enzymes over time, whereas increased gamma-glutamyl transferase was linked to a reduced likelihood of improvement [50].

As highlighted above, ALT is used for MASLD screening. In a study aiming to optimize ALT cutoffs for diagnosing MASLD, ALT 95th percentiles of 24–29 U/L were identified in girls and 29–32 U/L in boys aged 6–17 years. Differences from NHANES cutoffs highlight how reference criteria affect MASLD prevalence estimates. Age-, sex-, and puberty-specific cutoffs are preferable, especially in children <12 years. Since ALT may be normal despite MASLD, improved imaging and noninvasive diagnostics are needed to optimize screening and reduce unnecessary burden [51].

Lifestyle interventions focused on physical activity and nutrition are the cornerstone of treatment and should continue even if other therapies are introduced. The use of anti-obesity medications is recommended to aid weight reduction, and bariatric surgery is also an option for patients with MASLD and obesity. Early treatment is encouraged to help reduce the long-term economic and health burden of worsening metabolic disease [39].

3.3.2 Antropometric indices and dislipidemia in overweight and obese children

Children with high visceral adiposity often exhibit an atherogenic lipid profile – elevated triglycerides, low HDL cholesterol, and increased small dense LDL. These lipid disturbances tend to correlate more strongly with waist-based measures than with BMI [52–54].

Lipid disorders are a common problem in overweight and obese children and may significantly contribute to the increase in cardiovascular risk in the population of young adults [55, 56].

The age at which dyslipidemia is assessed in children is highly relevant. Puberty exerts a visible effect on lipid metabolism, characterized by a decrease in HDL-C, LDL-C, and total cholesterol, alongside an increase in triglycerides, when comparing pubertal with prepubertal children. These changes have been documented both in the general pediatric population and among children with obesity [57].

In a case-control study, it was shown that children with dyslipidemia were older and had elevated fundamental anthropometric measurements, such as waist circumference and BMI, compared to overweight and obese children without lipid abnormalities [58].

In an Indian cohort study on obese children, impaired LDL and HDL levels demonstrated a female predominance, whereas elevated triglyceride levels were observed more frequently among males [59]. In contrast, a large cohort study from Poland reported elevated triglyceride values among overweight and obese children, with a higher prevalence observed in girls [55].

In children and adolescents with type 1 diabetes, lipid disorders are common, particularly among those who are overweight or obese. These disorders involve not only quantitative abnormalities but also functional alterations in lipoprotein fractions. Notably, HDL loses its protective cardiovascular role in type 1 diabetes due to dysfunction, as its proteome exhibits an altered protein composition compared with that of healthy individuals [60].

In type 1 diabetes, obesity and hyperglycemia promote the early presence of oxLDL, its associated enzyme, and antibodies in the circulation, indicating their potential value as early biomarkers of cardiovascular disease (CVD) [61].

Dyslipidemia was more frequently observed in adolescents with well-controlled diabetes who were overweight or obese, compared to those with poorly controlled diabetes but normal body weight, which underscores the importance of assessing anthropometric indices associated with dyslipidemia [62].

3.3.3 Antropometric indices and insulin resistance in overweight and obese children

Visceral fat is a principal driver of insulin resistance in youth: the combined effects of FFA overflow, hypoadiponectinemia, and inflammation converge to impair insulin sensitivity and β-cell function, raising the risk of impaired glucose tolerance and early type 2 diabetes [28, 63].

In children and adolescents, waist circumference (WC) has proven to be a clinically meaningful measure of both overall and central adiposity, independent of BMI. Its strong associations with insulin resistance, proinsulin and fasting insulin underscore its predictive value for early metabolic dysfunction [64]. Similarly, previous studies have demonstrated that waist circumference is significantly correlated with insulin levels in obese children, thereby supporting its validity as a practical and reliable marker for the early identification of hyperinsulinemia [65].

Lipocalin-2, produced by adipose and immune cells, is associated with inflammation and may represent a link between obesity, insulin resistance, and cardiovascular disease. Lipocalin-2, serum insulin, and HOMA-IR were positively correlated with weight, BMI, and waist circumference. Thus, simple anthropometric measurements combined with serum lipocalin-2 can help predict insulin resistance in obese children, whereas serum adipsin and IL-10 showed no such association [66].

Disruptions in glucose and lipid regulation emerge early in obesity, increasing the risk of developing type 2 diabetes and cardiovascular disease at a young age. Some researchers recommend incorporating the oral glucose tolerance test into the routine evaluation of children with a BMI above 2 SDS [67].

Relatively recent, some researchers point out that current BMI and WC cut-offs do not adequately reflect regional fat depots, which vary by age and sex. Additionally, insulin resistance–based cut-offs increase with age from childhood to adulthood and should be adjusted accordingly [68]

Both waist circumference and BMI showed significant correlations with insulin resistance as measured by HOMA-IR. Waist circumference may serve as a practical clinical tool to identify children at risk [69], while HOMA-IR demonstrates a strong correlation with BMI and can be considered a surrogate marker of insulin resistance [70].

Although obesity in childhood clearly increases future metabolic risk, BMI alone is a limited measure of adiposity. Many studies have shown that Waist-based indices such as WC and waist-to-height ratio (WHtR) appear to capture metabolic risk more effectively, though the evidence in pediatric populations is still mixed [71–73]. But, most studies remain cross-sectional, underscoring the need for large, long-term cohorts to evaluate which measures best predict adult insulin resistance and related outcomes [71–73].

3.3.4 Other comorbidities in overweight and obese children

Central obesity is robustly linked with elevated blood pressure in pediatric populations. Mechanisms include sympathetic overactivity, salt retention, endothelial dysfunction, and vascular stiffness. Studies show that WC and WtHR outperform BMI in predicting hypertension in youth cohorts [74–76].

Elevated 8-iso-PGF2α levels in obese children are associated with high blood pressure, visceral adiposity, and increased insulin resistance, suggesting that this biomarker may play a role in the development of cardiovascular diseases and could serve as a sensitive tool for early diagnosis [77].

Seven-year follow-up assessments of obese children at 8 years of age showed that neither BMI nor waist circumference reliably predicted cardiovascular risk clustering when adiposity was excluded as a contributing factor [78].

In individuals with type 1 diabetes, carotid intima-media thickness (cIMT) demonstrates a significant association with waist circumference but not with BMI. This finding underscores the superior discriminatory value of waist circumference as an indicator of central adiposity and its related metabolic perturbations. Visceral fat accumulation, reflected more accurately by waist circumference, contributes to insulin resistance through elevated free fatty acid flux, dysregulated carbohydrate and lipid metabolism, and the pro-inflammatory and pro-coagulant milieu of chronic hyperglycemia. These mechanisms collectively promote early atherosclerotic progression, thereby explaining the stronger correlation between cIMT and waist circumference than with BMI [18].

4. Clinical and public health implications

4.1 Integrating WC in routine pediatric assessments

Despite compelling evidence linking waist circumference (WC) to visceral adiposity and early cardiometabolic dysfunction, it remains underutilized in pediatric settings compared with body mass index (BMI). Incorporating WC into routine visits for children and adolescents could substantially improve risk stratification, as the measurement is inexpensive, quick, and noninvasive, requiring minimal training and no specialized equipment. Regular monitoring of WC alongside BMI provides a more comprehensive picture of body fat distribution and its metabolic consequences [10]. In large pediatric cohorts, WC has demonstrated stronger associations than BMI with insulin resistance, elevated triglycerides, reduced HDL cholesterol, and early hypertension, supporting its value as an adjunct to BMI for earlier identification of high-risk children and for enabling timely intervention [74].

Advanced imaging methods, such as dual-energy X-ray absorptiometry (DXA) and air displacement plethysmography, provide more precise fat estimates, but their longitudinal predictive value in children has not yet been established. For now, simple anthropometric measures – particularly WC and WHtR – offer inexpensive, practical tools for improving early risk stratification beyond BMI alone [71].

However, looking ahead, it has been suggested that BMI and waist circumference should be replaced by more precise measures of body fat and regional fat depots, given their stronger associations with metabolic disturbances [68]. Other researchers hold the opposite view. They argue that dual-energy X-ray absorptiometry (DXA) for body composition analysis should remain limited to research settings, as it does not appear to provide additional or earlier insights into obesity-related metabolic complications [67].

4.2 Recommended cut-offs by WHO, IDF, AAP

Although international health bodies increasingly acknowledge the role of central adiposity, their recommendations remain fragmented and inconsistent. The World Health Organization (WHO) recognizes WC and waist-to-height ratio (WtHR) as useful markers of cardiometabolic risk in pediatric populations but highlights the absence of universal standards and emphasizes the need for population-specific reference data, which limits cross-regional comparability [1, 79]. The International Diabetes Federation (IDF) includes waist circumference (WC) as a necessary criterion in pediatric metabolic syndrome for children aged ten years and older, applying age – and sex-specific percentiles (e.g. WC ≥90th percentile) [80]. Nevertheless, these thresholds vary widely across cohorts, reflecting the lack of a harmonized methodology. Similarly, the American Academy of Pediatrics (AAP), in its 2023 clinical practice guideline, advocates for WC measurement as a complement to BMI when screening for comorbidities such as dyslipidemia, hypertension, and fatty liver disease. However, WC assessment is still rarely incorporated into electronic health record templates or preventive screening protocols, underscoring the persistent gap between recommendations and clinical implementation [15]. Taken together, these discrepancies highlight an urgent need for globally harmonized, evidence-based cut-offs for WC in pediatric populations. Without consensus, the utility of WC as a universal screening tool remains limited, and opportunities for early prevention of cardiometabolic disease are repeatedly missed.

4.3 Barriers to implementation

Several barriers continue to hinder the widespread adoption of WC in pediatric practice. One of the most fundamental is the absence of consensus on the anatomical site of measurement. While some protocols recommend using the midpoint between the iliac crest and the lowest rib, others measure at the umbilical level, producing inconsistencies that undermine comparability across studies and clinical care [81]. WC also lacks standardized, globally accepted percentile charts similar to those available for BMI. Instead, cut-off percentiles differ markedly by country, sex, age, and ethnicity; for example, recently published reference curves from Macao diverge substantially from European and North American data, highlighting the challenge of cross-population interpretation [10]. Finally, limited awareness and implementation exacerbate the problem: pediatricians are still primarily trained to rely on BMI, and WC measurement remains absent from many electronic health records and screening protocols, thereby widening the gap between evidence and practice [74].

4.4 Potential for combined use of WC and BMI

Emerging evidence suggests that the combination of BMI and WC may offer the strongest predictive utility. Children who present with both high BMI and elevated WC are at markedly higher risk of insulin resistance, dyslipidemia, and hypertension compared with those identified by BMI alone [82]. A pragmatic two-step approach has been proposed: BMI can serve as the initial screening tool to identify overweight and obese children, followed by WC or WtHR for risk stratification to capture central adiposity, even among those in the upper-normal BMI range. This dual strategy enhances early identification of children who require intervention and allows more efficient allocation of clinical and public health resources [18].

Ultimately, without standardized protocols and globally harmonized cut-offs, the integration of waist circumference into pediatric practice will remain fragmented, perpetuating underdiagnosis and delaying intervention. Bridging this gap between evidence and implementation is essential not only for optimizing individual patient care but also for advancing population-level strategies to curb the long-term cardiometabolic burden of childhood obesity.

5. Future research directions

Progress in understanding the relationship between central adiposity and cardiometabolic risk in children has been significant, but critical knowledge gaps remain. Future research must prioritize large-scale, ethnically diverse, and longitudinal cohorts that can map trajectories of adiposity and metabolic health from childhood into adulthood. Existing evidence is predominantly cross-sectional, limiting causal inference, and long-term follow-up studies are essential to determine whether waist circumference (WC) and waist-to-height ratio (WtHR) in childhood genuinely predict incident type 2 diabetes, hypertension, or cardiovascular events in adult life [71].

Another pressing need is the development of sex – and ethnicity-specific cut-offs. Current thresholds, often anchored to the 90th percentile, do not adequately reflect differences in body fat distribution between boys and girls, nor do they account for ethnic variations in cardiometabolic risk. Recent multinational analyses confirm that optimal WtHR cut-offs can differ significantly between populations, suggesting that a universal threshold may not be appropriate [20]. Establishing harmonized, population-specific reference values will be critical for improving both accuracy and equity in pediatric risk assessment.

Future research should also focus on integrating anthropometry with imaging and molecular biomarkers. Advanced imaging modalities such as MRI and DXA provide precise quantification of visceral and ectopic fat, while circulating biomarkers of inflammation (e.g., hs-CRP, IL-6), oxidative stress, and adipokine profiles (e.g., leptin, adiponectin) offer mechanistic insights. Combining WC or WtHR with these tools may yield more robust risk stratification models and help clarify causal pathways linking central adiposity to cardiometabolic dysfunction [83, 84]. However, the feasibility and cost-effectiveness of integrating such measures into routine pediatric care remain to be determined.

Finally, the emergence of artificial intelligence (AI) and machine learning (ML) models offers new opportunities for precision risk prediction. Algorithms that integrate anthropometrics, imaging, laboratory biomarkers, and electronic health record data have shown promise in predicting obesity-related complications in children with greater accuracy than traditional models. By leveraging large datasets, AI could help refine cut-offs, identify novel risk phenotypes, and personalize early interventions. Nevertheless, ethical concerns, algorithmic bias, and the need for external validation across diverse populations must be carefully addressed before widespread implementation.

In summary, future research should move beyond isolated anthropometric indicators toward a multidimensional approach that combines WC and WtHR with imaging, biomarkers, and predictive analytics. Such efforts will be pivotal in bridging the current gap between epidemiological evidence and clinical application, ultimately enabling more accurate, equitable, and personalized strategies for preventing cardiometabolic disease in children.

6. Conclusions

The evidence reviewed in this chapter demonstrates that waist circumference (WC) provides a superior reflection of central adiposity compared with body mass index (BMI) and is more strongly associated with early manifestations of cardiometabolic dysfunction in children and adolescents. Elevated WC consistently correlates with insulin resistance, dyslipidemia, hypertension, and ectopic fat deposition, whereas BMI, although useful for classifying general overweight and obesity, fails to capture these high-risk metabolic phenotypes.

Nevertheless, BMI remains valuable as an easily accessible, standardized, and globally recognized metric. Its simplicity and widespread use in surveillance and clinical practice ensure that it will remain an indispensable screening tool. Importantly, WC and BMI should not be viewed as competing measures but rather as complementary indicators that, when combined, provide a more comprehensive assessment of pediatric adiposity and associated risk. Children with elevated BMI but normal WC may have a more benign metabolic profile, whereas those with concurrent elevation of both indices are at particularly high risk for cardiometabolic complications.

The routine implementation of WC measurement in pediatric practice is therefore warranted. Its inclusion alongside BMI in both clinical workflows and public health surveillance would allow for earlier and more accurate identification of children at increased risk, facilitating timely interventions to prevent the progression to type 2 diabetes, cardiovascular disease, and other obesity-related disorders. This approach aligns with calls from the World Health Organization, the International Diabetes Federation, and the American Academy of Pediatrics, all of which emphasize the importance of assessing central adiposity, even though consensus on measurement techniques and cut-offs remains incomplete.

Moving forward, harmonization of WC protocols and reference values will be essential to maximize its clinical utility and ensure comparability across populations. In the meantime, pediatricians and public health professionals should not delay the integration of WC into routine assessments, given its low cost, ease of use, and added predictive power. The integration of WC into everyday practice represents not only a refinement of obesity screening but also a crucial step toward bridging the gap between epidemiological evidence and real-world prevention of cardiometabolic disease in the next generation.

Measuring the waist may prove as vital as weighing the child – only by combining both can we truly prevent the cardiometabolic diseases of tomorrow.

Author details

Maria-Zinaida Dobre[1], Bogdana Virgolici[1*], Andreea-Consuela Timnea-Florescu[2,3], Olivia Timnea[4] and Daciana Costina Andrada Stefan[1]

1 Department of Biochemistry, Carol Davila University of Medicine and Pharmacy, Bucharest, Romania

2 Grigore Alexandrescu Children's Hospital, Bucharest, Romania, and Titu Maiorescu Faculty of Medicine, Bucharest, Romania

3 Titu Maiorescu Faculty of Medicine, Bucharest, Romania

4 Romano-Americana University, Faculty of Sports and Kinetotherapy, Department of physiology, Bucharest, Romania

*Address all correspondence to: bogdana.virgolici@umfcd.ro

References

[1] World Health Organization. Obesity and Overweight – Key Facts. 2023. Available at: https://www.who.int/news-room/fact-sheets/detail/obesity-and-overweight [Accessed: 2025-September-27]

[2] Zhang X, Liu J, Ni Y, Yi C, Fang Y, Ning Q, Shen B, Zhang K, Liu Y, Yang L, Li K. Global prevalence of overweight and obesity in children and adolescents: A systematic review and meta-analysis. JAMA Pediatrics. 2024;**178**(8):800–813

[3] Obesity Evidence Hub. *Children – global context*. https://www.obesityevidencehub.org.au/collections/trends/children-global-contex [Accessed: 2025-September-27]

[4] Nahorna A, Baur H. Evaluating abdominal obesity by waist circumference, anthropometric indices and bioelectrical impedance analysis: A comparative pilot study. Obesity Science & Practice. 2025;**11**(3):e70078

[5] Zhou Y, Tang P, Wang Y, Tang Y, Yang Y. Joint association of weight-adjusted-waist index and physical activity with insulin resistance in adolescents: A cross-sectional study. BMC Endocrine Disorders. 2024;**24**(1):100

[6] Gordito Soler M, Tárraga López PJ, Áa L-G, Paublini H, Rifá E M-A, Vicente-Herrero MT, Ramírez-Manent JI. Is measuring BMI and waist circumference as good in assessing insulin resistance as using bioelectrical impedance to measure total body fat and visceral fat? Diabetology. 2025;**6**(4):32

[7] Agbaje AO. Waist-circumference-to-height-ratio had better longitudinal agreement with DEXA-measured fat mass than BMI in 7237 children. Pediatric Research. 2024;**96**(5):1369–1380

[8] Haapala EA. Identifying adolescents with increased cardiometabolic risk—Simple, but challenging. Jornal de Pediatria. 2025;**101**(1):1–3

[9] Jiang L, Zhang A, Tu C, Gao Y, He J, Pan X, Zhang X, Zhang Y. Study on reference value of waist circumference percentile curve and abdominal obesity cutoff points of children and adolescents aged 6–20 in Macao. BMC Public Health. 2025;**25**(1):1889

[10] National Academies of Sciences, Engineering, and Medicine; Health and Medicine; Division; Food and Nutrition Board; Roundtable on Obesity Solutions; Callahan EA, editor. Translating Knowledge of Foundational Drivers of Obesity into Practice: Proceedings of a Workshop Series. Washington (DC): National Academies Press (US); 2023 Jul 31. 10, The Science, Strengths, and Limitations of Body Mass Index.

[11] Freedman DS, Zemel BS, Weber DR, Dietz WH. The cross-sectional relation of body mass index to adiposity among 8-to 19-year-olds within several races and ethnicities. The Journal of Pediatrics. 2025;**277**:114375

[12] Vanderwall C, Randall Clark R, Eickhoff J, Carrel AL. BMI is a poor predictor of adiposity in young overweight and obese children. BMC Pediatrics. 2017;**17**(1):135

[13] Nevill AM, Reuter CP, Brand C, Gaya AR, Mota J, Renner JDP,

Duncan MJ. BMI fails to reflect the developmental changes in body fatness between boys and girls during adolescence. International Journal of Environmental Research and Public Health. 2021;**18**(15):7833

[14] Goran MI. Measurement issues related to studies of childhood obesity: Assessment of body composition, body fat distribution, physical activity, and food intake. Pediatrics. 1998;**101**(3 Pt 2):505–518

[15] Gomwe H, Phiri L, Marange CS. Waist-based anthropometric measures and central adiposity-related comorbidities in children. South African Family Practice. 2024;**66**(1):1–6

[16] Junior CA, Mocellin MC, Gonçalves EC, Silva DA, Trindade EB. Anthropometric indicators as body fat discriminators in children and adolescents: A systematic review and meta-analysis. Advances in Nutrition. 2017;**8**(5):718–727

[17] Eslami M, Pourghazi F, Khazdouz M, Tian J, Pourrostami K, Esmaeili-Abdar Z, Ejtahed HS, Qorbani M. Optimal cut-off value of waist circumference-to-height ratio to predict central obesity in children and adolescents: A systematic review and meta-analysis of diagnostic studies. Frontiers in Nutrition. 2023;**9**:985319

[18] Zong X, Kelishadi R, Hong YM, et al. Establishing international optimal cut-offs of waist-to-height ratio for predicting cardiometabolic risk in children and adolescents aged 6–18 years. BMC Medicine. 2023;**21**(1):442

[19] Verduin WM, Van Den Helder R, Doodeman HJ, Struijf E, Houdijk AP. Dexa body composition assessment in 10-11 year healthy children. PLoS One. 2016;**11**(10):e0165275

[20] Simoni P, Guglielmi R, Gómez MP. Imaging of body composition in children. Quantitative Imaging in Medicine and Surgery. 2020;**10**(8):1661

[21] Mahaffey R, Brown N, Cramp M, Morrison SC, Drechsler WI. Evaluation of bioelectrical impedance analysis in measuring body fat in 6-to-12-year-old boys compared with air displacement plethysmography. British Journal of Nutrition. 2023;**130**(6):1098–1104. DOI: 10.1017/JS0007114522004019

[22] Chen F, Wu L, Chen Y, Wang J, Liu J, Huang G, Hou D, Liao Z, Zhang T, Xie X, Liu G. A comparison of bioelectrical impedance analysis and air displacement plethysmography to assess body composition in children. Frontiers in Public Health. 2023;**11**:1164556. DOI: 10.3389/fpubh.2023.1164556

[23] Lemos T, Gallagher D. Current body composition measurement techniques. Current Opinion in Endocrinology, Diabetes and Obesity. 2017;**24**(5):310–314

[24] Nie MJ, Sun RZ, Fan CQ, Wang JJ, Fei X, Hu ZK, Li HJ. Diagnostic performance of anthropometric measurements for identifying obesity in high-altitude pediatric populations: Evidence from Tibet via bioelectrical impedance analysis. Lipids in Health and Disease. 2025;**24**(1):216

[25] Shetty S, Suvarna R, Bhattacharya S, Seetharaman K. Visceral adiposity and cardiometabolic risk: Clinical insights and assessment. Cardiology in Review. 2025. DOI: 10.1097/CRD.0000000000000984

[26] Dhokte S, Czaja K. Visceral adipose tissue: The hidden culprit for type 2 diabetes. Nutrients. 2024;**16**(7):1015. DOI: 10.3390/nu16071015

[27] Luo Y, Luo D, Li M, Tang B. Insulin resistance in pediatric obesity: From mechanisms to treatment strategies. Pediatric Diabetes. 2024:2298306. DOI: 10.1155/2024/2298306

[28] Chait A, Den Hartigh LJ. Adipose tissue distribution, inflammation and its metabolic consequences, including diabetes and cardiovascular disease. Frontiers in Cardiovascular Medicine. 2020;**7**:522637

[29] Singer K, Lumeng CN. The initiation of metabolic inflammation in childhood obesity. Journal of Clinical Investigation. 2017;**127**(1):65–73. DOI: 10.1172/JCI88882

[30] Kawai T, Autieri MV, Scalia R. Adipose tissue inflammation and metabolic dysfunction in obesity. American Journal of Physiology-Cell Physiology. 2021;**320**(3):C375–C391. DOI: 10.1152/ajpcell.00379.2020

[31] Vilahur G, Ben-Aicha S, Badimon L. New insights into the role of adipose tissue in thrombosis. Cardiovascular Research. 2017;**113**(9):1046–1054

[32] Badran M, Gozal D. PAI-1: A major player in the vascular dysfunction in obstructive sleep apnea? International Journal of Molecular Sciences. 2022;**23**(10):5516

[33] King RJ, Ajjan RA. Vascular risk in obesity: Facts, misconceptions and the unknown. Diabetes and Vascular Disease Research. 2017;**14**(1):2–13

[34] Geurtsen ML, Santos S, Felix JF, Duijts L, Vernooij MW, Gaillard R, Jaddoe VW. Liver fat and cardiometabolic risk factors among school-age children. Hepatology. 2020;**72**(1):119–129

[35] Schusterova I, Leenen FH, Jurko A, Sabol F, Takacova J. Epicardial adipose tissue and cardiometabolic risk factors in overweight and obese children and adolescents. Pediatric Obesity. 2014;**9**(1):63–70

[36] Goran MI, Gower BA. Relation between visceral fat and disease risk in children and adolescents. The American Journal of Clinical Nutrition. 1999;**70**(1):149S–156S

[37] Rinella ME, Lazarus JV, Ratziu V, Francque SM, Sanyal AJ, Kanwal F, Romero D, Abdelmalek MF, Anstee QM, Arab JP, Arrese M, Bataller R, Beuers U, Boursier J, Bugianesi E, Byrne CD, Castro Narro GE, Chowdhury A, Cortez-Pinto H, Cryer DR, Cusi K, El-Kassas M, Klein S, Eskridge W, Fan J, Gawrieh S, Guy CD, Harrison SA, Kim SU, Koot BG, Korenjak M, Kowdley KV, Lacaille F, Loomba R, Mitchell-Thain R, Morgan TR, Powell EE, Roden M, Romero-Gómez M, Silva M, Singh SP, Sookoian SC, Spearman CW, Tiniakos D, Valenti L, Vos MB, Wong VW-S, Xanthakos S, Yilmaz Y, Younossi Z, Hobbs A, Villota-Rivas M, Newsome PN, et al. A multisociety Delphi consensus statement on new fatty liver disease nomenclature. Journal of Hepatology. 2023;**79**:1542–1556

[38] Panganiban J, Kehar M, Ibrahim SH, Hartmann P, Sood S, Hassan S, Ramirez CM, Kohli R, Censani M, Mauney E, Cuda S, Karjoo S. Metabolic dysfunction-associated steatotic liver disease (MASLD) in children with obesity: An Obesity Medicine Association (OMA) and

expert joint perspective 2025. Obesity Pillars. 2025;**14**:100164. DOI: 10.1016/j.obpill.2025.100164

[39] Vos MB, Abrams SH, Barlow SE, et al. NASPGHAN clinical practice guideline for the diagnosis and treatment of nonalcoholic fatty liver disease in children. Journal of Pediatric Gastroenterology and Nutrition. 2017;**64**(2):319. DOI: 10.1097/mpg.0000000000001482

[40] Mari L, Lazzer S, Gatti A, D'Alleva M, Zaccaron S, Stafuzza J, Rejc E, Vandoni M, Bondesan A, Caroli D, Frigerio F, Abbruzzese L, Ventura E, Sartorio A. Visceral adiposity, anthropometric and liver function indexes for identifying Metabolic Dysfunction Associated Steatotic Liver Disease (MASLD) in adolescents with obesity: Which performs better? Journal of Clinical Medicine. 2025;**14**(6):2085. DOI: 10.3390/jcm14062085

[41] Welsh JA, Karpen S, Vos MB. Increasing prevalence of nonalcoholic fatty liver disease among United States adolescents, 1988-1994 to 2007-2010. The Journal of Pediatrics. 2014;**162**(3):496. DOI: 10.1016/j.jpeds.2012.08.043

[42] S TE, T OA, V SS, et al. Comparison of non-invasive liver fat scoring systems as markers of metabolic dysfunction-associated liver disease. Cureus. 2024;**16**(10):e72222. DOI: 10.7759/cureus.72222

[43] Pang Q, Zhang JY, Song SD, Qu K, Xu XS, SS L, Liu C. Central obesity and nonalcoholic fatty liver disease risk after adjusting for body mass index. World Journal of Gastroenterology. 2015;**21**(5):1650–1662

[44] Chao H-C, Lin H-Y. Comparison of body mass index and fat indices in predicting the severity of nonalcoholic fatty liver disease among children who are overweight and obese. Frontiers in Pediatrics. 2021;**9**:724426. DOI: 10.3389/fped.2021.724426

[45] Weng X, Xu J, Yang S. Association between the arm circumference and non-alcoholic fatty liver disease in American children and adolescence: A population-based analysis. Frontiers in Public Health. 2024;**12**:1323795. DOI: 10.3389/fpubh.2024.1323795

[46] Stroes ASR, Draijer L, Chegary M, Kreier F, van Os E, Goede J, Boonstra V, Westerbeek I, Bouma S, Kusters M, Roelants R, Beuers U, Holleboom AG, Benninga MA, Koot BGP. ALT is an effective screening tool for advanced metabolic dysfunction-associated steatotic liver disease in children with obesity and overweight. Clinical Gastroenterology and Hepatology. 2025. DOI: 10.1016/j.cgh.2025.05.011

[47] Li Y, Liu R, An Y, et al. Markers of body fat, the mediating role of alanine aminotransferase, and their association with the risk of metabolic dysfunction-associated steatotic liver disease. European Journal of Pediatrics. 2025;**184**:524

[48] Liu Y, Wang Y, Xing Y, Wolters M, Shi D, Zhang P, Dang J, Chen Z, Cai S, Wang Y, Liu J, Wang X, Zhou H, Xu M, Guo L, Li Y, Song J, Li J. Establishing a non-invasive model to screen metabolic dysfunction-associated steatotic liver disease in children aged 6–14 years in China and its applications in high-obesity-risk countries and regions. The Lancet Regional Health - Western Pacific. 2024;**49**:101150

[49] Xanthakos SA, Lavine JE, Yates KP, Schwimmer JB, Molleston JP, Rosenthal P, Murray KF, Vos MB, Jain AK, Scheimann AO, Miloh T, Fishbein M, Behling CA, Brunt EM, Sanyal AJ, Tonascia J; NASH Clinical Research Network. Progression of fatty liver disease in children receiving standard of care lifestyle advice. Gastroenterology. 2020;**159**(5): 1731–1751.e10. DOI: 10.1053/j.gastro.2020.07.034

[50] Aitokari L, Lahti S, Kivelä L, Riekki H, Hiltunen P, Vuorela N, Viitasalo A, Soininen S, Huhtala H, Lakka T, Kurppa K. Alanine aminotransferase cutoffs for the pediatric fatty liver disease: Major impact of the reference population. Journal of Personalized Medicine. 2023;**13**:12040. DOI: 10.1002/jpn3.12040

[51] Fernández-Aparicio Á, Mohatar-Barba M, Perona JS, Schmidt-riovalle J, Navarro-Pérez CF, González-Jiménez E. Discriminative capacity of visceral adiposity and triglyceride glucose-waist circumference indices for metabolic syndrome in Spanish adolescents: A cross-sectional study. Metabolites. 2025;**15**(8):535

[52] Abdelhaleem BA, Emam EK, Salem AM, Yacoub GE, Helal RA, Abdelhamed MH. The interplay between visceral adiposity and cardiometabolic risk in children with obesity. Cureus. 2025;**17**(5):e84062

[53] Baran R, Baran J, Leszczak J, Bartosiewicz A, Wyszyńska J. Lipid profile, obesity indicators and cardiometabolic risk factors in school-aged children and adolescents: Sex-specific associations. Journal of Clinical Medicine. 2025;**14**(18):6677. DOI: 10.3390/jcm14186677

[54] Brzeziński M, Metelska P, Myśliwiec M, et al. Lipid disorders in children living with overweight and obesity- large cohort study from Poland. Lipids in Health and Disease. 2020;**19**:47

[55] Bassali R, Waller JL, Gower B, Allison J, Davis CL. Utility of waist circumference percentile for risk evaluation in obese children. International Journal of Pediatric Obesity. 2010;**5**(1):97–101. DOI: 10.3109/17477160903111722

[56] Nielsen TRH, Lausten-Thomsen U, Fonvig CE, et al. Dyslipidemia and reference values for fasting plasma lipid concentrations in Danish/North-European White children and adolescents. BMC Pediatrics. 2017;**17**:116

[57] Altaan EA, Alsarraf Z, Alsarraf Z, Abow FH. The prevalence of dyslipidemia in pediatric obesity and its relation to lifestyle of obese children (prevalensi dislipidemia pada obesitas anak dan hubungannya dengan gaya hidup anak obesitas). Indonesian Journal on Health Science and Medicine. 2025;**2**(1). DOI: 10.21070/ijhsm.v2i1.63

[58] Jacob AS, G. R. Prevalence of metabolic comorbidities in obese children. International Journal of Contemporary Pediatrics 2017. 2017;**4**:1450–1455

[59] Noras K, Rusak E, Jarosz-Chobot P. The problem of abnormal body weight and dyslipidemia as risk factors for cardiovascular diseases in children and adolescents with Type 1 diabetes. Journal of Diabetes Research. 2021:5555149

[60] Omar NN, EL Hefnawy MH, EL Soda MF, Heider NM, Hamed HI.

Assessment of oxLDL, anti-oxLDL antibodies and lipoprotein-associated phospholipase A2 as cardiovascular risk markers in obese adolescents with and without T1DM. The Bulletin of Faculty of Pharmacy, Cairo University. 2017;**55**(2):325–331. DOI: 10.1016/j.bfopcu.2017.07.003

[61] Wysocka-Mincewicz M, Kołodziejczyk H, Wierzbicka E, Szalecki M. Overweight, obesity and lipids abnormalities in adolescents with type 1 diabetes. Pediatric Endocrinology, Diabetes, and Metabolism. 2015;**21**(2):70–81. DOI: 10.18544/PEDM-21.02.0027,2-s2.0-84988259151

[62] Caprio S, Perry R, Kursawe R. Adolescent obesity and insulin resistance: Roles of ectopic fat accumulation and adipose inflammation. Gastroenterology. 2017;**152**(7):1638–1646

[63] Lee S, Bacha F, Gungor N, Arslanian SA. Waist circumference is an independent predictor of insulin resistance in black and white youths. The Journal of Pediatrics. 2006;**148**(2):188–194. DOI: 10.1016/j.jpeds.2005.10.001

[64] Cempaka PMVP, Sidiartha GL. Waist circumference and insulin levels in obese children. Pediatrics Indonesia. 2017;**57**(4):194–197

[65] El Sehmawy AA, Diab FEA, Hassan DA, Mohammed DS, Gamal El Din Al Anany M, Eldesoky NA, Elamir RY. Utility of Adipokines and IL-10 in association with anthropometry in prediction of insulin resistance in obese children. diabetes, Metabolic Syndrome and Obesity: Targets and Therapy. 2022;**15**: 3231–3241. DOI: 10.2147/DMSO.S377072

[66] Elsedfy H, Amr NH, Hussein O, Kholy ME. Insulin resistance in obese pre-pubertal children: Relation to body composition. Egyptian Journal of Medical Human Genetics. 2014;**15**(3):249–255. DOI: 10.1016/j.ejmhg.2014.04.002

[67] Hübers M, Pourhassan M, Braun W, Geisler C, Müller MJ. Definition of new cut-offs of BMI and waist circumference based on body composition and insulin resistance: Differences between children, adolescents and adults. Obesity Science. 2017. DOI: 10.1002/osp4.121

[68] Hirschler V, Aranda C, Calcagno Mde L, Maccalini G, Jadzinsky M. Can waist circumference identify children with the metabolic syndrome? Archives of Pediatrics & Adolescent Medicine. 2005;**159**(8):740–744. DOI: 10.1001/archpedi.159.8.740

[69] Joseph CR, Kumar H, Bhat K. Cross-sectional observational study on correlation of obesity and overweight in children with insulin resistance based on HOMA-IR score. Open Journal of Pediatrics and Child Health. 2023;**8**(1):039–044. DOI: 10.17352/ojpch.000050

[70] DeLacey S, Josefson JL. A mini-review of pediatric anthropometrics as predictors of future insulin resistance. Frontiers in Endocrinology. 2022;**13**:826430. DOI: 10.3389/fendo.2022.826430

[71] Lee CM, Huxley RR, Wildman RP, Woodward M. Indices of abdominal obesity are better discriminators of cardiovascular risk factors than BMI: A meta-analysis. Journal of Clinical Epidemiology. 2008;**61**(7):646–653. DOI: 10.1016/j.jclinepi.2007.08.012

[72] Janssen I, Katzmarzyk PT, Ross R. Body mass indx, waist circumference, and health risk: Evidence in support of current national institutes of health guidelines. Archives of Internal Medicine. 2002;**162**(18):2074–2079. DOI: 10.1001/archinte.162.18.2074

[73] Nimkarn N, Sewarit A, Pirojsakul K, Paksi W, Chantarogh S, Saisawat P, Tangnararatchakit K. Waist-to-height-ratio is associated with sustained hypertension in children and adolescents with high office blood pressure. Frontiers in Cardiovascular Medicine. 2023;**9**:1026606

[74] Pazin DC, da Luz Kaestner Tl, Olandoski M, Baena CP, de Azevedo Abreu G, Kuschnir MC, Bloch KV, Faria-Neto JR. Association between abdominal waist circumference and blood pressure in Brazilian adolescents with normal body mass index: Waist circumference and blood pressure in adolescents. Global Heart. 2020;**15** (1):27

[75] Cruz NR, Cardoso PC, Frossard TN, Ferreira FD, Brener S, Gomides AF, Valente MA, Velloso-Rodrigues C. Waist circumference as high blood pressure predictor in school age children. Ciência & Saúde Coletiva. 2019;**24**:1885–1893

[76] Demirhan I, Oner E, Kurutas EB. Evaluation of the relationship between insulin resistance and 8-iso prostaglandin levels in obesity children. Folia Medica. 2023;**65**(4):589–596. DOI: 10.3897/folmed.65. e81316repetdelacey

[77] Garnett SP, Baur LA, Srinivasan S, Lee JW, Cowell CT. Body mass index and waist circumference in midchildhood and adverse cardiovascular disease risk clustering in adolescence. The American Journal of Clinical Nutrition. 2007;**86**(3):549–555

[78] Rathsman B, Rosfors S, Sjöholm A, Nyström T. Early signs of atherosclerosis are associated with insulin resistance in non-obese adolescent and young adults with type 1 diabetes. Cardiovascular Diabetology. 2012;**11**:145. DOI: 10.1186/1475-2840-11-145

[79] Zhang B, Shi H, Cai W, Yang B, Xiu W. Metabolic syndrome in children and adolescents: Definitions, epidemiology, pathophysiology, interventions, and challenges. Frontiers in Endocrinology. 2025;**16**:1512642

[80] Hampl SE, Hassink SG, Skinner AC, Armstrong SC, Barlow SE, Bolling CF, Avila Edwards KC, Eneli I, Hamre R, Joseph MM, Lunsford D. Clinical practice guideline for the evaluation and treatment of children and adolescents with obesity. Pediatrics. 2023;**151**(2):e2022060640

[81] Bibiloni MDM, Gallardo-Alfaro L, Gómez SF, Wärnberg J, Osés-Recalde M, González-Gross M, Gusi N, Aznar S, Marín-Cascales E, González-Valeiro M, Serra-Majem L, Terrados N, Segu M, Lassale C, Homs C, Benavente-Marín JC, Labayen I, Zapico AG, Sánchez-Gómez J, Jiménez-Zazo F, Alcaraz PE, Sevilla-Sánchez M, Herrera-Ramos E, Pulgar S, Sistac C, Schröder H, Bouzas C, Tur JA. Combined body mass index and waist-to-height ratio and its association with lifestyle and health factors among spanish children: The PASOS Study. Nutrients. 2022;**14**(2):234. DOI: 10.3390/nu14020234

[82] Kuciene R, Dulskiene V. Associations between body mass index, waist circumference, waist-to-height

ratio, and high blood pressure among adolescents: A cross-sectional study. Scientific Reports. 2019;**9**:9493. DOI: 10.1038/s41598-019-45956-9

[83] Neeland IJ, Yokoo T, Leinhard OD, Lavie CJ. 21st century advances in multimodality imaging of obesity for care of the cardiovascular patient. JACC: Cardiovascular Imaging. 2021;**14** (2):482–494

[84] Huang L, Huhulea EN, Abraham E, Bienenstock R, Aifuwa E, Hirani R, Schulhof A, Tiwari RK, Etienne M. The role of artificial intelligence in obesity risk prediction and management: Approaches, insights, and recommendations. Medicina. 2025;**61** (2):358

Section 3

Recent Developments in Obesity Assessments in Women and Elderly Populations

Chapter 5

Perspective Chapter: Beyond BMI – Rethinking Obesity Assessment in Women's Health

Tuğba Gürbüz and Oya Gökmen

Abstract

Body mass index (BMI) remains the most frequently used anthropometric index for classifying obesity in both clinical and public health settings. Despite its simplicity and utility, BMI fails to capture the heterogeneity of body composition and the unique physiological, hormonal, and metabolic conditions that affect women throughout their lifespan. The limitations of BMI are particularly evident in reproductive-aged, pregnant, and postmenopausal women, where factors such as fat distribution, muscle mass, and visceral adiposity play more critical roles in disease risk than total body weight alone. This chapter explores the historical context, methodological limitations, and clinical misapplications of BMI in women's health, emphasizing its inadequacy in capturing nuanced risk profiles. It further examines alternative assessment tools – including waist-to-hip ratio, body fat percentage, imaging modalities, and metabolic markers – and advocates for a multidimensional, individualized approach to obesity evaluation. Moving beyond BMI, this chapter aims to offer a comprehensive framework that aligns obesity assessment with precision medicine and sex-specific healthcare needs.

Keywords: body mass index (BMI), visceral adiposity, reproductive endocrinology, polycystic ovary syndrome (PCOS), metabolic health, precision medicine

1. Introduction

Obesity is a global health crisis with disproportionate implications for women across different stages of life, from adolescence and reproductive years to menopause and beyond. Traditionally, body mass index (BMI) has served as the primary tool for assessing obesity, largely due to its simplicity, reproducibility, and widespread use in population-level epidemiological studies. Calculated as weight in kilograms divided by height in meters squared (kg/m^2), BMI has long been considered a surrogate for adiposity and metabolic health risk. However, emerging evidence suggests that BMI may not be an accurate or sufficient indicator of health status in women, especially when viewed through the lens of reproductive endocrinology and maternal-fetal medicine [1, 2].

Women experience dynamic physiological changes – including hormonal fluctuations, shifts in fat distribution, and alterations in insulin sensitivity – that can significantly affect body composition without necessarily altering BMI. For instance, a woman with a BMI of 25 kg/m^2 may have vastly different health risks depending on whether her adiposity is predominantly subcutaneous or visceral [3]. These variations are particularly consequential during critical reproductive windows, such as preconception, pregnancy, and the postpartum period, where metabolic adaptations and inflammatory responses can profoundly influence outcomes [4].

Furthermore, BMI does not differentiate between lean mass and fat mass, nor does it account for ethnic differences in body composition or the phenomenon of "normal weight obesity (NWO)," where individuals exhibit cardiometabolic risk despite having a BMI within the normal range [5]. This diagnostic blind spot is especially problematic in clinical decisions regarding fertility treatment, polycystic ovary syndrome (PCOS), gestational diabetes mellitus (GDM), and hypertensive disorders of pregnancy. For example, BMI has limited utility in predicting ovulatory function or oocyte quality in assisted reproductive technologies (ARTs) [6].

The overreliance on BMI may also mask the need for timely intervention in women whose weight does not meet clinical thresholds for obesity but whose metabolic risk is significantly elevated. In this context, emerging diagnostic approaches – such as waist-to-hip ratio (WHR), dual-energy Xray absorptiometry (DEXA), and serum adipokine profiling – offer more nuanced, individualized risk stratification [7]. These tools reflect a growing recognition that effective obesity assessment in women must transcend a one-size-fits-all metric and instead embrace a multifactorial, sex-specific approach aligned with precision medicine.

In the following sections, this chapter will critically evaluate the conceptual and methodological limitations of BMI, present alternative and complementary tools for assessing obesity in women, and propose an integrated framework that enhances clinical decision-making in gynecology, obstetrics, and reproductive medicine.

2. Historical background and evolution of BMI

BMI was first conceptualized in the nineteenth century by Belgian mathematician and statistician Adolphe Quetelet, who introduced the Quetelet Index as a tool to describe the "average man" in anthropometric studies. His intent was not to measure health or adiposity but to develop a statistical model of human growth and morphology [8]. Despite its nonmedical origins, the Quetelet Index was later rebranded as BMI and adopted in clinical and epidemiological contexts during the mid-twentieth century, particularly following the work of Ancel Keys and colleagues in 1972, who validated its correlation with body fat and mortality in selected populations [9].

Over the decades, BMI has become the most commonly used metric to classify individuals into categories of underweight, normal weight, overweight, and obesity, with fixed cutoffs established by the World Health Organization (WHO). These thresholds – <18.5 kg/m^2 for underweight, 18.5–24.9 for normal, 25.0–29.9 for overweight, and ≥ 30.0 for obesity – have been adopted globally due to their ease of use and scalability in large populations [10]. The widespread institutionalization of BMI in public health policy, insurance systems, and clinical guidelines has further entrenched its dominance as the de facto standard for assessing adiposity.

However, the very simplicity that renders BMI attractive also underpins its fundamental weaknesses. As a two-dimensional index derived solely from weight and height, BMI makes no distinction between lean body mass and fat mass, nor does it account for fat distribution, bone density, age, sex, or ethnicity – all of which significantly influence metabolic risk [11]. In women, this becomes particularly problematic due to physiological variations in body fat composition across the menstrual cycle, pregnancy, and menopause, as well as differential patterns of fat accumulation, such as gynoid versus android obesity [12].

Moreover, the BMI thresholds currently in use were derived predominantly from studies in Western male populations and may not accurately reflect health risks in diverse global or sex-specific cohorts. Several studies have demonstrated that individuals of Asian descent, for example, are at increased cardiometabolic risk at lower BMI levels compared to their Caucasian counterparts, prompting the WHO to propose lower cutoff points for these populations [13]. In women, similar adjustments may be necessary, given the complex interplay between reproductive hormones, adipose tissue function, and metabolic regulation.

Despite these known limitations, BMI continues to exert disproportionate influence in clinical decision-making, often guiding interventions ranging from lifestyle modification to eligibility for fertility treatment or bariatric surgery. This reliance persists despite the availability of more precise diagnostic tools and a growing consensus in the medical literature that BMI should be used with caution – particularly in the context of individualized, sex-specific medicine [14].

As we transition toward precision healthcare models, it becomes imperative to reassess the historical inertia of BMI and critically evaluate its role in modern medicine. For women, in particular, the need for more sensitive and specific measures of adiposity and metabolic risk is not just a scientific imperative but an ethical one.

3. Limitations of BMI in women's health

While BMI has gained traction as a global standard for obesity classification, it has notable and clinically significant limitations – particularly in the context of women's health. These limitations arise from both its methodological simplicity and its inability to reflect the dynamic, hormonally driven physiology that characterizes the female body across the life course. In women, especially those in reproductive, gestational, and menopausal stages, BMI may provide misleading or incomplete assessments of body fat distribution, metabolic health, and disease risk [15].

One of the most critical shortcomings of BMI is its failure to distinguish between fat mass and lean body mass. Women typically possess a higher percentage of body fat than men at any given BMI, owing to sex-specific hormonal influences such as estrogen-mediated fat deposition [12]. This inherent biological variation results in the underestimation or overestimation of health risks when BMI is applied uniformly across sexes. For example, a physically active woman with high muscle mass may be erroneously classified as overweight or obese, while a sedentary woman with sarcopenic obesity – low muscle mass and high fat mass – may fall into the "normal" BMI range despite significant cardiometabolic risk [16].

Another limitation lies in BMI's insensitivity to fat distribution. Numerous studies have established that visceral fat – rather than total fat – is a stronger predictor of insulin resistance, type 2 diabetes, and cardiovascular disease, particularly in women [3, 17]. Because BMI is a global measure, it cannot account for variations in central adiposity, which becomes more prominent with advancing age and hormonal changes such as menopause [18]. This is especially problematic in the evaluation of postmenopausal women, who experience a shift from peripheral (gynoid) to central (android) fat accumulation, even in the absence of significant weight change.

The concept of "NWO" further underscores BMI's diagnostic limitations. NWO refers to individuals with a BMI within the normal range but with an elevated body fat percentage and metabolic abnormalities [5]. This phenotype is disproportionately observed in women and is associated with increased risks of dyslipidemia, hypertension, and infertility. The prevalence of NWO challenges the assumption that a "normal" BMI equates to metabolic health and underscores the need for more sophisticated screening in clinical settings, especially in gynecology and reproductive endocrinology.

Additionally, BMI does not adequately reflect the dynamic physiological changes during pregnancy. Weight gain, fluid retention, and changes in body composition during gestation can render BMI measurements obsolete or misleading [19]. For this reason, gestational weight gain charts and prepregnancy BMI classifications are often used in obstetric practice, though these too are subject to critique and population-specific variability [20].

In sum, BMI's lack of specificity, its poor correlation with visceral adiposity, and its inability to adapt to reproductive and hormonal milestones significantly reduce its utility in women's health. These limitations call for a more nuanced approach – one that incorporates sex-specific physiology, stage-of-life context, and emerging biomarkers into obesity assessment frameworks.

4. Alternative anthropometric and imaging-based tools

Given the well-documented limitations of BMI, particularly in the context of women's health, a range of alternative anthropometric and imaging-based tools has emerged to offer more accurate and individualized assessments of adiposity, metabolic risk, and disease burden. These methods address the dimensional gaps left by BMI – namely its inability to distinguish fat from lean mass and its failure to capture fat distribution, particularly visceral fat, which is a crucial determinant of metabolic dysfunction in women [3].

4.1 Waist circumference and waist-to-hip ratio

Waist circumference (WC) and WHR are widely recognized as superior indicators of central obesity compared to BMI. Numerous studies have demonstrated a strong correlation between WC/WHR and visceral adiposity, insulin resistance, and cardiovascular risk – especially in postmenopausal women, where android fat distribution becomes more pronounced [18, 21]. According to the WHO, a WC >88 cm or a WHR >0.85 in women is associated with a significantly increased risk of cardiometabolic diseases [22].

Unlike BMI, which provides a generalized index, WC and WHR reflect body fat distribution – a key mediator of adverse health outcomes in women with PCOS,

GDM, and metabolic syndrome. These tools are inexpensive, reproducible, and clinically actionable, yet remain underutilized in routine gynecological and reproductive care [23].

4.2 Body fat percentage and bioelectrical impedance analysis (BIA)

Direct measurement of body fat percentage provides greater insight into body composition than BMI alone. BIA and skinfold thickness measurements are among the most accessible methods to estimate total fat mass, although their accuracy can be influenced by hydration status, menstrual phase, and recent physical activity – all particularly relevant in women [24]. In reproductive endocrinology, higher body fat percentage has been associated with anovulation, poorer oocyte quality, and suboptimal IVF outcomes – even when BMI remains within the normal range [25].

4.3 Dual-energy Xray absorptiometry

DEXA is considered the gold standard for assessing body composition, offering precise measurements of total and regional fat mass, lean tissue, and bone mineral density. DEXA distinguishes android and gynoid fat depots and has demonstrated predictive value in assessing cardiovascular and metabolic risk, particularly in perimenopausal and postmenopausal women [26]. Although more expensive and less widely available than BMI or WC, DEXA is increasingly used in research settings and offers critical insight in high-risk or complex clinical scenarios.

4.4 Visceral adiposity index (VAI) and lipid accumulation product (LAP)

Composite indices, such as VAI and LAP, have gained attention for their ability to reflect both anatomical and functional aspects of adiposity. VAI incorporates WC, BMI, triglycerides, and HDL-C levels to estimate visceral fat dysfunction, while LAP is calculated using WC and fasting triglyceride levels. Both indices have shown strong correlations with insulin resistance and metabolic syndrome in women and are especially useful in identifying at-risk individuals with normal BMI but abnormal metabolic profiles [27, 28].

4.5 Magnetic resonance imaging (MRI) and computed tomography (CT)

While not routinely used in clinical practice due to cost and accessibility constraints, imaging modalities such as MRI and CT provide the most accurate assessments of visceral fat compartments. These tools have elucidated the pathophysiological role of ectopic fat deposition – intra-abdominal, hepatic, and even pericardial fat – in contributing to cardiometabolic disease in women, independent of BMI [29]. Their use is currently limited to specialized research and diagnostic centers but may become more prevalent as precision medicine evolves.

Collectively, these anthropometric and imaging-based methods represent a paradigm shift in the evaluation of obesity. By moving beyond BMI and incorporating these tools into clinical and research practice, particularly in the context of women's health, clinicians can better stratify risk, individualize care, and improve outcomes in gynecological and reproductive medicine.

5. BMI and women across life stages: Reproductive to postmenopausal

The physiological significance and clinical interpretation of BMI vary substantially across the distinct reproductive stages of a woman's life. From adolescence to reproductive age, pregnancy, perimenopause, and postmenopause, hormonal shifts, changes in fat distribution, and fluctuations in metabolic homeostasis complicate the use of BMI as a universal tool. Understanding the interaction between BMI and these life stages is essential for developing individualized approaches to weight management and risk assessment in women's health.

5.1 Adolescence and early reproductive age

During adolescence and early adulthood, the female body undergoes significant endocrinological and anthropometric changes that alter fat distribution and body composition. Estrogen promotes the deposition of subcutaneous fat, particularly in the gluteofemoral region, a pattern referred to as gynoid fat distribution [12]. While this may not dramatically impact BMI, it has profound implications for metabolic protection and fertility. Nonetheless, BMI remains the primary screening tool for undernutrition or early-onset obesity, both of which can disrupt menstrual function and ovarian reserve [30, 31].

In adolescents with PCOS, BMI often underrepresents the extent of visceral adiposity and insulin resistance. Even mildly elevated BMI values may be associated with subfertility, dyslipidemia, and hyperandrogenism in this population [32].

5.2 Pregnancy and the perinatal period

Pregnancy presents unique challenges for BMI interpretation. Prepregnancy BMI is commonly used to stratify obstetric risk and to guide recommendations for gestational weight gain. Women with prepregnancy BMI ≥ 30 kg/m^2 face significantly increased risks of GDM, hypertensive disorders of pregnancy, and cesarean delivery [4]. However, BMI does not account for differences in fat distribution or adipose tissue function that may influence placental development, insulin sensitivity, or fetal growth trajectories [33].

Additionally, excessive gestational weight gain among women with a normal BMI may still confer adverse perinatal outcomes, including fetal macrosomia and postpartum weight retention. Conversely, some overweight women may have metabolically healthy profiles, yet still face clinical bias due to BMI-based categorization [34].

5.3 Perimenopause and menopause

The menopausal transition is marked by declining estrogen levels, redistribution of adipose tissue from peripheral to central depots, and increased visceral fat accumulation – even in the absence of weight gain [18]. As a result, women may retain the same BMI throughout menopause while experiencing dramatic increases in cardiometabolic risk. BMI in this phase poorly reflects the underlying metabolic shifts, including increased inflammation, insulin resistance, and dyslipidemia [35].

This life stage also sees a rising prevalence of sarcopenic obesity – defined by a combination of reduced muscle mass and increased fat mass – which can occur even in women with normal or mildly elevated BMI. Sarcopenic obesity is associated with impaired mobility, osteoporosis, and frailty, emphasizing the need for body composition analysis rather than BMI alone [36].

5.4 Clinical implications across the lifespan

The application of static BMI cutoffs fails to consider the nonlinear relationship between adiposity and health across different female life stages. Clinicians should be cautious in interpreting BMI in isolation and must incorporate age-specific, reproductive-stage-specific, and ethnically tailored tools for risk stratification. This includes the complementary use of WC, DEXA scans, metabolic panels, and clinical context in gynecology, obstetrics, and reproductive medicine.

Ultimately, a woman-centered approach that aligns anthropometric interpretation with hormonal, reproductive, and metabolic realities is essential for advancing precision healthcare.

6. Toward a multidimensional obesity framework in women's health

The persistent reliance on BMI as a solitary metric for obesity classification is increasingly at odds with the principles of precision medicine and sex-specific healthcare. For women, whose physiological, reproductive, and metabolic profiles are uniquely dynamic, a multidimensional framework that transcends BMI is urgently required. This framework should integrate anatomical, biochemical, hormonal, behavioral, and contextual elements to provide a holistic understanding of adiposity and its consequences.

6.1 Incorporating body composition and fat distribution

Beyond total body weight, the distribution and function of adipose tissue are critical determinants of cardiometabolic risk. Visceral adiposity, for example, is more strongly associated with insulin resistance and endothelial dysfunction than subcutaneous fat, particularly in midlife and postmenopausal women [3, 17]. Tools such as DEXA, MRI, and CT imaging, though not universally available, provide gold-standard measurements of regional fat distribution and are essential in high-risk or research contexts. Simpler clinical surrogates – such as WC and waist-to-height ratio – can serve as proxies for visceral fat and are cost-effective for broader implementation [37].

6.2 Integrating metabolic and inflammatory markers

Obesity is not merely a disorder of energy imbalance but a complex, chronic inflammatory state. This is particularly relevant in women, in whom hormonal states (e.g., pregnancy, PCOS, menopause) interact with metabolic pathways to produce variable phenotypes of obesity. Therefore, a multidimensional framework should routinely include metabolic markers such as fasting glucose, insulin, triglycerides, HDL-C, HbA1c, HOMA-IR, and emerging adipokines (e.g., leptin, adiponectin) to assess metabolic health beyond body size [38]. In particular, the identification of "metabolically healthy obesity" (MHO) or "normal weight metabolic obesity" (NWMO) phenotypes can guide targeted interventions in reproductive medicine, endocrinology, and preventive care.

6.3 Life stage and hormonal milieu

A woman's stage of life and hormonal status are central to interpreting any obesity metric. Menstrual irregularities, pregnancy outcomes, and menopausal transitions are all modulated by the hormonal and inflammatory profile, which often diverges from BMI-based predictions [18, 35]. As such, a comprehensive obesity model must consider gonadal steroid levels, ovarian reserve markers (e.g., AMH, FSH), and stage-specific benchmarks when assessing risk. For example, the same BMI value may indicate entirely different clinical implications for an adolescent with PCOS versus a perimenopausal woman with sarcopenic obesity.

6.4 Psychosocial and behavioral context

Behavioral, socioeconomic, and cultural factors significantly shape obesity risk and response to treatment, particularly in women. Stress, sleep disturbances, trauma history, disordered eating, and weight stigma disproportionately affect women and influence both fat distribution and metabolic regulation [39]. Any effective framework must incorporate validated instruments to assess dietary intake, physical activity, sleep quality, and mental health, alongside traditional anthropometric data.

6.5 Translational models: From concept to clinical practice

Efforts to integrate these diverse domains have led to the development of composite indices and staging systems, such as the Edmonton Obesity Staging System (EOSS), which stratifies risk based on metabolic, physical, and psychological parameters rather than BMI alone [40]. In women's health, adapting such models with reproductive and gynecologic parameters could enhance risk prediction and treatment personalization in areas such as infertility, prenatal care, and menopausal health.

In summary, a truly multidimensional obesity framework in women's health must move beyond anthropometry and embrace a biopsychosocial model. This requires not only the inclusion of advanced diagnostics and biomarkers but also the contextualization of findings within a woman's life stage, reproductive status, and lived experience.

7. Clinical applications and future directions

Translating a multidimensional understanding of obesity into clinical practice requires a paradigm shift – one that prioritizes individualized, evidence-based, and sex-specific evaluation strategies. For women, whose adiposity-related health risks vary across life stages, hormonal contexts, and reproductive statuses, reliance on BMI alone not only limits diagnostic precision but also risks undertreatment or overtreatment. The integration of advanced anthropometric, metabolic, hormonal, and psychosocial assessments into routine care can profoundly enhance outcomes in gynecology, reproductive endocrinology, obstetrics, and preventive medicine.

7.1 Gynecology and reproductive medicine

In fertility care, the use of BMI thresholds to guide access to ARTs remains common but increasingly controversial. Evidence shows that high BMI is associated with reduced live birth rates and increased obstetric complications in ART cycles, yet a solely BMI-based exclusion criterion may ignore metabolically healthy individuals or falsely reassure those with normal BMI but elevated visceral adiposity or insulin resistance [6, 41]. Incorporating measures such as WC, metabolic panels, and body composition analysis can optimize preconception counseling and treatment personalization.

In PCOS, a condition where metabolic dysfunction often coexists with reproductive symptoms, BMI provides limited predictive value. Integrating tools such as HOMA-IR, lipid profiles, and DEXA-derived fat distribution indices can improve phenotypic characterization and therapeutic targeting [42].

7.2 Obstetric care

Preconception and antenatal risk stratification often rely on prepregnancy BMI, which correlates with gestational diabetes, hypertensive disorders, and fetal macrosomia [4]. However, many women with elevated BMI may remain metabolically healthy, and vice versa. A more nuanced approach – incorporating metabolic screening (e.g., HbA1c, fasting insulin), inflammatory markers, and individualized gestational weight gain goals – may improve both maternal and neonatal outcomes [43]. Furthermore, understanding the interaction between adiposity, placental function, and fetal programming requires a broader toolkit than BMI provides.

7.3 Menopausal health and chronic disease prevention

In midlife women, especially postmenopausal patients, central obesity is a major driver of cardiovascular disease, osteoporosis, and metabolic syndrome. Sarcopenic obesity, which often goes undetected by BMI, increases fall risk, frailty, and mortality [44]. Tools such as DEXA, handgrip strength testing, and frailty indices should be considered standard adjuncts to BMI in this population. Personalized lifestyle interventions, hormone replacement therapy consideration, and pharmacologic treatments should be informed by multidimensional risk stratification rather than BMI alone.

7.4 Future research and policy implications

There remains a critical need for longitudinal studies evaluating the predictive power of alternative obesity metrics in diverse female populations. Research should explore how combining anthropometric, biochemical, and psychosocial indicators can yield clinically actionable phenotypes. Additionally, healthcare policies must evolve to include and reimburse more precise tools – such as DEXA scans, insulin sensitivity assays, and behavioral risk screening – in women's health protocols.

Finally, medical education must be updated to move beyond BMI-centric paradigms. Clinicians should be trained in the interpretation and clinical integration of body composition data, metabolic markers, and life-stage-specific risks. Incorporating these elements into electronic health records, decision-support tools, and care pathways can standardize a more comprehensive, woman-centered approach.

8. Conclusion

The persistent reliance on BMI as a universal marker of obesity fails to capture the complexity of female physiology, particularly across different reproductive life stages. While BMI offers a convenient population-level screening tool, it is insufficient for individualized risk stratification in women's health. Its inability to differentiate between fat and lean mass, its disregard for fat distribution, and its failure to adapt to hormonal dynamics severely limit its clinical applicability – especially in contexts such as infertility, pregnancy, menopause, and metabolic disorders such as PCOS.

This chapter emphasizes the need for a multidimensional, sex-specific framework for obesity assessment. By integrating alternative anthropometric measures (e.g., WHR, DEXA), biochemical markers (e.g., insulin, adipokines), and life-stage-dependent considerations, clinicians can achieve a more precise understanding of health risks in women. Furthermore, incorporating psychosocial and behavioral dimensions aligns obesity evaluation with modern principles of precision medicine.

Future clinical practice and health policies must evolve beyond BMI-centric paradigms to embrace comprehensive, individualized models that reflect the unique metabolic and reproductive physiology of women. Such an approach is not only scientifically imperative but also ethically necessary to ensure equitable and effective care in women's health.

Conflict of interest

The authors declare no conflict of interest.

Nomenclature

BMI	Body mass index (kg/m^2)
WC	Waist circumference
WHR	Waist-to-hip ratio
DEXA	Dual-energy Xray absorptiometry
BIA	Bioelectrical impedance analysis
VAI	Visceral adiposity index
LAP	Lipid accumulation product
PCOS	Polycystic ovary syndrome
GDM	Gestational diabetes mellitus
HOMA-IR	Homeostatic model assessment of insulin Resistance
HDL-C	High-density lipoprotein cholesterol
TG	Triglyceride
MHO	Metabolically healthy obesity
NWO	Normal weight obesity
NWMO	Normal weight metabolic obesity

ART	Assisted reproductive technologies
EOSS	Edmonton obesity staging system
AMH	Anti-Müllerian hormone
FSH	Follicle-stimulating hormone

Appendix

As summarized in **Table A1**, various anthropometric and imaging-based tools are used to assess adiposity

Appendix A: Obesity assessment tools – summary table.

Tool/index	Measures	Advantages	Limitations
Body mass index (BMI)	Weight/height^2	Simple, widely used	Ignores fat distribution and lean mass
Waist circumference (WC)	Abdominal girth	Reflects central adiposity	Cutoffs vary by population
Waist-to-hip ratio (WHR)	Waist/hip circumference	Correlates with metabolic risk	Less accurate in extremely obese individuals
Dual-energy Xray absorptiometry (DEXA)	Total and regional fat, lean, bone mass	Gold standard for body composition	Expensive, limited availability
BIA	Body fat percentage	Noninvasive, quick	Affected by hydration and menstrual cycle
Visceral adiposity index (VAI)	WC, BMI, TG, HDL-C	Estimates visceral fat function	Complex calculation, not routinely used
Lipid accumulation product (LAP)	WC, triglyceride levels	Correlates with insulin resistance	Influenced by fasting state
Magnetic resonance imaging (MRI)	Visceral fat, ectopic fat	Highly accurate	Costly, not used in routine practice

Table A1.
Comparison of tools and indices used for assessing adiposity.

Author details

Tuğba Gürbüz* and Oya Gökmen
Department of Obstetrics, Gynecology, and Reproductive Medicine, Medistate Kavacık Hospital, Istanbul, Turkey

*Address all correspondence to: drtgurbuz@hotmail.com

References

[1] Rothman KJ. BMI-related errors in the measurement of obesity. International Journal of Obesity (London). 2008;**32 Suppl 3:S56–S59**. DOI: 10.1038/ijo.2008.87

[2] Hruby A, Hu FB. 2015. The epidemiology of obesity: A big picture. PharmacoEconomics. **33**(7):673–689. DOI: 10.1007/s40273-014-0243-x

[3] Després J-P. 2012. Body fat distribution and risk of cardiovascular disease: An update. Circulation. **126** (10):1301–1313. DOI: 10.1161/ CIRCULATIONAHA.111.067264

[4] Catalano PM, Shankar K. Obesity and pregnancy: Mechanisms of short term and long term adverse consequences for mother and child. BMJ. 2017;356:j1. DOI: 10.1136/bmj.j1

[5] Romero-Corral A, Somers VK, Sierra-Johnson J, et al. Normal weight obesity: A risk factor for cardiometabolic dysregulation and cardiovascular mortality. European Heart Journal. 2010;**31**(6):737–746. DOI: 10.1093/eurheartj/ehp487

[6] Luke B, Brown MB, Missmer SA, et al. The effect of increasing obesity on the response to and outcome of assisted reproductive technology: A national study. Fertility and Sterility. 2011;**96** (4):820–825. DOI: 10.1016/ j.fertnstert.2011.07.1100

[7] Ross R, Neeland IJ, Yamashita S, et al. Waist circumference as a vital sign in clinical practice: A consensus statement from the IAS and ICCR working group on visceral obesity. Nature Reviews Endocrinology. 2020;**16** (3):177–189. DOI: 10.1038/s41574-019-0310-7

[8] Eknoyan G. 2008. Adolphe Quetelet (1796–1874)—the average man and indices of obesity. Nephrology Dialysis Transplantation. **23**(1):47–51. DOI: 10.1093/ndt/gfm517

[9] Keys A, Fidanza F, Karvonen MJ, Kimura N, Taylor HL. 1972. Indices of relative weight and obesity. Journal of Chronic Diseases. **25** (6-7):329–343. DOI: 10.1016/0021-9681 (72)90027-6

[10] World Health Organization. Obesity: Preventing and Managing the Global Epidemic. Report of a WHO consultation. WHO Technical Report Series. 2000;894:i–253

[11] Nuttall FQ. 2015. Body mass index: Obesity, BMI, and health: A critical review. Nutrition Today. **50** (3):117–128. DOI: 10.1097/ NT.0000000000000092

[12] Wells JC. 2007. Sexual dimorphism of body composition. Best Practice & Research Clinical Endocrinology & Metabolism. **21**(3):415–430. DOI: 10.10 16/j.beem.2007.04.007

[13] WHO Expert Consultation. Appropriate body-mass index for Asian populations and its implications for policy and intervention strategies. The Lancet. 2004;**363**(9403):157–163. DOI: 10.1016/S0140-6736(03)15268-3

[14] Prentice AM, Jebb SA. 2001. Beyond body mass index. Obesity Reviews. **2**(3):141–147. DOI: 10.1046/ j.1467-789x.2001.00031.x

[15] Shah NR, Braverman ER. Measuring adiposity in patients: The utility of body mass index (BMI), percent body fat, and leptin. PLoS One. 2012;7(4):e33308. DOI: 10.1371/journal.pone.0033308

[16] Institute of Medicine. The Current State of Obesity Solutions in the United States: Workshop Summary. Washington (DC): National Academies Press (US); 2014

[17] Neeland IJ, Poirier P, Després J-P. 2018. Cardiovascular and metabolic heterogeneity of obesity: Clinical challenges and implications for management. Circulation. **137**(13): 1391–1406. DOI: 10.1161/ CIRCULATIONAHA.117.029617

[18] Lovejoy JC, Champagne CM, de Jonge L, et al. Increased visceral fat and decreased energy expenditure during the menopausal transition. International Journal of Obesity. 2008;**32**(6):949–958. DOI: 10.1038/ijo.2008.25

[19] Catalano PM, Ehrenberg HM. 2006. The short- and long-term implications of maternal obesity on the mother and her offspring.. BJOG: An International Journal of Obstetrics & Gynaecology. **113**(10):1126–1133. DOI: 10.1111/j.1471-0528.2006.00989.x

[20] Institute of Medicine. National Research Council. Weight Gain during Pregnancy: Reexamining the Guidelines. Washington (DC): National Academies Press (US); 2009

[21] Wajchenberg BL. 2000. Subcutaneous and visceral adipose tissue: Their relation to the metabolic syndrome. Endocrine Reviews. **21** (6):697–738. DOI: 10.1210/ edrv.21.6.0415

[22] World Health Organization. Waist Circumference and Waist–hip Ratio: Report of a WHO Expert Consultation. Geneva: WHO; 2011

[23] Sahakyan KR, Somers VK, Rodriguez-Escudero JP, et al. Normal-weight central obesity: Implications for total and cardiovascular mortality. Annals of Internal Medicine. 2015;**163** (11):827–835. DOI: 10.7326/M14-2525

[24] Lukaski HC. 2013. Evolution of bioimpedance: A circuitous journey from estimation of physiological function to assessment of body composition and a return to clinical research. European Journal of Clinical Nutrition. **67**(Suppl S1):S2–S9. DOI: 10.1038/ejcn.2012.149

[25] Chavarro JE, Ehrlich S, Colaci DS, et al. Body mass index and short-term weight change in relation to treatment outcomes in women undergoing assisted reproduction. Fertility and Sterility. 2012;**98**(1):109–116. DOI: 10.1016/ j.fertnstert.2012.04.012

[26] Nicklas BJ, Wang X, You T, et al. Effect of exercise intensity on abdominal fat loss during calorie restriction in overweight and obese postmenopausal women: A randomized, controlled trial. The American Journal of Clinical Nutrition. 2009;**89**(4): 1043–1052. DOI: 10.3945/ ajcn.2008.26938

[27] Amato MC, Giordano C, Galia M, et al. Visceral adiposity index: A reliable indicator of visceral fat function associated with cardiometabolic risk. Diabetes Care. 2010;**33**(4):920–922. DOI: 10.2337/dc09-1825

[28] Kahn HS. The "lipid accumulation product" performs better than the body

mass index for recognizing cardiovascular risk: A population-based comparison. BMC Cardiovascular Disorders. 2005;**5**:26. DOI: 10.1186/1471-2261-5-26

[29] Thomas EL, Frost G, Taylor-Robinson SD, Bell JD. 2012. Excess body fat in obese and normal-weight subjects. Nutrition Research Reviews. **25**(1): 150–161. DOI: 10.1017/S0954422412000054

[30] Rogol AD, Clark PA, Roemmich JN. 2000. Growth and pubertal development in children and adolescents: Effects of diet and physical activity. The American Journal of Clinical Nutrition. **72**(2):521S–528S. DOI: 10.1093/ajcn/72.2.521S

[31] Misra M, Klibanski A. 2014. Endocrine consequences of anorexia nervosa. The Lancet Diabetes & Endocrinology. **2**(7):581–592. DOI: 10.1016/S2213-8587(13)70180-3

[32] Carmina E, Lobo RA. 1999. Polycystic ovary syndrome (PCOS): Arguably the most common endocrinopathy is associated with significant morbidity in women. The Journal of Clinical Endocrinology & Metabolism. **84**(6):1897–1899. DOI: 10.1210/jcem.84.6.5803

[33] Barbour LA, McCurdy CE, Hernandez TL, et al. Cellular mechanisms for insulin resistance in normal pregnancy and gestational diabetes. Diabetes Care. 2007;**30 Suppl 2:S112–S119**. DOI: 10.2337/dc07-s202.

[34] Gaillard R, Welten M, Oddy WH, et al. Associations of maternal prepregnancy body mass index and gestational weight gain with cardio-metabolic risk factors in adolescent offspring: A prospective cohort study. BJOG: An International Journal of Obstetrics & Gynaecology. 2016;**123**(2):207–216. DOI: 10.1111/1471-0528.13700

[35] Matthews KA, Crawford SL, Chae CU, et al. Are changes in cardiovascular disease risk factors in midlife women due to chronological aging or to the menopausal transition? Journal of the American College of Cardiology. 2009;**54**(25): 2366–2373. DOI: 10.1016/j.jacc.2009.10.009

[36] Kammire DE, Walkup MP, Ambrosius WT, et al. Effect of weight change following intentional weight loss on bone health in older adults with obesity. Obesity. 2019;**27**(11): 1839–1845. DOI: 10.1002/oby.22604

[37] Ashwell M, Gibson S. Waist-to-height ratio as an indicator of 'early health risk': Simpler and more predictive than using a 'matrix' based on BMI and waist circumference. BMJ Open. 2016;**6**(3):e010159. DOI: 10.1136/bmjopen-2015-010159

[38] Blüher M. Metabolically healthy obesity. Endocrine Reviews. 2020;**41** (3):bnaa004. DOI: 10.1210/endrev/bnaa004

[39] Puhl R, Suh Y. 2015. Health consequences of weight stigma: Implications for obesity prevention and treatment. Current Obesity Reports. **4** (2):182–190. DOI: 10.1007/s13679-015-0153-z

[40] Padwal RS, Pajewski NM, Allison DB, Sharma AM. 2011. Using the Edmonton obesity staging system to predict mortality in a population-representative cohort of people with overweight and obesity. CMAJ : Canadian Medical Association

Journal = Journal de l'Association Medicale Canadienne. **183**(14): E1059–E1066. DOI: 10.1503/cmaj.110387

[41] Maheshwari A, Stofberg L, Bhattacharya S. 2007. Effect of overweight and obesity on assisted reproductive technology—a systematic review. Human Reproduction Update. **13**(5):433–444. DOI: 10.1093/humupd/dmm017

[42] Carmina E, Azziz R, Bergfeld W, et al. Female pattern hair loss and androgen excess: A report from the multidisciplinary androgen excess and PCOS committee. The Journal of Clinical Endocrinology & Metabolism. 2016;**101**(10):4525–4531. DOI: 10.1210/jc.2016-2136

[43] Gaillard R, Welten M, Oddy WH, et al. Associations of maternal prepregnancy body mass index and gestational weight gain with cardio-metabolic risk in adolescent offspring. JAMA Pediatrics. 2013;**167**(7):616–622. DOI: 10.1001/jamapediatrics.2013.105

[44] Rossi AP, Watson NL, Newman AB, et al. Effects of body composition, obesity, and weight loss on bone health in older adults. Current Osteoporosis Reports. 2020;**18**(5):556–564. DOI: 10.1007/s11914-020-00615-w

Chapter 6

Body Composition Characteristics in Aging Populations: Clinical Limitations of BMI and Implications for Chronic Metabolic Diseases

Yiting Zhao, Jiangbo Ye, Wansu Yu, Qian Du and Donghui Liu

Abstract

Decades of research confirm body mass index (BMI) as a primary obesity metric and predictor of chronic metabolic diseases (diabetes, cardiovascular diseases). However, its clinical utility demonstrates pronounced limitations in elderly populations due to aging-related comorbidities like sarcopenia and osteoporosis. Adipose accumulation in aging individuals often fails to correlate with BMI elevation, as age-related muscle atrophy and bone loss may mask fat deposition despite normal or subnormal BMI ranges. Structural remodeling, coupled with functional dysregulation of adipose tissue, characterized by ectopic visceral redistribution, lipid metabolic dysregulation, and chronic inflammation, further diminishes BMI's sensitivity for metabolic risk stratification. Emerging evidence advocates integrating BMI with waist circumference (WC), visceral adiposity index (VAI), and triglyceride-glucose (TyG) index to enhance predictive efficacy for metabolic disease risks, particularly in elderly adults. This review systematically delineates aging-specific body composition profiles and diagnostic limitations of BMI, offering actionable insights to refine clinical metrics and advance precision-based clinical paradigms for aging demographics.

Keywords: body mass index, adipose tissue, obesity, sarcopenia, chronic metabolic diseases, elderly people

1. Introduction

The World Health Organization (WHO) defines obesity as a chronic metabolic disorder characterized by abnormal or excessive adipose fat accumulation, posing significant health risks [1]. This pathological condition arises from interactions across multiple systems throughout the body. In recent years, the epidemic of overweight and obesity has emerged as a global public health challenge. The global adult

IntechOpen

prevalence of overweight and obesity reached two billion cases by 2021, with China, India, and the United States of America bearing the highest burden. Projections indicate that, without effective interventions, global obesity cases may reach 3.8 billion by 2050 [2].

2. Obesity-related pathophysiology

2.1 Chronic inflammation in obesity

Adipose tissue, especially visceral adipose tissue (VAT), is a key factor driving chronic inflammation in obesity [3–5]. Studies show that adipocytes undergo pathological hypertrophy, hyperplasia, and functional dysregulation under nutrient excess, excessively producing free fatty acids (FFA), reactive oxygen species (ROS), and pro-inflammatory cytokines (e.g., interleukin-6 [IL-6], tumor necrosis factor-α [TNF-α]) [6]. These factors drive adipose immune cell (macrophages and lymphocytes) infiltration and complex "immune cell–adipocyte" crosstalk, inducing systemic chronic inflammation [3]. Under persistent inflammatory conditions, adipocytes further activate NOD-like receptor thermal protein domain-associated protein 3 (NLRP3) inflammasome, inhibiting proliferator-activated receptor gamma coactivator-1α (PGC-1α)/ sirtuin 1 (SIRT1)-mediated mitochondrial biogenesis and blocking PTEN-induced kinase 1 (PINK1)-Parkin-dependent mitophagy. This upregulates dynamin-related protein 1 (Drp1) and downregulates mitofusin-2 (MFN2) expression in mitochondria, ultimately inducing mitochondrial membrane potential collapse, mitochondrial DNA (mtDNA) leakage, and energy metabolism disorders. This cascade culminates in skeletal muscle cell apoptosis and myocardial dysfunction, forming an "inflammation–mitochondrial injury–tissue apoptosis" vicious cycle [7].

Additionally, obesity is linked to pathological overactivation of leptin, resistin, and insulin-like growth factor-1 (IGF-1) signaling pathways. Adipose-derived extracellular vesicles (EVs) and their pro-inflammatory factors (e.g., interleukin-1β (IL-1β)) increase, coupled with n-6/n-3 polyunsaturated fatty acid (PUFA) metabolite imbalance, collectively impairing immune cell function. These changes not only exacerbate chronic inflammation but also promote autoimmune tendencies while weakening immune surveillance [8]. Meanwhile, ectopic lipid deposition in skeletal muscle induces a lipotoxic milieu, inhibits β-oxidation, and promotes pro-inflammatory myokine secretion, driving a positive feedback loop of adipose-skeletal muscle inflammation [9].

2.2 Effects of aging on adipose tissue

Adipocyte aging drives chronic inflammation and insulin resistance through phenotypic remodeling, secretory dysregulation, and insulin signaling impairment, exacerbating metabolic comorbidities [10, 11]. Concurrently, aging promotes thermogenesis weakness, adipose redistribution from subcutaneous to visceral regions, ectopic fat infiltration in bone marrow, and skeletal muscle atrophy [12]. Evidence implicates adipose dysfunction as a central driver of organismal aging and age-related pathologies [12, 13].

2.3 Obesity-related complications

Obesity acts as a pivotal risk factor for metabolic disorders, strongly linked to type 2 diabetes mellitus (T2DM), hypertension, dyslipidemia, and obstructive sleep apnea (OSA). These conditions cluster in metabolic syndrome (MS), collectively heightening cardiovascular disease (CVD) risk [14]. Adipose dysfunction in obesity drives adipokine dysregulation. Pro-inflammatory adipokines (e.g., leptin, resistin) are upregulated, while antiinflammatory adipokines (e.g., adiponectin, omentin-1) are downregulated [13, 15]. This adipokine imbalance, combined with insulin resistance, triggers vascular remodeling and endothelial dysfunction, accelerating T2DM and CVD progression [16–18].

2.3.1 Obesity and T2DM

Obesity-driven chronic inflammation disrupts glucose homeostasis through adipose tissue infiltration by M1 macrophages and $CD8^+$ T cells, triggering pro-inflammatory cytokine (TNF-α, IL-6) release that impairs peroxisome proliferator-activated receptor γ (PPAR-γ) activation and insulin signaling pathways [19, 20]. Excessive release of FFA induces lipotoxicity in hepatocytes and skeletal muscle cells via mitochondrial dysfunction and endoplasmic reticulum (ER) stress, impairing the insulin signaling pathway and causing insulin resistance in the liver and skeletal muscle. In addition, prolonged hyperglycemia and overloaded FFA in pancreatic β-cells promote dedifferentiation and apoptosis, impairing insulin secretion capacity [20–22].

Notably, a subset of obese individuals (BMI ≥30 kg/m^2) exhibit metabolically healthy obesity (MHO), characterized by preserved adiponectin levels in plasma and reduced oxidative stress and ceramide accumulation in skeletal muscle compared to metabolically unhealthy obesity (MUO) counterparts [23]. This MHO phenotype is associated with attenuated adipose inflammation, moderated lipolytic activity, and maintained mitochondrial integrity, potentially underpinning enhanced insulin sensitivity and β-cell function [23].

2.3.2 Obesity and hypertension

In obesity, VAT secretes pro-inflammatory cytokines (TNF-α, IL-6) and activates macrophages and $CD8^+$ T-cells, driving endothelial dysfunction [16, 23]. VAT also upregulates angiotensinogen (AGT) expression, stimulates vascular smooth muscle cell (VSMC) contraction via angiotensin II (Ang II), and promotes extracellular matrix deposition, accelerating vascular remodeling [24, 25]. Furthermore, VAT enhances aldosterone production through renin-angiotensin-aldosterone system (RAAS) activation, induces sodium reabsorption via the serum/glucocorticoid-regulated kinase 1 (SGK1) – epithelial sodium channel (ENaC) signaling pathway, and promotes VSMC proliferation and collagen deposition, ultimately causing sodium retention and vascular fibrosis [26]. Particularly, perivascular adipose tissue (PVAT) in obesity elevates M1-macrophage infiltration and pro-inflammatory factor (TNF-α, IL-6) secretion, shifting vessels from a dilated to a constricted and inflamed state [18]. PVAT-derived Ang II further inhibits endothelial dilation through paracrine mechanisms and accelerates vascular fibrosis [16]. Thus, systemic and local pathologies synergistically drive hypertension pathogenesis.

2.3.3 Obesity and atherosclerosis

Chronic adipose inflammation, particularly in VAT and epicardial adipose tissue (EAT), promotes atherogenesis [27]. VAT and EAT release pro-inflammatory cytokines (TNF-α, IL-6) and adipokines (leptin, resistin) that impair the insulin signaling pathway and exacerbate metabolic dysregulation and atherosclerosis risk [28, 29]. These pro-inflammatory factors upregulate vascular cell adhesion molecule-1 (VCAM-1) and intercellular adhesion molecule-1 (ICAM-1) to recruit monocytes, promoting atherosclerotic plaque formation [30]. In addition, pro-inflammatory factors also induce mitochondrial dysfunction and NADPH oxidase (NOX) activation in endothelial cells, which increase ROS production, disrupt endothelial nitric oxide (NO) synthase (eNOS) activity, and induce vasoconstriction and thrombosis, further accelerating atherogenesis progression [29, 30].

2.3.4 Obesity and heart failure

In obesity, insulin resistance-caused hyperinsulinemia drives sympathetic activation and RAAS overactivity, promoting hypertension progression and sodium retention [14, 16]. Ang II, generated via RAAS activation, elevates blood pressure through vasoconstriction, and aldosterone-mediated sodium-water retention further exacerbates cardiac preload [16, 31]. Insulin resistance also disrupts myocardial energy homeostasis by impairing glucose transporter 4 (GLUT4) membrane translocation in cardiomyocytes, predisposing to heart failure [32]. Sustained preload elevation from obesity-induced hypervolemia triggers left ventricular hypertrophy and dilation, culminating in hemodynamic dysfunction and heart failure with preserved ejection fraction (HFpEF) [33, 34].

3. Limitations of BMI in clinical application

BMI, as a primary diagnostic indicator for obesity recommended by the WHO, exhibits significant limitations in accurately assessing adiposity. While the WHO defines obesity as BMI ≥30 kg/m^2 (≥28 kg/m^2 for Chinese populations), BMI fails to distinguish body compositions (e.g., adipose, muscle, and bone ratios) or capture adipose distribution patterns and associated metabolic dysregulation [1, 35]. These clinical limitations are particularly critical in aging populations, where BMI values may fall within normal or even subnormal ranges due to muscle atrophy and bone loss obscuring adipose accumulation, thereby impeding timely therapeutic interventions [36, 37]. Emerging evidence highlights that two paradoxical obesity phenotypes may be misclassified merely based on BMI values, leading to underestimation or misjudgment of health risks. One is termed normal weight obesity (NWO). These individuals, with normal BMI but pathological VAT, exhibit heightened risks of T2DM and CVD compared to metabolically healthy counterparts [38, 39]. The other is termed MHO. Despite BMI-defined obesity, these individuals display attenuated adipose inflammation and reduced metabolic complications, challenging the notion that obesity universally predicts adverse outcomes [23].

3.1 Limitations of BMI in differentiating muscle and fat mass: Clinical implications of sarcopenic obesity

Emerging evidence demonstrates a robust positive association between lean body mass (LBM) and metabolic homeostasis, with higher skeletal muscle mass correlating with improved insulin sensitivity and reduced all-cause mortality. Conversely, adipose tissue mass, especially VAT, serves as a critical predictor of insulin resistance and CVD [40, 41]. Sarcopenic obesity represents a clinically distinct syndrome, characterized by concurrent skeletal muscle depletion and pathological adipose accumulation [42, 43]. Aging and obesity synergistically drive VAT into a pro-inflammatory phenotype, triggering systemic chronic inflammation and insulin resistance via TNF-α and IL-6 release [36, 44, 45]. These pro-inflammatory cytokines disrupt the balance between muscle protein synthesis and degradation, impair myocyte autophagic processes, and promote muscle atrophy and abnormal fatty infiltration in muscle tissue, thereby disrupting skeletal muscle function and accelerating sarcopenia [43, 44, 46]. Meanwhile, progressive aging and obesity also drive aberrant mitochondrial fission and excessive ROS accumulation in skeletal muscle, further inhibiting skeletal muscle cell proliferation and differentiation [47]. Abnormal accumulation of intermuscular adipose tissue (IMAT) directly contributes to sarcopenic obesity by inducing chronic inflammation, activating the ubiquitin-proteasome-mediated muscle degradation, and suppressing the insulin signaling pathway [36, 48].

BMI shows limited utility in detecting muscle quantity and quality reductions, rendering it ineffective for sarcopenic obesity diagnosis and resulting in significant diagnostic omissions [37]. Studies reveal that sarcopenic obesity prevalence rises sharply with aging, independently predicting mortality and cardiovascular events despite normal BMI ranges [41, 49, 50]. Notably, community-based Chinese cohorts demonstrated that BMI-based obesity screening achieves <30% sensitivity for sarcopenic obesity detection [51].

3.2 Limitations of BMI to differentiate depot-specific fat distribution: Clinical implications of visceral versus subcutaneous adiposity

Human adipose tissue is anatomically distinguished into subcutaneous adipose tissue (SAT) and VAT, exhibiting divergent biological behaviors and metabolic roles. SAT primarily functions as an energy reservoir, sequestering excess lipids to prevent ectopic deposition in metabolically active organs like the liver, heart, and skeletal muscle [3, 52]. Conversely, VAT heightens inflammatory activity due to immune cell infiltration and elevates glucocorticoid receptor expression and catecholamine-induced lipolysis, amplifying systemic insulin resistance and CVD risk [52, 53]. Furthermore, ectopic lipid accumulation in nonadipose tissues, such as the liver, heart, and skeletal muscle, represents an independent risk for obesity-associated cardiovascular complications through hepatic lipid overload, lipoprotein overproduction, and atherosclerotic plaque formation [3, 54].

Aging-related adipose tissue redistribution remains inadequately captured by BMI metrics. Epidemiological evidence demonstrates that elderly individuals classified as "normal weight" by BMI often exhibit elevated VAT levels, correlating with heightened risks for T2DM onset, CVD events, and all-cause mortality compared to those in higher BMI categories [55–57]. This paradox is particularly evident in T2DM patients, where ectopic fat deposition shows direct pathogenic links to cardiometabolic complications and microvascular impairment [58].

3.3 Limitations of BMI to capture obesity-induced osteometabolic dysregulation: Clinical implications of the adipose-muscle-bone axis

Obesity increases skeletal deterioration and fracture risk [59]. Osteoporosis is a metabolic bone disease characterized by decreased bone strength and mass, significantly increasing fracture susceptibility. Bone marrow adipose tissue (BMAT) is a critical regulator of bone microenvironment dynamics and systemic metabolism. Increased BMAT adiposity in obesity and T2DM correlates with heightened bone fragility risk, mediated through pro-inflammatory cytokine (TNF-α, IL-6) secretion and adipokine dysregulation (leptin elevation, adiponectin reduction) [60]. In obesity, gut microbiota-derived lipopolysaccharides (LPS) induce grancalcin (GCA) secretion and bone marrow macrophage (BMM) senescence through Toll-like receptor 4 (TLR4) activation, thereby exacerbating bone resorption and skeletal deterioration [61]. Concurrently, skeletal muscle in obesity secretes excessive myostatin, which inhibits osteoblast activity and accelerates osteoclast production by blocking the Wnt signaling pathway and upregulating receptor activator of nuclear factor-κB ligand (RANKL) expression, thereby leading to osteoporosis [62]. Irisin, a myokine critical for bone anabolism, is significantly decreased in obese individuals, further exacerbating bone mineral density (BMD) reduction and osteoporosis progression [63].

Vitamin D, in its active form of 1,25-$(OH)_2D_3$, regulates calcium/phosphorus metabolism in vivo, affecting bone development and homeostasis. Obese individuals, especially elderly populations with obesity, frequently demonstrate reduced plasma 1,25-$(OH)_2D_3$ levels, which are negatively correlated with body weight, BMI, and adipose mass [64]. Vitamin D dysregulation impairs myofunction by disrupting calcium handling in skeletal muscle, heightening fall risk, and exacerbating osteosarcopenic obesity susceptibility [65, 66]. Meanwhile, vitamin D deficiency also promotes secondary hyperparathyroidism, which accelerates bone destruction and BMD reduction, leading to osteoporosis and osteoporotic fractures [67, 68].

BMI fails to accurately capture bone mass and quality in obese populations, leading to the underestimation of fracture susceptibility and missed identification of high-risk individuals requiring targeted interventions [69, 70]. Individuals with normal BMI but elevated adiposity mass exhibit heightened risks of low BMD; however, BMI cannot differentiate muscle-bone-fat composition, obscuring the coexistence of sarcopenia and osteoporosis in these subjects [71]. In addition, sarcopenic obesity patients have substantially elevated fracture risks compared to nonsarcopenic counterparts, while BMI is ineffective for early risk stratification [72, 73].

4. Beyond BMI: Advancing obesity diagnosis through multidimensional assessment

As a conventional diagnostic tool for obesity, BMI demonstrates significant limitations in elderly populations, including its failure to differentiate skeletal muscle and bone mass from adipose tissue, its limited capacity to reflect adipose tissue distribution patterns, and its insufficient sensitivity in metabolic risk assessment. These deficiencies may result in biased risk stratification and delayed clinical interventions. Therefore, developing multidimensional obesity assessment frameworks and hierarchical diagnostic criteria has emerged as a critical priority in both clinical practice and research. Here, we summarize advancing obesity assessment methods based on anthropometry, imaging, and biomarkers, aiming to provide a theoretical basis and practical framework for precise obesity phenotyping and risk stratification [74].

4.1 Integrated diagnostic metrics and novel measurement tools: Multidimensional risk assessment

Comprehensive integration of anthropometric and metabolic biomarkers exhibits superior efficacy in assessing fat distribution patterns, skeletal muscle mass, and metabolic dysregulation in adipose tissue, thereby enhancing the diagnostic evaluation for ectopic adipose deposition and the predictive accuracy for obesity-related complication risks.

4.1.1 Waist circumference (WC)

Waist circumference (WC), measured as the midabdominal circumference at the iliac crest-lower rib margin midpoint, serves as a key anthropometric indicator for indirect VAT assessment. Compared to BMI, WC demonstrates its superior prognostic value for all-cause mortality in middle-aged and elderly populations. Notably, WC alone cannot resolve the anatomical distribution between SAT and VAT compartments, limiting its utility in metabolic risk stratification [75, 76].

4.1.2 A body shape index (ABSI)

A body shape index (ABSI), calculated as $ABSI = \frac{WC(cm)}{\left(BMI\left(kg/m^2\right)^{\frac{2}{3}} \times height(cm)^{\frac{1}{2}}\right)}$, is an innovative metric which integrates BMI and WC and simultaneously captures both generalized adiposity and VAT deposition [77]. Elevated ABSI values specifically indicate pronounced VAT deposition and independently predict myocardial infarction incidence, major adverse cardiovascular events, and all-cause mortality risk [78, 79].

4.1.3 Weight-adjusted waist index (WWI)

Weight-adjusted waist index (WWI) is calculated as $WWI\left(\frac{cm}{\sqrt{kg}}\right) = \frac{WC(cm)}{\sqrt{weight\left(kg\right)}}$ an index that integrates WC and body weight and provides a comprehensive evaluation of VAT accumulation, skeletal muscle mass, and BMD [80]. Increased WWI values reflect adverse adiposity patterns characterized by reduced skeletal muscle mass, diminished BMD, and elevated adipose tissue deposition, which demonstrate positive associations with hypertension, T2DM, dyslipidemia, and sarcopenia [81, 82]. This index exhibits its clinical utility in identifying sarcopenic obesity phenotypes.

4.1.4 Visceral adiposity index (VAI)

Visceral adiposity index (VAI) integrates WC (cm), BMI (kg/m^2), triglycerides (TG) (mmol/L), and high-density lipoprotein cholesterol (HDL-C) (mmol/L), which accurately reflects VAT dysfunction and insulin resistance. This composite index provides a valuable tool for evaluating adipose dysfunction and metabolic dysregulation [80]. The calculation formula of VAI is as follows: Males:
$VAI = \left(\frac{WC}{39.68+(1.88\times BMI)}\right) \times \left(\frac{TG}{1.03}\right) \times \left(\frac{1.31}{HDL-C}\right)$;
Females: $VAI = \left(\frac{WC}{36.58+(1.89\times BMI)}\right) \times \left(\frac{TG}{0.81}\right) \times \left(\frac{1.52}{HDL-C}\right)$.

4.1.5 Triglyceride-glucose (TyG) index

Triglyceride-glucose (TyG) index, calculated as
$TyG\, index = ln[fasting\, TG\,(mg/dl) \times fasting\, glucose\,(mg/dl)/2]$, is used as a straightforward surrogate marker for insulin resistance, effectively reflecting both systemic inflammation and metabolic dysfunction [83]. Elevated TyG index values correlate positively with increased risks of dyslipidemia, T2DM, hypertension, and CVD, concurrent with pronounced prognostic implications for patient outcomes [84, 85].

4.1.6 Bioelectrical impedance analysis (BIA)

Bioelectrical impedance analysis (BIA) enables accurate body composition evaluation through quantification of tissue-specific electrical impedance, deriving critical parameters such as fat mass, LBM and phase angle (PA) [86]. BIA quantifies total body impedance (Z), representing the combined opposition to alternating current (AC) flow through biological tissues [87]. This impedance comprises resistance (R) and reactance (Xc), governed by the fundamental equation: $Z^2 = R^2 + Xc^2$. Notably, BIA effectively reflects muscle quality (mass, density, architecture) and demonstrates high diagnostic accuracy in detecting sarcopenia [88]. Studies also prove that elevated fat mass significantly correlates with increased CVD incidence through BIA assessment, whereas higher LBM demonstrates a protective effect against CVD risk [89].

4.2 Advanced medical imaging modalities: Volumetric quantification of adipose tissue and skeletal muscle

Medical imaging modalities capitalize on tissue-specific attenuation characteristics (adipose tissue, skeletal muscle, bone) via X-ray and magnetic field interactions, enabling high-fidelity visualization of adipose distribution, skeletal muscle mass, and bone microarchitectural parameters.

4.2.1 Dual-energy X-ray absorptiometry (DXA)

Dual-energy X-ray absorptiometry (DXA) employs differential attenuation of X-ray energies by adipose tissue, skeletal muscle, and bone to quantify regional fat distribution and total adipose mass. It effectively stratifies sarcopenic obesity risk through VAT assessment. Leveraging low-dose X-ray technology, DXA enables comprehensive body composition profiling, including fat mass, LBM, and BMD [90, 91].

4.2.2 Computed tomography (CT)

Computed Tomography (CT) can accurately distinguish the distribution and changes of VAT, SAT, and skeletal muscle through tissue-specific attenuation patterns, facilitating comprehensive body composition assessment [92]. Myosteatosis, characterized by ectopic adipose infiltration within skeletal muscle, has emerged as a critical prognostic marker for mortality risk in asymptomatic populations. Diagnostic evaluation of myosteatosis relies on quantifying muscle radiodensity at the L3 vertebral level via CT, where diminished attenuation values correlate with lipid accumulation and metabolic dysregulation [93, 94]. Advanced CT analysis protocols permit simultaneous quantification of VAT, SAT, skeletal muscle mass, IMAT, BMD, and hepatic fat fraction (HFF), establishing their utility in identifying risk stratification for sarcopenia, nonalcoholic fatty liver disease (NAFLD), T2DM and CVD [95, 96].

4.2.3 Magnetic resonance imaging (MRI)

Magnetic resonance imaging (MRI) employs chemical shift imaging to discriminate between adipose tissue and water signals, enabling precise fat quantification through proton density fat fraction (PDFF) calculation $\left(fat\,signal/(fat + water)signal\right)$ [97]. Advanced water-fat separation MRI protocols facilitate differential analysis of SAT and VAT, alongside longitudinal tracking of visceral fat dynamics [98]. MRI also detects skeletal muscle atrophy and ectopic adipose infiltration, supporting sarcopenia diagnosis [99]. Cross-sectional studies validate MRI-derived PDFF as a robust biomarker for T2DM risk, correlating with VAT accumulation and hepatic fat deposition [100]. Furthermore, whole-body MRI can identify distinct body composition phenotypes, predicting graded cardiometabolic risk and all-cause mortality [101, 102].

4.3 Biochemical biomarkers: Dynamic assessment of metabolic disease risk

The pathophysiological cornerstone of obesity lies in chronic inflammation-driven metabolic dysregulation. Biomarker profiling reveals critical distinctions between MHO and MUO: elevated adiponectin and HDL-C levels contrast with reduced plasminogen activator inhibitor-1 (PAI-1), small dense low-density lipoprotein (sdLDL), apolipoprotein B (ApoB), 24-hour glucose, FFA, TG, and urinary 8-iso-prostaglandin in MHO [23]. These parameters collectively reflect insulin sensitivity, lipid homeostasis, and inflammatory status. Isthmin-1 (ISM1) demonstrates utility in quantifying SAT/VAT ratios, enabling abdominal fat distribution assessment and metabolic risk stratification [103]. Analysis of Mendelian randomization also shows that VAT mass is significantly correlated with leptin, hepatocyte growth factor, and interleukin-16 (IL-16), which mediate the occurrence of coronary artery disease, heart failure, and stroke [104].

5. Conclusion

Obesity, a chronic metabolic disorder driven by systemic inflammation, significantly elevates risks for T2DM, hypertension, atherosclerosis, and heart failure. Conventional BMI-based diagnosis demonstrates limited sensitivity in detecting obesity subtypes, such as sarcopenic obesity, NWO, and MHO, leading to misclassification and underdiagnosis in high-risk populations, especially in elderly populations. A multidimensional evaluation framework integrating anthropometric, imaging, and biochemical metrics facilitates early detection and risk stratification of obesity and enhances the predictive accuracy of obesity-associated complications.

Appendices and Nomenclature

ABSI	A body shape index
AGT	Angiotensinogen
Ang II	Angiotensin II
ApoB	Apolipoprotein B
BFP	Body fat percentage
BIA	Bioelectrical impedance analysis
BMD	Bone mineral density
BMI	Body mass index
BMM	Bone marrow macrophage
Drp1	Dynamin-related protein 1
CT	Computed Tomography
CVD	Cardiovascular disease
DXA	Dual-energy X-ray absorptiometry
EAT	Epicardial adipose tissue
ENaC	Epithelial sodium channel
eNOS	Endothelial NO synthase
ER	Endoplasmic reticulum
EVs	Extracellular vesicles
FFA	Free fatty acid
GCA	Grancalcin
GLUT4	Glucose transporter 4
HDL-C	High-density lipoprotein cholesterol
HFF	Hepatic fat fraction
HFpEF	Heart failure with preserved ejection fraction
ICAM-1	Intercellular adhesion molecule-1
IGF-1	Insulin-like growth factor-1
IL-1β	Interleukin-1β
IL-6	Interleukin-6
IL-16	Interleukin-16
IMAT	Intermuscular adipose tissue
LBM	Lean body mass
LPS	Lipopolysaccharide
MFN2	Mitofusin-2
MHO	Metabolically healthy obesity
MRI	Magnetic resonance imaging

MS	Metabolic syndrome
mtDNA	Mitochondrial DNA
MUO	Metabolically unhealthy obesity
NAFLD	Nonalcoholic fatty liver disease
NLRP3	NOD-like receptor thermal protein domain associated protein 3
NO	Nitric oxide
NOX	NADPH oxidase
NOW	Normal weight obesity
OSA	Obstructive sleep apnea
PA	Phase angle
PAI-1	Plasminogen activator inhibitor-1
PDFF	Proton density fat fraction
PGC-1α	Proliferator-activated receptor gamma coactivator-1α
PINK1	PTEN-induced kinase 1
PVAT	Perivascular adipose tissue
PUFA	Polyunsaturated fatty acid
RAAS	Renin-angiotensin-aldosterone system
RANKL	Receptor activator of nuclear factor-κ B ligand
ROS	Reactive oxygen species
SAT	Subcutaneous adipose tissue
sdLDL	Small dense low-density lipoprotein
SGK1	Serum/glucocorticoid-regulated kinase 1
SIRT1	Sirtuin 1
T2DM	Type 2 diabetes mellitus
TG	Triglycerides
TLR4	Toll-like receptor 4
TNF-α	Tumor necrosis factor-α
TyG	Triglyceride-glucose
VAI	Visceral adiposity index
VAT	Visceral adipose tissue
VCAM-1	Vascular cell adhesion molecule-1
VSMC	Vascular smooth muscle cell
WC	Waist circumference
WHO	World Health Organization
WWI	Weight-adjusted waist index

Acknowledgments

This project was supported by Grant 32171174 from the National Natural Science Foundation of China; by Grant 2023A03J0531 and 2024A03J0658 from the Joint Funds from Guangzhou Science and Technology Project.

Conflict of Interest

The author declares that there is no conflict of interest.

Author details

Yiting Zhao[1], Jiangbo Ye[2], Wansu Yu[3], Qian Du[1*] and Donghui Liu[3*]

1 Department of Cardiology, Guangzhou Red Cross Hospital, Medical College, Jinan University, Guangzhou, China.

2 Department of Cardiology, Ziyun County People's Hospital, Anshun, China.

3 Department of Geriatrics, Guangzhou First People's Hospital, School of Medicine, South China University of Technology, Guangzhou, China.

*Address correspondence to: eyliudh@scut.edu.cn; duqian1213@126.com

References

[1] Bluher M. Obesity: global epidemiology and pathogenesis. Nature Reviews Endocrinology. 2019;**15**(5):288–298

[2] Gbdab C. Global, regional, and national prevalence of adult overweight and obesity, 1990-2021, with forecasts to 2050: a forecasting study for the Global Burden of Disease Study 2021. Lancet. 2025;**405**(10481):813–838

[3] Hagberg CE, Spalding KL. White adipocyte dysfunction and obesity-associated pathologies in humans. Nature Reviews Molecular Cell Biology. 2024;**25**(4):270–289

[4] Ouchi N, Parker JL, Lugus JJ, Walsh K. Adipokines in inflammation and metabolic disease. Nature Reviews Immunology. 2011;**11**(2):85–97

[5] Saltiel AR, Olefsky JM. Inflammatory mechanisms linking obesity and metabolic disease. Journal of Clinical Investigation. 2017;**127**(1):1–4

[6] Ahmed B, Sultana R, Greene MW. Adipose tissue and insulin resistance in obese. Biomedicine & Pharmacotherapy. 2021;**137**:111315

[7] Livshits G, Kalinkovich A. Inflammaging as a common ground for the development and maintenance of sarcopenia, obesity, cardiomyopathy and dysbiosis. Ageing research reviews. 2019;**56**:100980

[8] Shaikh SR, Beck MA, Alwarawrah Y, MacIver NJ. Emerging mechanisms of obesity-associated immune dysfunction. Nature Reviews Endocrinology. 2024;**20**(3):136–148

[9] Kalinkovich A, Livshits G. Sarcopenic obesity or obese sarcopenia: A cross talk between age-associated adipose tissue and skeletal muscle inflammation as a main mechanism of the pathogenesis. Ageing research reviews. 2017;**35**:200–221

[10] Rubio-Tomas T, Rueda-Robles A, Plaza-Diaz J, Alvarez-Mercado AI. Nutrition and cellular senescence in obesity-related disorders. The Journal of Nutritional Biochemistry. 2022;**99**:108861

[11] Stout MB, Justice JN, Nicklas BJ, Kirkland JL. Physiological Aging: Links Among Adipose Tissue Dysfunction, Diabetes, and Frailty. Physiology (Bethesda, Md.). 2017;**32**(1):9–19

[12] Nguyen TT, Corvera S. Adipose tissue as a linchpin of organismal ageing. Nature Metabolism. 2024;**6**(5):793–807

[13] Frasca D, Blomberg BB. Adipose tissue, immune aging, and cellular senescence. Seminars in Immunopathology. 2020;**42**(5):573–587

[14] Koskinas KC, Van Craenenbroeck EM, Antoniades C, Bluher M, Gorter TM, Hanssen H, et al. Obesity and cardiovascular disease: an ESC clinical consensus statement. European heart journal 2024;**45**:4063–4098

[15] Fuster JJ, Ouchi N, Gokce N, Walsh K. Obesity-Induced Changes in

Adipose Tissue Microenvironment and Their Impact on Cardiovascular Disease. Circulation Research. 2016;**118**(11):1786–1807

[16] Koenen M, Hill MA, Cohen P, Obesity SJR. Adipose Tissue and Vascular Dysfunction. Circulation Research. 2021;**128**(7):951–968

[17] Queiroz M, Sena CM. Perivascular adipose tissue in age-related vascular disease. Ageing Research Reviews. 2020;**59**:101040

[18] Hu H, Garcia-Barrio M, Jiang Z-S, Chen YE, Chang L. Roles of Perivascular Adipose Tissue in Hypertension and Atherosclerosis. Antioxidants & Redox Signaling. 2021;**34**(9):951–968

[19] Auger C, Kajimura S. Adipose Tissue Remodeling in Pathophysiology. Annual Review of Pathology: Mechanisms of Disease. 2023;**18**:71–93

[20] Sawalha K, Asad O, Tadisina S, Alalawi L, Mahmood M, Alkhatib D, et al. Obesity-Induced Hyperglycemia and Heart Failure Preserved Ejection Fraction: Uncharted Territories to Remission. Cureus. 2023;**15**(11):e49178

[21] Jin X, Qiu T, Li L, Yu R, Chen X, Li C, et al. Pathophysiology of obesity and its associated diseases. Acta pharmaceutica Sinica. B 2023;**13**:2403–2424

[22] Klein S, Gastaldelli A, Yki-Jarvinen H, Scherer PE. Why does obesity cause diabetes?. Cell Metabolism. 2022;**34**(1):11–20

[23] Petersen MC, Smith GI, Palacios HH, Farabi SS, Yoshino M, Yoshino J, et al. Cardiometabolic characteristics of people with metabolically healthy and unhealthy obesity. Cell Metabolism 2024; **36**:745–61e5

[24] Skov J, Persson F, Frokiaer J, Christiansen JS. Tissue Renin–Angiotensin Systems: A Unifying Hypothesis of Metabolic Disease. Frontiers in Endocrinology. 2014;**5**:23

[25] Pothen L, Verdoy R, De Mulder D, Esfahani H, Farah C, Michel LYM, et al. Sustained Downregulation of Vascular Smooth Muscle Acta2 After Transient Angiotensin II Infusion: A New Model of "Vascular Memory". Frontiers in Cardiovascular Medicine. 2022;**9**:854361

[26] Galiana-Simal A, Olivares-Alvaro E, Klett-Mingo M, Ruiz-Roso MB, Ballesteros S, de Las Heras N, et al. Proanthocyanidins block aldosterone-dependent up-regulation of cardiac gamma ENaC and Nedd4-2 inactivation via SGK1. The Journal of Nutritional Biochemistry. 2016;**37**:13–19

[27] Powell-Wiley TM, Poirier P, Burke LE, Despres J-P, Gordon-Larsen P, Lavie CJ, Lear SA, Ndumele CE, Neeland IJ, Sanders P, St-Onge M-P, et al. Obesity and Cardiovascular Disease: A Scientific Statement From the American Heart Association. Circulation 2021;**143**:e984–e1010

[28] Iacobellis G. Epicardial adipose tissue in contemporary cardiology. Nature Reviews Cardiology. 2022;**19**(9):593–606

[29] Wang X, He B. Endothelial dysfunction: molecular mechanisms and clinical implications. MedComm. 2024;**5**(8):e651

[30] Kong Y, Yang H, Nie R, Zhang X, Zuo F, Zhang H, et al. Obesity:

pathophysiology and therapeutic interventions. Molecular biomedicine 2025;**6**:25

[31] Haidar A, Obesity HT. Cardiorespiratory Fitness, and Cardiovascular Disease. Current Cardiology Reports. 2023;**25**(11): 1565–1571

[32] Patel TP, Rawal K, Bagchi AK, Akolkar G, Bernardes N, Dias DDS, et al. Insulin resistance: an additional risk factor in the pathogenesis of cardiovascular disease in type 2 diabetes. Heart Failure Reviews 2016;**21**:11–23

[33] Savji N, Meijers WC, Bartz TM, Bhambhani V, Cushman M, Nayor M, et al. The Association of Obesity and Cardiometabolic Traits With Incident HFpEF and HFrEF. JACC: Heart Failure 2018;**6**:701–709

[34] Borlaug BA, Jensen MD, Kitzman DW, Lam CSP, Obokata M, Rider OJ. Obesity and heart failure with preserved ejection fraction: new insights and pathophysiological targets. Cardiovascular Research. 2023;**118** (18):3434–3450

[35] Rubino F, Cummings DE, Eckel RH, Cohen RV, Wilding JPH, Brown WA, et al. Definition and diagnostic criteria of clinical obesity. The Lancet Diabetes & Endocrinology 2025;**13**:221–262

[36] Damluji AA, Alfaraidhy M, AlHajri N, Rohant NN, Kumar M, Al Malouf C, et al. Sarcopenia and Cardiovascular Diseases. Circulation 2023;**147**:1534–1553

[37] Barber TM, Kabisch S, Pfeiffer AFH, Weickert MO. Optimised Skeletal Muscle Mass as a Key Strategy for Obesity Management. Metabolites. 2025;**15**(2):85

[38] Losev V, Lu C, Tahasildar S, Senevirathne DS, Inglese P, Bai W, et al. Sex-specific body fat distribution predicts cardiovascular ageing. European Heart Journal. 2025: ehaf553

[39] Mohammadian Khonsari N, Khashayar P, Shahrestanaki E, Kelishadi R, Mohammadpoor Nami S, Heidari-Beni M, et al. Normal Weight Obesity and Cardiometabolic Risk Factors: A Systematic Review and Meta-Analysis. Frontiers in Endocrinology. 2022;**13**:857930

[40] Wannamethee SG, Atkins JL. Muscle loss and obesity: the health implications of sarcopenia and sarcopenic obesity. Proceedings of the Nutrition Society. 2015;**74**(4):405–412

[41] Lee H, Chung HS, Kim YJ, Choi MK, Roh YK, Yu JM, et al. Association between body composition and the risk of mortality in the obese population in the United States. Frontiers in Endocrinology. 2023;**14**:1257902

[42] Chen TP, Kao HH, Ogawa W, Arai H, Tahapary DL, Assantachai P, et al. The Asia-Oceania consensus: Definitions and diagnostic criteria for sarcopenic obesity. Obesity Research & Clinical Practice 2025;**19**:185–192

[43] Prado CM, Batsis JA, Donini LM, Gonzalez MC, Siervo M. Sarcopenic obesity in older adults: a clinical overview. Nature Reviews Endocrinology. 2024;**20**(5):261–277

[44] Li CW, Yu K, Shyh-Chang N, Jiang Z, Liu T, Ma S, et al. Pathogenesis of sarcopenia and the relationship with

fat mass: descriptive review. Journal of Cachexia, Sarcopenia and Muscle 2022;**13**:781–794

[45] Mirzai S, Carbone S, Batsis JA, Kritchevsky SB, Kitzman DW, Shapiro MD. Sarcopenic Obesity and Cardiovascular Disease: An Overlooked but High-Risk Syndrome. Current Obesity Reports. 2024;**13**(3):532–544

[46] Kitada M, Koya D. Autophagy in metabolic disease and ageing. Nature Reviews Endocrinology. 2021;**17** (11):647–661

[47] Axelrod CL, Dantas WS, Kirwan JP. Sarcopenic obesity: emerging mechanisms and therapeutic potential. Metabolism. 2023;**146**:155639

[48] Flores-Opazo M, Kopinke D, Helmbacher F, Fernandez-Verdejo R, Tunon-Suarez M, Lynch GS, et al. Fibro-adipogenic progenitors in physiological adipogenesis and intermuscular adipose tissue remodeling. . Molecular aspects of medicine. 2024;**97**:101277

[49] Benz E, Pinel A, Guillet C, Capel F, Pereira B, De Antonio M, et al. Sarcopenia and Sarcopenic Obesity and Mortality Among Older People. JAMA Network Open. 2024;7(3): e243604

[50] Peng L, Xiang Q, Jia G, Yin R. Association between sarcopenic obesity and dementia in the Chinese elderly using different definitions of obesity: evidence from the CHARLS. Frontiers in Aging Neuroscience. 2025;**17**:1540272

[51] Mo YH, Yang C, Su YD, Dong X, Deng WY, Liu BB, et al. Prevalence and diagnostic agreement of sarcopenic obesity with different definitions among Chinese community-dwelling older adults. Age and Ageing. 2022;**51**(1):afab272

[52] Ibrahim MM. Subcutaneous and visceral adipose tissue: structural and functional differences. Obesity Reviews. 2010;**11**(1):11–18

[53] Polkinghorne MD, West HW, Antoniades C. Adipose Tissue in Cardiovascular Disease: From Basic Science to Clinical Translation. Annual Review of Physiology. 2024;**86**:175–198

[54] Cheng X, Jiang S, Pan B, Xie W, Meng J. Ectopic and visceral fat deposition in aging, obesity, and idiopathic pulmonary fibrosis: an interconnected role. Lipids in Health and Disease. 2023;**22**(1):201

[55] Sun Y, Liu B, Snetselaar LG, Wallace RB, Caan BJ, Rohan TE, et al. Association of Normal-Weight Central Obesity With All-Cause and Cause-Specific Mortality Among Postmenopausal Women. JAMA Network Open. 2019;**2**(7):e197337

[56] Chen GC, Arthur R, Iyengar NM, Kamensky V, Xue X, Wassertheil-Smoller S, et al. Association between regional body fat and cardiovascular disease risk among postmenopausal women with normal body mass index. European Heart Journal 2019;**40**: 2849–2855

[57] Zheng J, Hu Y, Xu H, Lei Y, Zhang J, Zheng Q, et al. Normal-weight visceral obesity promotes a higher 10-year atherosclerotic cardiovascular disease risk in patients with type 2 diabetes mellitus-a multicenter study in China. Cardiovascular Diabetology 2023;**22**:137

[58] Zhong P, Tan S, Zhu Z, Zhu Z, Liang Y, Huang W, et al. Normal-weight central obesity and risk of cardiovascular and microvascular events in adults with prediabetes or diabetes: Chinese and British cohorts. Diabetes/Metabolism Research and Reviews. 2023;**39**(8):e3707

[59] Yang G, Jiang H, Xie D, Yuan S, Wu J, Zhang J, et al. Association of obesity with osteoporotic fracture risk in individuals with bone metabolism-related conditions: a cross sectional analysis. Frontiers in Nutrition. 2024;**11**:1365587

[60] Guimaraes GC, Coelho JBC, Silva JGO, de Sant'ana ACC, de Sa CAC, Moreno JM, et al. Obesity, diabetes and risk of bone fragility: How BMAT behavior is affected by metabolic disturbances and its influence on bone health. Osteoporosis International 2024;**35**:575–588

[61] Huang M, Huang M, Liu L, Yang F, He C, Sun YC, et al. Gut Microbiota Modulates Obesity-Associated Skeletal Deterioration Through Macrophage Aging and Grancalcin Secretion. Advanced Science. 2025;**12**(28): e2502634

[62] Kirk B, Feehan J, Lombardi G, Muscle DG. Bone, and Fat Crosstalk: the Biological Role of Myokines, Osteokines, and Adipokines. Current Osteoporosis Reports. 2020;**18**(4):388–400

[63] Colaianni G, Mongelli T, Colucci S, Cinti S, Grano M. Crosstalk Between Muscle and Bone Via the Muscle-Myokine Irisin. Current Osteoporosis Reports. 2016;**14**(4):132–137

[64] Hou J, He C, He W, Yang M, Luo X, Li C. Obesity and Bone Health: A Complex Link. Frontiers in Cell and Developmental Biology. 2020;**8**:600181

[65] Girgis CM, Baldock PA, Downes M. Vitamin D, muscle and bone: Integrating effects in development, aging and injury. Molecular and Cellular Endocrinology. 2015;**410**:3–10

[66] Kim J, Lee Y, Kye S, Chung Y-S, Lee O. Association of serum vitamin D with osteosarcopenic obesity: Korea National Health and Nutrition Examination Survey 2008–2010. Journal of Cachexia, Sarcopenia and Muscle. 2017;**8**(2):259–266

[67] Bouillon R, Marcocci C, Carmeliet G, Bikle D, White JH, Dawson-Hughes B, et al. Skeletal and Extraskeletal Actions of Vitamin D: Current Evidence and Outstanding Questions. Endocrine reviews 2019;**40**:1109–1151

[68] Bouillon R, LeBoff MS, Neale RE. Health Effects of Vitamin D Supplementation: Lessons Learned From Randomized Controlled Trials and Mendelian Randomization Studies. Journal of Bone and Mineral Research. 2023;**38**(10):1391–1403

[69] Kim J, Kang S, Kang H. Association between normal-weight obesity and bone mineral density in older Korean adults: A population-based cross-sectional study. Maturitas. 2024;**180**:107891

[70] Zhao X, He L, Wu X, Zhang L, Xiao J, Xiao C, et al. Disentangling the divergent causal pathways underlying the association between body mass index and bone mineral density: a comprehensive Mendelian randomization study. BMC Medicine 2025;**23**:305

[71] Kirk B, Zanker J, Duque G. Osteosarcopenia: epidemiology, diagnosis, and treatment—facts and numbers. Journal of Cachexia, Sarcopenia and Muscle. 2020;**11** (3):609–618

[72] Scott D, Seibel M, Cumming R, Naganathan V, Blyth F, Le Couteur DG, et al. Sarcopenic Obesity and Its Temporal Associations With Changes in Bone Mineral Density, Incident Falls, and Fractures in Older Men: The Concord Health and Ageing in Men Project. Journal of Bone and Mineral Research 2017;**32**:575–583

[73] Gandham A, Mesinovic J, Jansons P, Zengin A, Bonham MP, Ebeling PR, et al. Falls, fractures, and areal bone mineral density in older adults with sarcopenic obesity: A systematic review and meta-analysis. Obesity Reviews. 2021;**22**(5):e13187

[74] Thomas DM, Crofford I, Scudder J, Oletti B, Deb A, Heymsfield SB. Updates on Methods for Body Composition Analysis: Implications for Clinical Practice. Current Obesity Reports. 2025;**14**(1):8

[75] Amato MC, Giordano C, Galia M, Criscimanna A, Vitabile S, Midiri M, et al. Visceral Adiposity Index: a reliable indicator of visceral fat function associated with cardiometabolic risk. Diabetes Care 2010;**33**:920–922

[76] Tseng LY, Liang CK, Peng LN, Lin MH, Loh CH, Lee WJ, et al. The distinct impacts of sarcopenic and dynapenic obesity on mortality in middle-aged and older adults based on different adiposity metrics: Results from I-Lan Longitudinal Aging Study. Clinical Nutrition 2024;**43**:1892–1899

[77] Sweatt K, Garvey WT, Martins C. Strengths and Limitations of BMI in the Diagnosis of Obesity: What is the Path Forward?. Current Obesity Reports. 2024;**13**(3):584–595

[78] Wei S, Jiang W, Zheng H, Zhang J, Yang J, Wang Y, et al. The combined impact of BMI and ABSI on all-cause mortality among American adults with diabetes. Diabetology & Metabolic Syndrome 2025;**17**:48

[79] Xu W, He F, Huang H, Yang Z, Xiao Z, Zhou Y, et al. A body shape index for visceral fat and its changes predict cardiovascular outcomes of heart failure with preserved ejection fraction. European Heart Journal - Quality of Care and Clinical Outcomes. 2025;**11**:qcaf005

[80] Kim KJ, Son S, Kim KJ, Kim SG, Kim NH. Weight-adjusted waist as an integrated index for fat, muscle and bone health in adults. Journal of Cachexia, Sarcopenia and Muscle. 2023;**14**(5):2196–2203

[81] Kim JY, Choi J, Vella CA, Criqui MH, Allison MA, Kim NH. Associations between Weight-Adjusted Waist Index and Abdominal Fat and Muscle Mass: Multi-Ethnic Study of Atherosclerosis. Diabetes & Metabolism Journal. 2022;**46**(5):747–755

[82] Zhou H, Su H, Gong Y, Chen L, Xu L, Chen G, et al. The association between weight-adjusted-waist index and sarcopenia in adults: a population-based study. Scientific Reports. 2024;**14**(1):10943

[83] Tao L-C, Xu J-N, Wang T-T, Hua F, Li J-J. Triglyceride-glucose index as a marker in cardiovascular diseases: landscape and limitations.

Cardiovascular Diabetology. 2022;**21**(1):68

[84] Yang Y, Li S, Ren Q, Qiu Y, Pan M, Liu G, et al. The interaction between triglyceride-glucose index and visceral adiposity in cardiovascular disease risk: findings from a nationwide Chinese cohort. Cardiovascular Diabetology 2024;**23**:427

[85] Che B, Zhong C, Zhang R, Pu L, Zhao T, Zhang Y, et al. Triglyceride-glucose index and triglyceride to high-density lipoprotein cholesterol ratio as potential cardiovascular disease risk factors: an analysis of UK biobank data. Cardiovascular Diabetology 2023;**22**:34

[86] Son JW, Han B-D, Bennett JP, Heymsfield S, Lim S. Development and clinical application of bioelectrical impedance analysis method for body composition assessment. Obesity Reviews. 2025;**26**(1):e13844

[87] Akamatsu Y, Kusakabe T, Arai H, Yamamoto Y, Nakao K, Ikeue K, et al. Phase angle from bioelectrical impedance analysis is a useful indicator of muscle quality. Journal of Cachexia, Sarcopenia and Muscle 2022;**13**:180–189

[88] Luo M, Duan Z, Li Y, Wang Y, Chen L, Gao J, et al. Bioelectrical impedance analysis for sarcopenia: a systematic review and meta-analysis of diagnostic accuracy. Age and Ageing. 2025;**54**(6):afaf181

[89] Haidar A, Kronmal R, Allison M, Watson K, Srikanthan P, Horwich T. Examining the Relationship Between Anthropometric and Body Composition measures with Coronary Heart Disease Events: The Multi-Ethnic Study of Atherosclerosis. European Journal of Preventive Cardiology; 2025. p. zwaf212

[90] De Lorenzo A, Itani L, El Ghoch M, Frank G, De Santis GL, Gualtieri P, et al. The Association between Sarcopenic Obesity and DXA-Derived Visceral Adipose Tissue (VAT) in Adults. Nutrients 2024;**16**:1645

[91] Song X, Wu H, Zhang W, Wang B, Sun H. Equations for predicting DXA-measured visceral adipose tissue mass based on BMI or weight in adults. Lipids in Health and Disease. 2022;**21**(1):45

[92] Mazonakis M, Damilakis J. Computed tomography: What and how does it measure?. European Journal of Radiology. 2016;**85**(8):1499–1504

[93] Nachit M, Horsmans Y, Summers RM, Leclercq IA, Pickhardt PJ. AI-based CT Body Composition Identifies Myosteatosis as Key Mortality Predictor in Asymptomatic Adults. Radiology. 2023;**307**(5):e222008

[94] Ahn H, Kim DW, Ko Y, Ha J, Shin YB, Lee J, et al. Updated systematic review and meta-analysis on diagnostic issues and the prognostic impact of myosteatosis: A new paradigm beyond sarcopenia. Ageing Research Reviews. 2021;**70**:101398

[95] Kuriyama K, Matsui Y, Suzuki Y, Mizuno T, Watanabe T, Takemura M, et al. Relationship between sarcopenia classification and thigh muscle mass, fat area, muscle CT value and osteoporosis in middle-aged and older Japanese adults. Bone. 2022;**163**:116487

[96] Chang Y, Yoon SH, Kwon R, Kang J, YH K, JM K, et al. Automated Comprehensive CT Assessment of the

Risk of Diabetes and Associated Cardiometabolic Conditions. Radiology. 2024;**312**(2):e233410

[97] Nikiforaki K, Marias K. MRI Methods to Visualize and Quantify Adipose Tissue in Health and Disease. Biomedicines. 2023;**11**(12):3179

[98] Shen J, Baum T, Cordes C, Ott B, Skurk T, Kooijman H, et al. Automatic segmentation of abdominal organs and adipose tissue compartments in water-fat MRI: Application to weight-loss in obesity. European Journal of Radiology 2016;**85**:1613–1621

[99] Klickovic U, Zampedri L, Sinclair CDJ, Wastling SJ, Trimmel K, Howard RS, et al. Skeletal muscle MRI differentiates SBMA and ALS and correlates with disease severity. Neurology 2019;**93**:e895–e907

[100] An Q, Zhang QH, Wang Y, Zhang HY, Liu YH, Zhang ZT, et al. Association between type 2 diabetes mellitus and body composition based on MRI fat fraction mapping. Frontiers in Public Health. 2024;**12**:1332346

[101] Grune E, Nattenmuller J, Kiefer LS, Machann J, Peters A, Bamberg F, et al. Subphenotypes of body composition and their association with cardiometabolic risk - Magnetic resonance imaging in a population-based sample. Metabolism. 2025;**164**:156130

[102] Jung M, Raghu VK, Reisert M, Rieder H, Rospleszcz S, Pischon T, et al. Deep learning-based body composition analysis from whole-body magnetic resonance imaging to predict all-cause mortality in a large western population. EBioMedicine. 2024;**110**:105467

[103] Lopez-Yus M, Casamayor C, Soriano-Godes JJ, Borlan S, Gonzalez-Irazabal Y, Garcia-Sobreviela MP, et al. Isthmin-1 (ISM1), a novel adipokine that reflects abdominal adipose tissue distribution in individuals with obesity. Cardiovascular Diabetology 2023;**22**:335

[104] Huang Y, Liu Y, Ma Y, Tu T, Liu N, Bai F, et al. Associations of Visceral Adipose Tissue, Circulating Protein Biomarkers, and Risk of Cardiovascular Diseases: A Mendelian Randomization Analysis. Frontiers in Cell and Developmental Biology. 2022;**10**:840866

Section 4

BMI from Behavioral Health Perspectives

Chapter 7

Mental Health Perspectives on the BMI Paradox

Stephen Amarjeet Jiwanmall and Dheeraj Kattula

Abstract

The body mass index (BMI) paradox challenges the conventional understanding of the relationship between body weight and health outcomes. Sometimes, people who are overweight or slightly obese have better health and live longer than those with a normal BMI. This can be due to factors like weight stigma, biases, cultural views, financial issues, stress, and eating disorders. Weight stigma can have profound psychological impacts on individuals, leading to increased stress, anxiety, depression, and maladaptive coping mechanisms. Cognitive biases in BMI interpretation can result in misdiagnosis and inappropriate treatment decisions. Cultural and economic factors greatly influence how people view body weight and health. Stress affects BMI in complicated ways; it can sometimes protect people but also increase health risks for others. The link between eating disorders and obesity makes the BMI paradox more complex. This means treatment should consider trauma and include all body types. The body positivity movement supports accepting all body shapes; however, more research is needed to understand its effect on health. The BMI paradox underscores the need for a holistic, individualized approach to health assessment and treatment, focusing on developing more refined health measures beyond BMI and exploring the intricate relationships between physical and mental well-being.

Keywords: body mass index (BMI), weight stigma, psychological stress, eating disorders, body positivity, mental well-being, health assessment

1. Introduction

Body mass index (BMI) is a readily measurable and cost-effective metric. It is characterized by standardized thresholds for categorizing overweight and obesity and demonstrates a strong correlation with body fat levels as determined by the most precise methods. However, BMI is imperfect, as it does not directly evaluate body fat [1].

The BMI paradox refers to the observation that individuals categorized as overweight or mildly obese according to their BMI occasionally exhibit superior health outcomes and reduced mortality rates compared to those within the normal BMI range. This phenomenon challenges the conventional understanding of the relationship between body weight and health. Several factors may

IntechOpen

contribute to this discrepancy, including the limitations of BMI as a health indicator, the potential protective effects of additional body fat in certain conditions, and the impact of fitness levels independent of weight [2]. Furthermore, this underscores the complex interplay between physical and mental health, as psychological factors such as stress resilience and body image can influence overall well-being irrespective of BMI classification. To fully understand the discrepancy in BMI measures, we must look at health from many angles, not just weight. BMI also has significant aspects to consider from a mental health perspective.

2. Psychological impact of weight stigma

Weight stigma can have profound psychological impacts on individuals, regardless of their actual body size or health status. This form of discrimination can lead to increased stress, anxiety, and depression, as well as lower self-esteem and body dissatisfaction [3–5].

People who face weight stigma might start to believe negative views about themselves. This can lead to self-blame and feelings of worthlessness. They might cope in unhealthy ways, such as developing disordered eating habits or avoiding healthy behaviors. The pressure to fit into society's body ideals can cause a cycle of dieting and weight changes, which may increase mental distress.

Weight stigma is crucial in the relationship between BMI and self-reported health [6]. Additionally, findings suggest that worries about potential future stigma act as a mediator between perceived past discrimination experiences and both psychological and physical health [6].

Weight stigma is likely to contribute to weight gain and deteriorating health; therefore, it should be eliminated [7]. The pervasive nature of weight stigma in various settings, including healthcare, education, and employment, can also lead to social isolation and a reduced quality of life. Addressing weight stigma is crucial for promoting overall mental well-being and fostering a more inclusive society that values health at every size [8].

The revised classification presents a more detailed perspective on obesity, which can aid in lessening the adverse effects of weight stigma [9]. By prioritizing health over mere weight, it promotes a more empathetic and supportive attitude toward individuals with obesity. This change in emphasis can help mitigate the damaging consequences of weight bias and discrimination. For instance, healthcare professionals can concentrate on enhancing metabolic health and addressing specific health concerns related to obesity, rather than just focusing on weight reduction [10].

3. Cognitive biases in BMI interpretation

Cognitive biases, which are systematic thinking errors that affect our judgments and decisions, can significantly influence how people, including healthcare professionals, interpret and apply BMI results [11].

Cognitive biases can significantly influence the interpretation of BMI.

Weight bias/stigma: Negative stereotypes and attitudes toward individuals with elevated BMI, often rooted in societal norms and media portrayals, can influence healthcare providers' perceptions and actions. This bias may lead to:

A. Underestimation of health risks in individuals with "normal" BMI: Healthcare providers might overlook potential health issues, such as high visceral fat (fat surrounding internal organs), which increases the risk of conditions like Type 2 diabetes and heart disease if a patient falls within a "normal" BMI range [12].

B. Emphasis on weight loss as a primary solution: An overemphasis on weight loss as the primary intervention, driven by weight bias, may detract from addressing other important factors, such as health behaviors and patient-centered goals [13, 14].

C. Framing effect: How information about BMI and its implications is presented can influence perceptions and subsequent actions. For instance, framing BMI as a categorical measure (underweight, normal, overweight, and obese) can create a rigid perception of health, potentially overshadowing the complex reality of individual health and well-being [15, 16]. The use of stigmatizing language, such as "obese," instead of person-centered terms like "larger bodies," can also negatively impact patient engagement and communication.

D. Anchoring bias: The tendency to heavily rely on the initial piece of information presented, even if later information contradicts it, can affect BMI interpretation [17]. For example, once a patient is labeled with a particular BMI category, it can become challenging to objectively consider other factors that might challenge that initial assessment, potentially leading to the overlooking of alternative diagnoses or treatment approaches.

E. Availability bias: Judging the likelihood of a diagnosis or health outcome based on the ease with which examples come to mind can influence BMI interpretation [18]. Suppose healthcare providers frequently encounter patients in certain BMI categories developing specific health conditions; in that case, they might be more likely to assume the same for other patients, potentially overlooking other relevant information. In essence, cognitive biases can contribute to misdiagnosis, inappropriate treatment decisions, and compromised patient care when BMI is relied upon as the sole or primary indicator of health.

To reduce these biases, healthcare providers should:

1. **Be aware of personal and hidden biases**: Understand how personal experiences, societal norms, and cultural factors affect your BMI judgments.

2. **Use a person-centered approach**: Look at the individual's unique health profile, including body composition, lifestyle, and other health markers – not just the BMI number.

3. **Keep learning and training**: Learn about different thinking biases and ways to lessen their impact on clinical decisions.

4. **Practice reflective reasoning and critical thinking**: Question assumptions, consider other explanations, and actively seek information that might challenge first impressions.

5. **Use cognitive aids and decision support systems**: Utilize tools and checklists to improve objective assessment and reduce reliance on gut feelings.

6. **Prioritize open communication and empathy**: Have respectful and nonjudgmental conversations with patients about their weight, health goals, and concerns.

By actively addressing these cognitive biases, healthcare professionals can move toward a more nuanced and individualized interpretation of BMI, thereby improving patient care and promoting more equitable health outcomes [19].

4. Cultural perspectives on body weight

Cultural perspectives on body weight exhibit considerable variation across different societies and historical periods, reflecting various values, beliefs, and historical contexts. In numerous Western cultures, thinness has been idealized as a beauty standard, particularly for women, resulting in widespread dieting and body dissatisfaction [20].

This ideal, however, stands in stark contrast to certain non-Western cultures, where fuller figures are traditionally associated with prosperity, health, and fertility. For example, in some African, Arab, and Pacific Island societies, larger body sizes are often perceived positively as indicators of wealth and status [21]. In certain Asian cultures, a complex relationship exists with body weight, where thinness is valued, yet plumpness in children is regarded as a sign of health. A multifaceted interplay of demographic, cultural, and economic factors influences the prevalence of obesity in South Asia. Although BMI is a widely utilized metric, it proves inadequate for accurately assessing obesity within this population [22].

Different cultures have different views on body weight. These views can affect how people feel about themselves, their eating habits, and their mental health. Globalization has mixed these views, bringing new challenges as old ideas meet new ones. We need to understand these cultural views to help people with health, body image, and weight. To effectively comprehend and address the escalating obesity epidemic in South Asia, it is imperative to develop more refined and context-specific measures [22].

5. Socio-economic factors affecting the BMI

Several socio-economic factors affect BMI and are directly related to mental health outcomes as well:

1. **Financial status**: Lower-income populations often have limited access to nutritious food and healthcare services, potentially leading to higher BMI but poorer overall health outcomes [23].

2. **Education levels**: Individuals with lower educational attainment may have less knowledge about healthy lifestyle choices and nutrition, which impacts their BMI and health status.

To begin with, individuals with lower educational attainment tend to follow diets high in carbohydrates and low in fiber. Additionally, they are more likely to consume sweets and red meats, while those with higher education levels are more inclined to eat fruits, vegetables, and fish. Furthermore, areas with a well-educated populace exhibit greater nutritional variety and lower calorie consumption. Lastly, the influence extends to neighboring communities, which should be considered when formulating public health strategies and interventions [24].

3. **Food deserts**: Areas with limited access to affordable, healthy food options can contribute to higher BMI among residents, while negatively affecting their overall health.

4. **Occupational factors**: Physically demanding jobs may result in higher muscle mass and BMI without necessarily indicating poor health, while sedentary occupations may lead to weight gain and associated health risks.

5. **Healthcare access**: Limited access to preventive care and medical services can result in undiagnosed or untreated health conditions, affecting the relationship between BMI and health outcomes.

6. **Stress levels**: Chronic stress, often associated with lower socio-economic status, can impact BMI and overall health through physiological and behavioral mechanisms.

7. **Environmental factors**: Neighborhood characteristics, such as the availability of green spaces and recreational facilities, can affect BMI and overall health outcomes.

8. **Social support networks**: The presence or absence of supportive social networks can impact health behaviors and outcomes, potentially contributing to the discrepancy in BMI.

Understanding these socio-economic factors is crucial for developing targeted interventions and policies to address the conundrum and improve public health outcomes.

6. Role of psychological stress in BMI

The allostatic load model of chronic stress emphasizes the role of glucocorticoid dysregulation within a "network of allostasis" that includes autonomic, endocrine, metabolic, and immune mediators [25].

6.1 Stress and weight gain

Chronic stress can lead to weight gain through various mechanisms, including increased cortisol production and stress-induced eating behaviors.

This may contribute to the development of overweight or mild obesity in some individuals. Living in stressful environments can lead to the development of different physical characteristics. Individuals known as "non-habituals," who encounter such environments, tend to develop a "lean-but-wide-waisted" body type, which is associated with a high risk of cardiovascular mortality. On the other hand, "habituators" in similar conditions tend to develop a "corpulent-but -narrow-waisted" body type, which is linked to a lower risk of cardiovascular mortality [25]. Additionally, there are also transitional or mixed body types.

Stress reactivity exhibits differential modifications, categorizing individuals into "habituators" and "non-habituators." "Habituators" are characterized by a reduced response (neuroendocrine, cardiovascular, neuroenergetic, and emotional) due to repeated exposure to a threatening environment, ultimately developing low stress reactivity. Conversely, "non-habituation" maintains high stress reactivity, as they do not exhibit such response modifications under continuous exposure to unsafe conditions. Empirical evidence from repeated experimental stress challenges indicates that subjects may habituate or fail to habituate in their cortisol response [26].

6.2 Stress resilience

Individuals with higher psychological resilience tend to have a higher BMI, while those with lower resilience scores are more likely to be underweight, particularly among women. This underscores the intricate relationship between psychological resilience and weight management, highlighting the need for specific interventions to address the varied effects of psychological factors on weight outcomes [27].

6.3 Metabolic adaptations

Chronic stress exposure may lead to metabolic adaptations in individuals with higher BMI, potentially offering protective effects against certain health risks, as explained earlier as "habituators."

6.4 Inflammation and stress

Obesity is associated with chronic low-grade inflammation, which may interact with stress responses in complex ways. This interaction could potentially modulate health outcomes in overweight or mildly obese individuals.

Often assessed through C-reactive protein (CRP) indicators, inflammation can significantly influence health outcomes. Research indicates that the beneficial effect of a higher BMI might only be apparent in those with increased inflammation levels. A higher BMI may not offer the same survival benefits without inflammation and could be linked to worse outcomes [28].

6.5 Psychosocial factors

Overweight individuals may face various social pressures and expectations. These factors can affect their stress levels and health behaviors, possibly contributing to the observed health disparity outcomes.

6.6 Stress and disease progression

Psychological stress can influence the progression and outcomes of different medical conditions. The connection between stress, BMI, and disease outcomes may help clarify the anomalous findings in specific patient groups.

6.7 Neuroendocrine responses

Variations in neuroendocrine responses to stress between normal-weight and overweight individuals may play a role in this discrepancy. These differences could impact health outcomes across various medical conditions.

More research is necessary to better understand the role of psychological stress in impacting BMI and its implications for clinical practice and public health efforts.

7. Eating disorders and the BMI

People with obesity have a higher risk of developing eating disorders (EDs), such as binge eating disorder (BED), bulimia nervosa (BN), and other specified feeding or eating disorders (OSFED). These disorders are typically associated with:

1. **Compensatory behaviors**: Some people with obesity may resort to compensatory actions, such as restricting calories or exercising excessively, to cope with feelings of guilt or shame about their weight.

2. **Loss of control**: Individuals with BED or BN often feel a loss of control over their food intake, which societal expectations regarding weight and body shape can worsen.

Understanding EDs in the context of BMI disparity requires a deeper grasp of the complex relationships among weight, body image, and mental health. Here are several important points to consider:

1. **Reframing ED beyond mere weight measurement**: EDs go beyond simple weight loss or gain. They are complex mental health issues marked by disordered eating patterns, body image concerns, and emotional regulation difficulties.

2. **Weight-inclusive perspective**: Focusing on the person's relationship with food and their body is crucial rather than focusing only on weight-related outcomes.

3. **Intersection of trauma, mental health, and weight**: Recognizing that EDs often coexist with other mental health issues (such as depression and anxiety) is important. They may also arise from traumatic experiences or societal pressures.

4. **Societal expectations around body shape and size**: Acknowledging how societal norms about thinness, beauty standards, and weight affect EDs is vital.

5. **Weight-related stigma and shame**: Individuals with higher BMIs may experience internalized shame, low self-esteem, anxiety, and depression due to societal expectations regarding beauty standards.

6. **Disordered eating behaviors as coping mechanisms**: It is important to understand how some people may use disordered eating behaviors (like restrictive eating and bingeing) to cope with stress, emotions, or body image issues.

7. **A weight-inclusive, trauma-informed approach focuses on overall health and well-being:** It emphasizes meeting a person's physical and mental health needs, rather than just pursuing weight loss. It also provides a safe, nonjudgmental environment for individuals to share their experiences while recognizing the possible effects of trauma on eating habits and body image. Lastly, fostering cooperation among healthcare providers, mental health professionals, and other experts is essential for comprehensive care.

8. Body positivity movement

The body positivity movement is an important social and cultural movement advocating for acceptance, self-love, and inclusivity across various body shapes, sizes, ages, abilities, and appearances. In the context of BMI disparity, body positivity plays a key role in addressing the complex interactions between weight, health, and body image [29].

Key aspects of the impact of the body positivity movement include:

1. **Challenging weight stigma**: The movement aims to decrease weight-based discrimination and stigma, which can have harmful effects on mental health. Promoting acceptance of all body types may help lessen the adverse psychological effects linked to weight stigma.

2. **Improving body image and self-esteem**: The movement encourages people to value their bodies, regardless of size or shape. This can lead to a better body image and higher self-esteem, which may help protect against mental health issues that often accompany poor body image.

3. **Shifting focus from weight to overall health**: Body positivity promotes a broader view of health, highlighting factors beyond BMI or weight. This

perspective acknowledges that health outcomes are not determined solely by body size.

4. **Promoting health-seeking behaviors**: By reducing shame and stigma surrounding body size, the movement may encourage individuals to pursue health-promoting actions and seek medical help without fear of judgment.

5. **Addressing disordered eating**: Body positivity can help prevent the development of disordered eating patterns by fostering a healthier relationship with food and body image.

6. **Influencing healthcare practices**: The movement has generated discussions about weight bias in healthcare, potentially leading to more compassionate and effective care for people across the weight spectrum.

7. **Mental health resilience**: By promoting self-acceptance and community support, body positivity may enhance mental health resilience, affecting how individuals navigate health challenges, regardless of their BMI.

8. **Intersectionality**: The movement recognizes the connections between body size and other identity factors, such as race, gender, and disability, promoting a more detailed understanding of health and well-being.

9. **Media representation**: Increased visibility of diverse body types in the media can help normalize body diversity and ease the psychological pressure to fit unrealistic ideals.

10. **Stress reduction**: By encouraging self-acceptance, body positivity may help decrease chronic stress related to body dissatisfaction, potentially influencing the complex interactions between stress, weight, and health observed in the BMI disparity.

While the body positivity movement offers many potential benefits, its influence on BMI is complex and not entirely understood. More research is needed to clarify how changing societal views on body size and promoting body positivity affect the relationship between BMI and health outcomes [30]. Additionally, critics argue that the movement should not dissuade individuals from engaging in health-promoting activities or seeking medical help when necessary.

In summary, the body positivity movement changes how we view body size and health. It emphasizes acceptance, mental well-being, and overall health. This disparity in BMI shows that we need a deeper understanding of how body size, mental health, and physical health are connected.

9. Conclusion

The discrepancy in BMI in different groups highlights the complicated relationship between body weight, health outcomes, and mental well-being. This phenomenon challenges the traditional view of obesity and points to the need for a more detailed approach to health assessment. Various factors, such as weight stigma, cognitive biases, cultural views, socioeconomic elements, psychological stress, and EDs, all influence the discrepancy.

Weight stigma significantly affects mental health and potentially leads to stress, anxiety, and depression. Cognitive biases in interpreting BMI can result in misdiagnosis and inappropriate treatment choices. Cultural and economic factors greatly influence how people view body weight and health. Stress affects BMI in many ways; it can protect some people but increase health risks for others. The link between EDs and obesity makes the BMI issue more complex. This highlights the need for a treatment approach that considers trauma and includes all body types.

The body positivity movement has arisen as a response to these challenges, promoting acceptance and inclusion among various body types. While it offers potential mental health and self-esteem benefits, more research is required to understand its effects on physical health outcomes.

The BMI disparity emphasizes the importance of a comprehensive and individualized approach to health assessment and treatment. Future research should aim to develop more precise health measures beyond BMI and explore the intricate connections between physical and mental well-being. Healthcare professionals must understand these complexities to provide effective, compassionate care addressing health and body weight.

Acknowledgments

I acknowledge using AI (Paperpal) for literature search and "Grammarly" software for language editing.

I acknowledge "SUN PHARMACEUTICALS (SYNASTRA)" for sponsoring the chapter processing charges.

Conflict of interest

The authors declare no conflicts of interest.

Author details

Stephen Amarjeet Jiwanmall* and Dheeraj Kattula
Department of Psychiatry, Christian Medical College, Vellore, India

*Address all correspondence to: stephenjiwanmall@yahoo.com; stephen76@cmcvellore.ac.in

References

[1] AMA. Use of BMI alone is an imperfect clinical measure. American Medical Association [Internet]. Available from: https://www.ama-assn.org/delivering-care/public-health/ama-use-bmi-alone-imperfect-clinical-measure [Accessed: 2025-July-9]

[2] Callahan, Emily A. National Academies of Sciences E, Division H, M BF, N SROO, Callahan EA the science, strengths, and limitations of body mass index. In: Translating Knowledge of Foundational Drivers of Obesity into Practice: Proceedings of a Workshop Series. ; National Academies Press (US); 2023. Available from: https://www.ncbi.nlm.nih.gov/books/NBK594362/ [Accessed: 2025-July-9]

[3] Rm P. Weight stigma and barriers to effective obesity care. Gastroenterology Clinics of North America. 2023;**52** (2):418–424 Available from: https://pubmed.ncbi.nlm.nih.gov/37197883/

[4] Rr B. Weight stigma and bias: Standards of care in overweight and obesity-2025. BMJ Open Diabetes Research & Care. 2025;**13**(Suppl 1):2–6 Available from: https://pubmed.ncbi.nlm.nih.gov/40379436/

[5] Rm P, Ms H, Rl P. Weight stigma as a psychosocial contributor to obesity. The American Psychologist. 2020;**75** (2):274–289 Available from: https://pubmed.ncbi.nlm.nih.gov/32053000/

[6] Jm H, and Brenda M. Weight stigma mediates the association between BMI and self-reported health. Health Psychology : Official Journal of the Division of Health Psychology, American Psychological Association. 2015;**34**(2):172–175 Available from: https://pubmed.ncbi.nlm.nih.gov/25133837/

[7] Tomiyama AJ, Carr D, Granberg EM, Major B, Robinson E, Sutin AR, et al. How and why weight stigma drives the obesity 'epidemic' and harms health. BMC Medicine. 2018;**16**:123

[8] Sa J, K D, Mb N, P S, K R, J F, et al. Weight stigma in patients with obesity and its clinical correlates: A perspective from an indian bariatric clinic. Cureus. 2022;**14** 2–7. Available from: https://pubmed.ncbi.nlm.nih.gov/35974866/

[9] Rubino F, Cummings DE, Eckel RH, Cohen RV, Wilding JPH, Brown WA, et al. Definition and diagnostic criteria of clinical obesity. The Lancet Diabetes & Endocrinology. 2025;**13**:221–262

[10] Guglielmi G. New obesity definition sidelines BMI to focus on health. Nature. 2025;**637**(8047):773–774

[11] Saposnik G, Redelmeier D, Ruff CC. Cognitive biases associated with medical decisions: A systematic review. BMC Medical Informatics and Decision Making. 2025. Available from: https://bmcmedinformdecismak.biomedcentral.com/articles/10.1186/s12911-016-0377-1

[12] Yale medicine [Internet]. Why You Shouldn't Rely on BMI Alone. Available from: https://www.yalemedicine.org/news/why-you-shouldnt-rely-on-bmi-alone [Accessed: 2025-July-21]

[13] Puhl RM, Phelan SM, Nadglowski J, Kyle TK. Overcoming weight bias in the

management of patients with diabetes and obesity. Clinical Diabetes. 2016;**34** (1):44–50

[14] Fruh SM, Graves RJ, Hauff C, Williams SG, Hall HR. Weight bias and stigma. Nursing Clinics of North America. 2021;**56**(4):479–493

[15] Westbury S, Oyebode O, van Rens T, Barber TM. Obesity stigma: Causes, consequences, and potential solutions. Current Obesity Reports. 2023;**12**(1):10–23

[16] Brown A, Flint SW, Batterham RL. Pervasiveness, impact and implications of weight stigma. eClinicalMedicine. 2022;**47**:101408

[17] Ra C, R J, T M, B J, Kb A, C N, et al. Influencing weight bias: The impact of biased questionnaire anchors on stereotype beliefs and judgments. Obesity Research & Clinical Practice. 2015;**9**. Available from: https://pubmed.ncbi.nlm.nih.gov/25726506/

[18] Biases in obesity research: Identify, correct, endorse, or abandon effort? - Ioannidis - 2016 - Obesity - Wiley Online Library [Internet]. Available from: https://onlinelibrary.wiley.com/doi/full/10.1002/oby.21457 [Accessed: 2025-July-21]

[19] Bannuru RR. Weight stigma and bias: Standards of care in overweight and obesity—2025. BMJ Open Diabetes Research & Care. 2025;**13**(Suppl 1): e004962 Available from: https://drc.bmj.com/content/13/Suppl_1/e004962

[20] Lee A, Cardel M, Donahoo WT. Social and environmental factors influencing obesity. In: Feingold KR, Ahmed SF, Anawalt B, Blackman MR, Boyce A, Chrousos G, et al. editors. Endotext. South Dartmouth (MA): MDText.com, Inc; 2000. p. 25. Available from: http://www.ncbi.nlm.nih.gov/books/NBK278977/

[21] Naigaga DA, Jahanlu D, Claudius HM, Gjerlaug AK, Barikmo I, Henjum S. Body size perceptions and preferences favor overweight in adult Saharawi refugees. Nutrition Journal. 2018;**17**:17

[22] Beyond BMI. Exploring obesity trends in the south Asian region. Obesity Pillars. 2025;**13**:100156

[23] L C, Z Z, W B, M T, L C, Z X. Global health impacts of high BMI: A 30-Year analysis of trends and disparities across regions and Demographics. Diabetes Research and Clinical Practice. 2024;**217**. Available from: https://pubmed.ncbi.nlm.nih.gov/39368489/

[24] Azizi Fard N, De Francisci Morales G, Mejova Y, Schifanella R. On the interplay between educational attainment and nutrition: A spatially-aware perspective. EPJ Data Science. 2021;**10**(1):1–21

[25] Peters A, McEwen BS. Stress habituation, body shape and cardiovascular mortality. Neuroscience & Biobehavioral Reviews. 2015; **56**:139–150

[26] Kirschbaum C, Prussner JC, Stone AA, Federenko I, Gaab J, Lintz D, et al. Persistent high cortisol responses to repeated psychological stress in a subpopulation of healthy men. Biopsychosocial Science and Medicine. 1995;**57**:468

[27] Zheng N, Zhuang M, Zhu Y, Wang Y, Ye M, Zhang Y, et al. Association between psychological

resilience and body mass index in a community-based population: A cross-sectional study. Obesity Science & Practice. 2024;**10**:e761

[28] Drechsler C, Wanner C. The obesity paradox and the role of inflammation. Journal of the American Society of Nephrology. 2016;**27**(5):1270

[29] Cohen R, Irwin L, Newton-John T, Slater A. #bodypositivity: A content analysis of body positive accounts on Instagram. Body Image. 2019;**29**:47–57

[30] Harriger JA, Wick MR, Sherline CM, Kunz AL. The body positivity movement is not all that positive on TikTok: A content analysis of body positive TikTok videos. Body Image. 2023;**46**:256–264

Chapter 8

Psychiatric, Behavioral, and Familial Risk Factors in Adolescent BMI

Esen Öksüzoğlu Makbule

Abstract

This chapter examines the psychiatric and psychological mechanisms underlying elevated BMI in adolescents, emphasizing the contribution of internalizing disorders (such as anxiety and depression), emotion dysregulation, and related psychopathological traits. These conditions not only co-occur with excess weight but may also act as driving forces through maladaptive coping strategies and altered reward sensitivity. In particular, impulsivity and disordered eating behaviors – including emotional, external, and restrictive eating – are highlighted as core behavioral risk factors. Moreover, maternal characteristics, such as impulsivity, psychological distress, and problematic eating attitudes, significantly shape adolescents' emotional and behavioral responses to food, often through intergenerational pathways such as modeling and emotion contagion. Framed within developmental psychopathology and family systems theory, this chapter calls for psychobehavioral risk screening in obesity assessments and underscores the need for culturally sensitive, family-based interventions tailored to address both psychological vulnerability and obesogenic dynamics in the home environment.

Keywords: psychopathology, eating behaviors, impulsivity, emotion regulation, intergenerational transmission, adolescent obesity, body mass index, internalizing symptoms, maternal influences

1. Introduction

Adolescent obesity has become a critical and pressing public health concern worldwide. According to the World Health Organization, the prevalence of obesity among children and adolescents aged 5–19 increased from 4% in 1975 to more than 18% in 2016 [1]. More recent meta-analytic evidence indicates that one in five young people now live with overweight or obesity, with prevalence rates particularly high in high-income countries [2]. Adolescent obesity is associated with a broad spectrum of adverse outcomes, including metabolic complications leading to increased mortality and an elevated risk of psychiatric disorders, particularly internalizing disorders such as depression and anxiety.

While obesity is medically defined using age- and sex-specific BMI percentiles, this definition only captures the physical manifestation of a broader, multifactorial condition. Beyond caloric imbalance, adolescent obesity reflects the interplay of psychological traits, neurobiological mechanisms, and familial environments [3]. Traits such as impulsivity, difficulties in emotion regulation, and internalizing symptoms are strongly implicated in unhealthy weight trajectories [4, 5]. Disordered eating behaviors – including emotional eating, external eating, and binge eating – often serve as maladaptive coping strategies, reinforcing the cycle of distress and weight gain [6]. Neurobiological findings support this perspective, with evidence pointing to altered stress reactivity, reduced inhibitory control, and heightened reward sensitivity as underlying mechanisms [6, 7].

Psychological vulnerabilities seldom operate in isolation. Family dynamics, particularly maternal psychological distress and disordered eating, also shape adolescents' emotional development and eating behaviors [8, 9]. Maternal modeling and feeding practices provide important pathways through which risks may be transmitted across generations, although these influences interact with broader social and cultural factors.

In sum, these findings highlight adolescent obesity as a developmentally embedded and psychologically mediated condition. The following sections synthesize evidence on psychiatric, behavioral, and familial risk factors, with particular attention to intergenerational processes. Particular attention will be given to psychosocial factors such as self-esteem and body image, as these represent crucial pathways linking obesity with long-term psychological adjustment.

2. Psychiatric risk factors and related disorders

A growing body of evidence highlights the close and bidirectional relationship between psychiatric disorders and obesity in adolescence. Rather than a simple cause–and–effect relationship, these conditions often codevelop and reinforce one another through intertwined psychological, behavioral, and biological mechanisms [10–12]. Psychiatric conditions may predispose adolescents to obesity by fostering maladaptive coping strategies such as emotional eating, avoidance, or reduced physical activity. Psychotropic medications – including antidepressants, antipsychotics, and mood stabilizers – can further contribute to weight gain [13]. Conversely, the psychosocial burden of obesity – marked by weight stigma, discrimination, and body dissatisfaction – has been consistently associated with depression, anxiety, and other internalizing symptoms [14, 15].

This reciprocal interplay illustrates obesity as both a potential cause and consequence of psychiatric disorders. Adolescents with obesity are at increased risk of peer victimization and social exclusion, processes that erode self-esteem and exacerbate internalizing distress. At the same time, psychiatric symptoms disrupt healthy routines around diet, sleep, and physical activity, creating a self-reinforcing cycle of psychological and physical health problems. As noted earlier, adolescence may represent a particularly sensitive period, as rapid biological changes intersect with increasing social pressures. Identifying and addressing psychiatric comorbidities is therefore essential not only for improving mental health but also for enhancing the effectiveness of weight-related interventions.

2.1 Eating disorders

Among psychiatric comorbidities, eating disorders show the most direct overlap with adolescent obesity. Binge eating disorder (BED) is the most prevalent form, characterized by recurrent episodes of uncontrolled food intake, often triggered by emotional distress, and strongly associated with obesity [16, 17]. Estimates suggest that up to 40–70% of individuals with BED also meet the criteria for obesity [18]. Bulimia nervosa (BN), although less frequent, contributes to weight dysregulation through cycles of restrictive dieting, binge eating, and compensatory behaviors such as vomiting or excessive exercise [19]. Night eating syndrome (NES) is also more common in youth with obesity, with prevalence rates between 6% and 16% [20, 21]. NES is frequently comorbid with depressive symptoms, compounding the psychological burden [22, 23].

Despite distinct clinical features, these disorders share common mechanisms with obesity – particularly body dissatisfaction, low self-esteem, and reliance on food as an emotion-regulation strategy [24]. As discussed earlier, this overlap suggests that obesity and eating disorders represent points on a spectrum of disordered eating [25]. Clinically, this underscores the need for integrated interventions combining nutritional guidance with psychotherapy – including cognitive-behavioral and family-based therapies – which are more effective than dietary strategies alone in reducing both weight and psychiatric symptoms [26].

2.2 Mood disorders

Mood disorders, particularly major depressive disorder (MDD) and bipolar affective disorder (BD), are associated with obesity. Longitudinal studies show that adolescents with MDD have up to a 50% greater risk of developing obesity, while childhood depression predicts higher BMI in adulthood [27, 28]. Atypical depressive features – hypersomnia, increased appetite, rejection sensitivity – are especially linked to excess weight [29, 30]. The relationship between obesity and BD is similarly complex. Adolescents with BD and obesity often present more severe depressive episodes, longer illness duration, and poorer treatment response. Obesity has also been linked to higher hospitalization rates and reduced efficacy of mood stabilizers, particularly lithium and valproate [31, 32]. Depression itself can undermine behavioral and pharmacological weight loss efforts, perpetuating obesity [33].

Shared mechanisms – such as HPA axis dysregulation, low-grade inflammation, and metabolic disturbances – appear common to both obesity and mood disorders [34]. Genetic vulnerabilities, including variants of the fat mass and obesity-associated (FTO) gene, predispose individuals to both higher BMI and depression [35]. Environmental stressors, including childhood adversity and maternal depression, further amplify risk [36]. Recent neuroimaging studies suggest that obesity may exacerbate structural brain changes in BD, particularly white matter disruptions, whereas lithium appears to mitigate these effects [37].

When considered together, these findings highlight the bidirectional and multifactorial nature of the obesity–mood disorder relationship, underscoring the need for integrated biopsychosocial interventions.

2.3 Anxiety disorders

Anxiety disorders, including social anxiety disorder (SAD), panic disorder (PD), specific phobias, and generalized anxiety disorder (GAD) – are consistently more prevalent in adolescents with obesity [10, 38]. Psychosocial mechanisms include weight stigma, teasing, and exclusion, which foster anxiety symptoms; conversely, anxiety may promote maladaptive coping, such as emotional eating, avoidance of physical activity, and sedentary behaviors [39]. Sex-specific trends have been observed: girls with obesity are more likely to develop SAD, GAD, and specific phobias, whereas boys show higher rates of PD [40]. Longitudinal studies confirm that childhood obesity increases the risk of anxiety disorders later in life, with stronger effects in females. As discussed earlier, stigma and body dissatisfaction are likely key psychological mediators of this link.

Shared biological mechanisms – such as HPA axis dysregulation, autonomic hyperarousal, and systemic inflammation – further explain the overlap between obesity and anxiety [41]. Beyond anxiety disorders, obsessive–compulsive disorder (OCD) and posttraumatic stress disorder (PTSD) have also been associated with higher obesity risk, potentially through compulsive eating rituals, stress-related hormonal changes, and sleep disruption [42].

Overall, these findings highlight the importance of early screening and treatment of anxiety symptoms in adolescents with obesity. Interventions that concurrently address anxiety and weight-related behaviors may prevent the escalation of self-reinforcing cycles of distress and maladaptive coping.

2.4 Attention-deficit/hyperactivity disorder (ADHD)

ADHD is increasingly recognized as an important risk factor for obesity. Core features such as impulsivity, inattention, and executive dysfunction undermine eating regulation, adherence to routines, and engagement in physical activity [43]. Meta-analyses suggest that youth with ADHD are approximately 40% more likely to develop obesity [44]. Binge and emotional eating are particularly common in this group, reflecting shared deficits in impulse control and reward processing [45]. Disrupted sleep, also frequent in ADHD, compounds these risks by altering appetite-regulating hormones and circadian rhythms. In turn, obesity can exacerbate ADHD-related impairments, including attention difficulties and executive dysfunction, creating a vicious cycle.

Neurobiological research suggests that shared dopaminergic dysfunction underlies both impulsivity and heightened food cue sensitivity [44]. Importantly, ADHD and obesity may also exhibit common developmental origins in early self-regulation difficulties, echoing themes discussed earlier regarding impulsivity and emotion dysregulation. Medication effects add complexity: stimulants often suppress appetite, whereas adjunctive antipsychotics or mood stabilizers may promote significant weight gain. Longitudinal findings indicate that inconsistent medication use, combined with poor sleep and impulsive eating, may heighten obesity risk over time.

In summary, ADHD contributes to obesity through behavioral dysregulation, neurobiological vulnerability, and treatment-related factors. Interventions should, therefore, integrate training in impulse control, structured daily routines, sleep hygiene, and careful pharmacological monitoring. Embedding these strategies within family-based approaches may improve both weight and psychiatric outcomes.

3. Behavioral and psychological risk factors

Adolescent obesity cannot be fully explained by caloric imbalance alone. A substantial body of research highlights the role of behavioral and psychological processes – particularly disordered eating behaviors, impulsivity, emotion dysregulation, internalizing symptoms, and self-esteem and body image disturbances – as critical drivers of elevated BMI [46–48]. These vulnerabilities often co-occur, creating reinforcing cycles of emotional distress, maladaptive eating, and weight gain. Importantly, they reflect developmental challenges in self-regulation, identity formation, and coping, which are shaped by both individual traits and family environments.

A wide range of studies further underscores these mechanisms. Disordered eating behaviors, such as emotional eating, external eating, night eating, and eating in the absence of hunger (EAH), consistently predict the onset and persistence of obesity and are linked to later eating disorders [46, 49]. Impulsivity, marked by difficulties with inhibitory control and delayed gratification, increases susceptibility to overeating in emotionally charged or cue-rich contexts and interacts with emotional distress to accelerate dysregulated eating [4, 50]. Emotion regulation problems often precede weight gain, with poor early self-regulation predicting higher BMI in adolescence; youth with obesity also rely more on maladaptive strategies like rumination or avoidance while underusing adaptive strategies such as cognitive reappraisal [51–53]. Internalizing symptoms, particularly anxiety and depression, are highly comorbid with obesity and show a bidirectional relationship, as demonstrated in longitudinal and cross-lagged studies [54, 55]. Finally, low self-esteem and negative body image emerge as salient vulnerabilities: stigma, bullying, and social comparison pressures erode self-worth, reinforce maladaptive eating, and predict long-term psychological distress and persistent obesity [56, 57].

All in all, behavioral and psychological risk factors constitute a closely interconnected system that sustains obesity across adolescence, underscoring the need to address not only caloric intake but also self-regulation, emotional well-being, self-esteem, and family dynamics in prevention and treatment efforts.

3.1 Disordered eating behaviors

Disordered eating behaviors encompass a spectrum of maladaptive eating patterns that do not always meet the criteria for clinical eating disorders but still carry significant risks for both weight gain and psychological distress [46, 47]. These behaviors are particularly prevalent among adolescents with elevated BMI and are recognized as central mechanisms in the onset and persistence of obesity. Importantly, they often emerge as coping responses to negative emotions or environmental cues and can serve as precursors to more severe eating disorders in later adolescence [49].

Several dimensions of disordered eating hold particular relevance in adolescence. Emotional eating – the tendency to eat in response to sadness, anxiety, or loneliness rather than hunger – has long been recognized as a strong predictor of weight gain and is closely associated with emotion regulation difficulties and internalizing symptoms [58, 59]. External eating, in contrast, describes eating prompted by sensory cues such as the sight or smell of food, a pattern especially common in obesogenic environments saturated with high-calorie options [60]. Restrained eating refers to deliberate attempts to control food intake to manage weight; paradoxically, excessive restraint often leads to heightened preoccupation with food and eventual overeating [61, 62].

Other patterns further illustrate the complexity of disordered eating. Loss-of-control eating involves a subjective inability to stop eating, typically accompanied by guilt and shame, and is closely tied to impulsivity and mood disturbances [63]. NES, characterized by excessive evening or nocturnal food intake, has been linked to circadian rhythm disruption, poor sleep, and depressive symptoms [64]. Similarly, EAH refers to food intake despite satiety, often reflecting poor interoceptive awareness and family patterns that encourage eating as a coping mechanism [59]. Finally, the construct of food addiction – though not formally recognized in DSM-5 [65] – has gained increasing attention. It describes addictive-like responses to highly processed foods and has been associated with impulsivity, low self-esteem, depression, and anxiety [66, 67].

These behaviors rarely emerge in isolation. Longitudinal studies suggest that exposure to parental emotional eating, inconsistent family routines, or the use of food as a coping strategy fosters the development of similar maladaptive patterns in children [68, 69]. Biological mechanisms provide additional insight: alterations in the HPA axis have been associated with stress-induced cravings and atypical hunger cues, reinforcing links between emotional distress and overeating [70]. Although often considered subclinical, disordered eating behaviors are associated with significant psychological burden, increased risk of eating disorder onset, metabolic complications, and resistance to conventional weight-loss interventions [59]. For this reason, early recognition and intervention are critical. Programs that strengthen emotion regulation, impulse control, interoceptive awareness, and structured family routines have shown effectiveness in disrupting maladaptive eating cycles [71]. By addressing the underlying emotional and behavioral drivers of disordered eating, prevention and treatment approaches can more effectively mitigate both the psychological and metabolic consequences of adolescent obesity.

3.2 Impulsivity and self-regulation

Impulsivity, broadly defined as a tendency to act quickly without adequate forethought, has emerged as a central transdiagnostic psychological risk factor in adolescent obesity. Adolescents with elevated impulsivity often exhibit difficulties in delayed gratification, motor inhibition, and emotional regulation in stressful contexts [50]. These difficulties increase vulnerability to overeating, preference for calorie-dense foods, and challenges in maintaining structured routines that support healthy weight control [4]. Recent evidence indicates that impulsivity is not only associated with unhealthy eating behaviors but also predicts BMI trajectories. In a structural equation modeling study, impulsivity emerged as one of the strongest predictors of adolescent BMI, both directly and indirectly through disordered eating patterns [72]. Similarly, population-based studies have shown that impulsivity traits, such as disinhibition and impulsive decision-making, are linked with higher snack consumption and reduced dietary restraint [73].

Impulsivity further undermines the effectiveness of weight management interventions. In a longitudinal study, obese children with higher impulsivity were less likely to achieve sustained weight loss and more prone to relapse following behavioral treatment, underscoring the importance of self-regulatory capacities in sustaining behavioral change [74]. Neuroimaging research further supports these findings, with adolescents with obesity frequently showing altered activation in reward- and control-related brain regions, particularly the orbitofrontal cortex and striatum. These alterations may explain heightened responsiveness to palatable foods and reduced inhibitory control [6, 75]. Importantly, impulsivity seldom operates in isolation. It frequently co-occurs with emotion dysregulation, anxiety, and depressive symptoms, creating a cumulative burden on psychological functioning. Environmental stressors, such as family conflict or inconsistent parenting, may exacerbate impulsive tendencies by limiting opportunities to practice self-regulation [4]. Intergenerational studies also demonstrate that parental – particularly maternal – impulsivity is correlated with adolescents' impulsivity and BMI, suggesting the joint influence of genetic predispositions and modeling processes [9].

Overall, impulsivity represents a transdiagnostic vulnerability that bridges psychological, neurobiological, and familial risk pathways. Interventions targeting impulse control and executive functioning – such as cognitive training, behavioral reinforcement, and mindfulness-based approaches – are promising in mitigating its negative impact. Moreover, structuring home and school environments to reduce exposure to high-calorie food cues and promote structured daily routines can support adolescents in strengthening regulatory skills. Addressing both individual traits and family dynamics is, therefore, essential for improving the effectiveness of obesity prevention and treatment strategies in this vulnerable group.

3.3 Internalizing symptoms

The association between elevated BMI and internalizing symptoms, such as anxiety and depression, has been widely documented, with both conditions representing significant contributors to adolescent morbidity [55]. Importantly, these associations do not emerge uniformly across development but become increasingly pronounced from middle childhood into adolescence. For example, data from the UK Millennium Cohort Study demonstrated that, while obesity and internalizing problems rarely co-occur in early childhood, they increasingly converge during adolescence, with obesity nearly doubling the risk of depressive and anxious symptoms by age 14 [54]. This convergence reflects bidirectional influences. Cross-lagged longitudinal models suggest that higher BMI in childhood predicts subsequent increases in depressive symptoms, whereas adolescent psychological distress predicts later weight gain [54]. These pathways remain significant even after controlling for socioeconomic adversity, suggesting that both environmental stressors and direct psychosocial mechanisms contribute to the reciprocal link.

Disordered eating behaviors are key mediators of this association. Early signs – such as calorie restriction, binge eating, or excessive exercise – often emerge in preadolescence and strongly predict both later eating disorder onset and emotional difficulties [49, 76, 77]. Rather than being transient, these behaviors tend to persist and escalate, reinforcing cycles of distress and weight gain. Shared vulnerabilities, including maladaptive coping strategies, anxiety sensitivity, and harm-avoidant cognitions, help explain why internalizing symptoms and disordered eating frequently co-occur [78, 79]. Social and cultural processes further intensify these risks. Experiences of weight-based stigma and peer exclusion are strongly associated with depressive symptoms, with body dissatisfaction emerging as a central mediator [80, 81]. Attempts to control weight through dieting often exacerbate psychological distress, as cycles of dietary restraint and failure undermine mood and self-esteem, increasing vulnerability to both depression and disordered eating [82, 83].

Biological mechanisms complement these psychosocial pathways. Dysregulation of the HPA axis, alterations in stress-related metabolic processes, and heightened inflammatory responses have all been implicated in linking obesity with internalizing psychopathology [84]. Genetic studies similarly point to shared heritability between depression, anxiety, and disordered eating, reinforcing the view of overlapping vulnerability pathways [85].

In summary, internalizing symptoms are not merely secondary outcomes of obesity but integral to its developmental and psychosocial context. From preadolescence onward, obesity and emotional disorders increasingly codevelop, sustained by cycles of stigma, body dissatisfaction, disordered eating, and maladaptive coping. Preventive interventions that integrate weight-related and psychological components – by enhancing emotion regulation skills, reducing stigma, and supporting adaptive coping – may help disrupt these reinforcing cycles and improve both mental health and weight outcomes [49, 54].

3.4 Self-esteem and body image

Low self-esteem and body dissatisfaction, which are closely related to internalizing difficulties, represent particularly salient psychosocial vulnerabilities in adolescents with obesity. Large-scale studies consistently demonstrate that overweight and obese youth report lower levels of self-esteem compared to their normal-weight peers, with adolescent girls disproportionately affected [56]. Low self-esteem not only contributes to negative body image but also predicts depressive symptoms, frequently driving maladaptive coping strategies such as emotional or binge eating [57]. This cycle of negative affect, overeating, and subsequent weight gain reinforces the reciprocal relationship between obesity and psychological distress. Population-based surveys provide further nuance. In an Australian cohort, obese children reported significantly lower competence across domains such as athletic performance and physical appearance, with obese girls being particularly vulnerable: two-thirds reported low appearance competence, and one in five endorsed low global self-worth [56]. Longitudinal studies confirm that childhood obesity nearly doubles the risk of developing low self-esteem in adolescence, even after accounting for baseline levels of self-esteem and other confounders [57]. These findings highlight how weight problems exert long-term developmental effects on adolescents' self-concept.

The developmental trajectory of self-esteem also plays a critical role in later psychological outcomes. Prospective research has shown that self-perceived attractiveness and social popularity in early adolescence serve as protective factors against disordered eating in young adulthood, whereas peer-rated likability was unexpectedly associated with increased vulnerability, underscoring that not all social evaluations function as protective influences [86]. Such findings suggest that specific self-esteem domains may be more predictive of subsequent maladaptive outcomes than global self-esteem alone. Cultural and social processes magnify these risks.

Adolescents with obesity are frequently subjected to teasing, bullying, and stigma – experiences that erode self-worth and heighten body dissatisfaction. Social comparison processes – especially in peer and media environments that idealize thinness and emphasize appearance – further exacerbate these vulnerabilities, fostering maladaptive eating behaviors and negative self-image. Over time, chronic exposure to such pressures has been shown to predict poorer mental health, reduced quality of life, and the persistence of obesity into adulthood [56, 86].

These findings underscore the importance of interventions directly addressing self-esteem and body image in the prevention and treatment of adolescent obesity. Programs that foster resilience, promote positive body image, and reduce weight-related stigma – particularly when implemented in school, family, and community contexts – are especially promising. When combined with behavioral and nutritional support, such approaches not only promote psychological well-being but also enhance the effectiveness of obesity prevention and treatment efforts.

3.5 Emotion regulation difficulties

Self-esteem and body image reflect the social-cognitive aspects of adolescent vulnerability, whereas emotion regulation difficulties underscore the affective and self-regulatory processes through which distress contributes to maladaptive eating. Emotion regulation refers to the capacity to monitor, evaluate, and modify emotional experiences, and deficits in this domain have been consistently identified as transdiagnostic risk factors for both obesity and associated psychopathology [52, 87]. Adolescents with overweight and obesity, particularly those who engage in binge or emotional eating, often struggle to identify, express, and manage emotions effectively [88]. Importantly, these difficulties are not merely secondary to excess weight but often originate early in development. For example, toddlers with poor self-regulation skills are more likely to develop higher BMI later in childhood [51], and maternal emotional dysregulation during pregnancy has been linked to obesity risk and disordered eating in offspring by preschool age [89]. Such findings suggest that emotion regulation difficulties represent early developmental vulnerabilities that contribute to later weight problems. In adolescence, reliance on maladaptive coping strategies such as rumination, suppression, or avoidance is particularly common, while adaptive strategies – such as cognitive reappraisal or problem-solving – are underutilized [90]. This reliance not only increases the likelihood of emotional eating in the short term but also heightens vulnerability to depressive and anxious symptoms, thereby reinforcing cycles of psychological distress and weight gain [53].

Neurobiological evidence complements these psychosocial findings. HPA axis dysregulation and heightened cortisol reactivity to stress have been associated with increased hunger and food cravings, contrary to normative stress responses, which typically involve appetite suppression [91]. In addition, deficits in interoceptive awareness – difficulty recognizing internal cues such as hunger and satiety – have been consistently observed among adolescents with obesity, further increasing vulnerability to emotional eating [92, 93]. Family and environmental contexts significantly influence these regulatory difficulties. Children exposed to inconsistent emotional support, intrusive feeding practices, or neglect are more likely to develop alexithymia, poor emotional awareness, and reliance on food as a primary coping strategy [94, 95]. Evidence suggests that disruptions in attachment relationships contribute to the intergenerational transmission of maladaptive emotion regulation and eating behaviors [87]. Gender differences add another layer of complexity: adolescent girls are more prone to suppression-related overeating and body dissatisfaction, while boys appear less consistently affected by sociocultural pressures tied to thinness [96, 97].

Finally, emotion regulation difficulties should be conceptualized as developmental vulnerabilities that intersect with biological, psychological, and social risk pathways. Interventions that strengthen these skills – including cognitive-behavioral therapy (CBT), dialectical behavior therapy for adolescents (DBT-A), and mindfulness-based approaches – have shown promise in reducing emotional eating and improving psychological well-being [98]. Preventive programs initiated early in life, focusing on emotional awareness and adaptive regulation strategies, may offer long-term protection against the concurrent development of obesity and related psychopathology.

4. Familial risk factors

Adolescents' psychological development and health behaviors, including eating patterns and emotion regulation, are strongly shaped by the family environment, with maternal factors receiving particular attention due to mothers' central role in caregiving, modeling, and coregulation [8]. Maternal psychological distress, disordered eating, and impulsivity directly and indirectly increase obesity risk by fostering emotional dysregulation, maladaptive eating, and higher BMI in offspring [8, 99–101]. Maternal eating behaviors, such as emotional or binge eating and using food as a reward, represent important intergenerational influences transmitted through modeling and family dynamics [102]. Maternal impulsivity further undermines routines and has stronger effects on daughters' BMI, suggesting gender-specific pathways [4, 9, 50].

The dyadic mother–child relationship is central to emotion socialization. Maternal difficulties in emotion regulation may foster maladaptive coping, leading adolescents to develop emotional eating, depressive symptoms, and elevated BMI [6, 72]. Gender differences are evident: girls tend to mirror maternal affective states, whereas boys may express distress through impulsive overeating or conduct problems [73, 86]. In addition, maternal weight status before and during pregnancy is among the strongest predictors of offspring obesity, reflecting the combined influence of biological predispositions and early feeding environments [103, 104].

Overall, maternal influences operate within a broader family system, underscoring the need for prevention and intervention programs that support maternal mental health, address impulsivity, and reshape eating behaviors alongside adolescent-focused treatments.

4.1 Maternal psychological distress

Maternal psychological distress – including depression, anxiety, and broader emotional difficulties – has been consistently associated with adverse developmental outcomes in children and adolescents. These outcomes include heightened emotional dysregulation, maladaptive eating behaviors, and an elevated risk of overweight and obesity [8, 99]. Mothers experiencing significant distress often struggle to maintain consistent routines, provide stable emotional support, or model adaptive coping strategies, thereby transmitting emotional vulnerabilities to their children [105]. Clinical research highlights a strong relationship between maternal affective symptoms and adolescents' psychological adjustment and obesity-related outcomes. Higher maternal depression and anxiety scores have been linked with increased adolescent BMI and emotional eating, highlighting the impact of maternal functioning on the family environment and children's regulatory capacities [99]. When maternal psychopathology co-occurs with disordered eating in the child, risks are magnified: maternal emotional difficulties are among the strongest predictors of bulimic behaviors in obese adolescents [106].

Beyond direct mood symptoms, maternal personality traits and attachment styles also play a role. Mothers of children with obesity more frequently report high anxiety, obsessiveness, and low self-esteem compared to mothers of lean children, pointing to a broader psychosocial profile of vulnerability [8]. Attachment research similarly shows that insecure maternal attachment styles are more common in this group [100]. Furthermore, low maternal conscientiousness has been linked to inconsistent or restrictive feeding practices, both of which may inadvertently foster weight gain in children [101]. Psychological distress also undermines mothers' ability to sustain healthy routines around meals, physical activity, and sleep – routines critical for weight regulation [9]. Parenting-role stress and general parental stress have been systematically linked to greater obesity risk in offspring [107]. Importantly, the relationship between maternal and adolescent distress is bidirectional: adolescents' internalizing or behavioral problems can heighten maternal stress, reinforcing cycles of vulnerability across generations [108].

Taken together, maternal psychological distress rarely acts in isolation. Instead, it interacts with personality traits, parenting stress, and family dynamics, shaping children's emotional development and eating behaviors in complex ways. Addressing maternal mental health within obesity prevention and intervention programs is, therefore, essential. Supporting mothers through targeted mental health care, stress management, and parenting interventions not only enhances maternal well-being but also reduces the intergenerational transmission of obesity-related risk.

4.2 Maternal disordered eating and impulsivity

Maternal eating behaviors exert a powerful influence on children's dietary habits and long-term relationships with food. Mothers who engage in emotional eating, binge eating, or restrictive practices often transmit these patterns intergenerationally through modeling, shared emotional climates, and feeding strategies [102]. In certain households, food functions as a coping mechanism or reward, contributing to the consolidation of maladaptive patterns and increasing the likelihood of persistence into adolescence. Maternal impulsivity compounds these risks. Defined by difficulties in self-control, a preference for immediate rewards, and challenges in delayed gratification, impulsivity undermines consistent parenting practices [4]. Maternal impulsivity has been associated with difficulties in regulating emotions, enforcing mealtime routines, and maintaining healthy limits, thereby reducing opportunities for children to develop self-regulation skills. Intergenerational pathways are both genetic and observational: children of impulsive mothers tend to show greater impulsivity themselves, which, in turn, predisposes them to obesity [50].

Empirical evidence supports the centrality of maternal pathways. Maternal impulsivity, more strongly than paternal impulsivity, has been linked with both children's impulsivity and BMI [9]. Gender-specific effects have also been observed: maternal impulsivity is particularly predictive of daughters' BMI, suggesting heightened sensitivity among girls. Longitudinal studies further demonstrate that when impulsive child temperament co-occurs with low maternal sensitivity, obesity risk is significantly amplified [109, 110]. Children with obesity frequently display impulsivity-linked eating behaviors, such as disinhibition, excessive snacking, and heightened responsiveness to external food cues [73, 111]. These findings suggest that impulsivity contributes to higher BMI both directly and indirectly by shaping maladaptive eating styles and self-regulatory failures [112, 113].

In sum, maternal disordered eating and impulsivity reinforce one another within mother–child dyads, creating a cycle of dysregulation that operates across behavioral, emotional, and relational domains. Addressing maternal vulnerabilities is, therefore, critical for effective prevention and treatment. Family-based programs that promote maternal self-regulation, encourage adaptive feeding practices, and support healthier coping mechanisms may disrupt these intergenerational pathways and mitigate adolescents' obesity risk [72].

4.3 Intergenerational modeling and emotion coregulation

The mother–child relationship provides a central context for the socialization of emotions and eating behaviors. Emotion coregulation refers to the ways in which caregivers guide children in recognizing, expressing, and managing emotions. When mothers themselves struggle with emotional regulation, they may unintentionally model maladaptive responses – such as emotional eating, withdrawal, or avoidance – while failing to scaffold adaptive strategies [6]. Over time, these dynamics strengthen the association between negative affect and food consumption, reinforcing adolescents' vulnerability to both psychological distress and obesity. Adolescents with obesity appear especially sensitive to maternal emotional and behavioral functioning. Studies show that maternal emotional instability, disordered eating, and impulsivity are linked with higher levels of adolescent emotional eating, depressive symptoms, and elevated BMI. Structural modeling further demonstrates that maternal impulsivity and maladaptive eating influence adolescent BMI indirectly through adolescents' own impulsivity and eating behaviors, highlighting the interactive nature of these parent–child pathways [72].

Gender-specific effects provide additional nuance. Girls are more likely to mirror maternal emotional states and eating patterns, whereas boys often externalize distress through impulsive overeating or behavioral difficulties [73, 86]. These findings align with broader developmental research indicating that females tend to internalize stress and body image concerns, while males are more prone to externalizing behaviors. In addition, maternal weight status and dietary behaviors contribute substantially to intergenerational risk. Maternal obesity before and during pregnancy strongly predicts obesity in offspring, with effects persisting into adolescence [103, 104]. Moreover, mothers shape the home food environment by establishing cultural and familial scripts around food use as comfort or reward, embedding regulatory strategies within daily practices [102].

Overall, intergenerational modeling and emotion coregulation illustrate how maternal vulnerabilities become embedded in the family system. Adolescents not only inherit biological predispositions but also internalize behavioral and emotional patterns through ongoing interaction. Effective interventions must, therefore, target both maternal and adolescent functioning – supporting maternal mental health, enhancing parental modeling of adaptive coping, and fostering healthier emotion regulation strategies within families. By addressing these dyadic dynamics, prevention and treatment efforts can more effectively disrupt cycles of maladaptive eating and obesity across generations.

5. Clinical implications

Effective management of adolescent obesity requires moving beyond traditional diet- and exercise-focused models to include psychiatric, behavioral, and familial dimensions. Routine screening for psychiatric comorbidities – such as depression, anxiety, ADHD, and eating disorders – should be incorporated into obesity assessments. Early identification of these vulnerabilities allows clinicians to address psychological mechanisms that sustain weight gain and complicate treatment. Integrating validated mental health measures into pediatric and adolescent obesity programs can prevent underdiagnosis and support individualized care.

Interventions that target self-regulatory capacities are particularly critical. CBT, DBT-A, and mindfulness-based approaches have shown promising efficacy in reducing impulsivity, strengthening emotion regulation, and addressing maladaptive eating patterns. Preventive programs initiated in childhood – focusing on frustration tolerance, adaptive coping, and impulse control – may provide long-term protection against the codevelopment of obesity and psychopathology.

Equally important is the role of the family environment, particularly maternal functioning. Treating maternal depression and anxiety, improving parenting practices, and fostering consistent routines around sleep, meals, and activity can reduce intergenerational risk. Family-based interventions that emphasize both feeding practices and emotion coregulation have shown promise in reshaping the relational context of adolescent development. Given observed gender differences – girls being more vulnerable to maternal modeling and boys more prone to externalizing distress – gender-sensitive tailoring of interventions may further increase their effectiveness.

At a broader level, public health strategies should complement clinical efforts. School-based programs to reduce stigma and promote positive body image, community initiatives supporting parental mental health, and culturally sensitive interventions targeting at-risk families can help disrupt cycles of vulnerability. Combining individual, family, and societal approaches is essential for achieving sustainable outcomes.

6. Conclusion

Adolescent obesity is best understood as a complex condition shaped by the intersection of psychiatric vulnerabilities, maladaptive behavioral patterns, and family dynamics. Rather than being a simple result of caloric imbalance, it is closely intertwined with depression, anxiety, ADHD, and eating disorders – each reinforcing cycles of distress and excess weight. Psychological factors such as impulsivity, low self-esteem, and emotion regulation difficulties further magnify vulnerability, highlighting the central role of self-regulatory capacities in weight trajectories.

Maternal functioning emerges as a particularly influential factor, with psychological distress, disordered eating, and impulsivity transmitting risk across generations through modeling and emotion coregulation. However, these influences operate within a broader biopsychosocial system that includes genetic, developmental, and sociocultural pathways. Addressing adolescent obesity, therefore, requires interventions that simultaneously target individual traits, familial processes, and social contexts.

Taken together, the evidence calls for integrated prevention and treatment strategies that combine psychiatric care, behavioral training, family-based interventions, and stigma reduction at the community level. By tackling the psychological and familial roots of obesity alongside lifestyle modification, such approaches hold the potential to reduce prevalence rates and mitigate the long-term psychological and health consequences across the lifespan.

Acknowledgments

The authors extend their sincere gratitude to Dr. Hande Günal Okumuş for her academic contributions to the development of this chapter. Appreciation is also expressed to colleagues and collaborators whose insights supported the preparation of this work.

Conflict of interest

The authors declare no conflict of interest. This chapter is intended for academic and educational purposes. No external funding was received for its preparation.

Author details

Esen Öksüzoğlu Makbule
Department of Child and Adolescent Psychiatry, Kastamonu University Faculty of Medicine, Kastamonu, Türkiye

*Address all correspondence to: esenmakbule@gmail.com

References

[1] NCD Risk Factor Collaboration (NCD-RisC). Worldwide trends in body-mass index, underweight, overweight, and obesity from 1975 to 2016: A pooled analysis of 2416 population-based measurement studies in 128.9 million children, adolescents, and adults. The Lancet (London, England). 2017;**390**(10113):2627–2644. DOI: 10.1016/S0140-6736(17)32129-3

[2] Zhang X, Liu J, Ni Y, Yi C, Fang Y, Ning Q, Shen B, Zhang K, Liu Y, Yang L, Li K, Liu Y, Huang R, Li Z. Global prevalence of overweight and obesity in children and adolescents: A systematic review and meta-analysis. Journal of the American Medical Association Pediatrics. 2024;**178**(8):800–813. DOI: 10.1001/jamapediatrics.2024.1576

[3] Dębski J, Przybyłowski J, Skibiak K, Czerwińska M, Walędziak M, Różańska-Walędziak A. Depression and obesity - do we know everything about it? A narrative review. Nutrients. 2024;**16**(19):3383. DOI: 10.3390/nu16193383

[4] Kidd C, Loxton NJ. A narrative review of reward sensitivity, rash impulsivity, and food addiction in adolescents. Progress in Neuro-Psychopharmacology and Biological Psychiatry. 2021;**109**:110265. DOI: 10.1016/j.pnpbp.2021.110265

[5] Granero R, Krug I, Reivan Ortiz GG. Editorial: The role of emotion regulation on the developmental course of eating disorders, obesity and food addiction. Frontiers in Psychiatry. 2024;**15**:1436479. DOI: 10.3389/fpsyt.2024.1436479

[6] Davis C. From passive overeating to "food addiction": A spectrum of compulsion and severity. International Scholarly Research Network Obesity. 2013;**2013**:435027. DOI: 10.1155/2013/435027

[7] Kalon E, Hong JY, Tobin C, Schulte T. Psychological and neurobiological correlates of food addiction. International Review of Neurobiology. 2016;**129**:85–110. DOI: 10.1016/bs.irn.2016.06.003

[8] Precenzano F, Smirni D, Vetri L, Marzuillo P, Lanzara V, Bitetti I, Siciliano M, Miraglia Del Giudice E, Esposito M, Santoro N, Carotenuto M. Childhood obesity and maternal personality traits: A new point of view on obesity behavioural aspects. Pediatric Reports. 2021;**13**(3):538–545. DOI: 10.3390/pediatric13030063

[9] Sleddens EF, Ten Hoor GA, Kok G, Kremers SP. Associations between parental impulsivity and child body mass index. SpringerPlus. 2016;**5**(1):1422. DOI: 10.1186/s40064-016-3048-x

[10] Rankin J, Matthews L, Cobley S, Han A, Sanders R, Wiltshire HD, Baker JS. Psychological consequences of childhood obesity: Psychiatric comorbidity and prevention. Adolescent Health, Medicine and Therapeutics. 2016;**7**:125–146. DOI: 10.2147/AHMT.S101631

[11] Stabouli S, Erdine S, Suurorg L, Jankauskienė A, Lurbe E. Obesity and eating disorders in children and adolescents: The bidirectional link. Nutrients. 2021;**13**(12):4321. DOI: 10.3390/nu13124321

[12] Chen W, Feng J, Jiang S, Guo J, Zhang X, Zhang X, Wang C, Ma Y,

Dong Z. Mendelian randomization analyses identify bidirectional causal relationships of obesity with psychiatric disorders. Journal of Affective Disorders. 2023;**339**:807–814. DOI: 10.1016/j.jad.2023.07.044

[13] Kokka I, Mourikis I, Bacopoulou F. Psychiatric disorders and obesity in childhood and adolescence: A systematic review of cross-sectional studies. Children (Basel, Switzerland). 2023;**10**(2):285. DOI: 10.3390/children10020285

[14] Tevie J, Shaya FT. Association between mental health and comorbid obesity and hypertension among children and adolescents in the US. European Child & Adolescent Psychiatry. 2015;**24**(5):497–502. DOI: 10.1007/s00787-014-0598-8

[15] Logan NE, Ward-Ritacco CL. The developing brain: Considering the multifactorial effects of obesity, physical activity & mental wellbeing in childhood and adolescence. Children (Basel, Switzerland). 2022;**9**(12):1802. DOI: 10.3390/children9121802

[16] Giel KE, Teufel M, Junne F, Zipfel S, Schag K. Food-related impulsivity in obesity and binge eating disorder: A systematic update of the evidence. Nutrients. 2017;**9**(11):1170. DOI: 10.3390/nu9111170

[17] Brockmeyer T, Skunde M, Wu M, Bresslein E, Rudofsky G, Herzog W, Friederich HC. Difficulties in emotion regulation across the spectrum of eating disorders. Comprehensive Psychiatry. 2014;**55**(3):565–571. DOI: 10.1016/j.comppsych.2013.12.001

[18] Kessler RC, Berglund PA, Chiu WT, Deitz AC, Hudson JI, Shahly V, Aguilar-Gaxiola S, Alonso J, Angermeyer MC, Benjet C, Bruffaerts R, de Girolamo G, de Graaf R, Haro JM, Kovess-Masfety V, O'Neill S, Posada-Villa J, Sasu C, Scott K, Viana MC, Xavier M. The prevalence and correlates of binge eating disorder in the World Health Organization World Mental Health Surveys. Biological Psychiatry. 2013;**73**(9):904–914. DOI: 10.1016/j.biopsych.2012.11.020

[19] Jebeile H, Lister NB, Baur LA, Garnett SP, Paxton SJ. Eating disorder risk in adolescents with obesity. Obesity Reviews. 2021;**22**(5):e13173. DOI: 10.1111/obr.13173

[20] Kaur J, Dang AB, Gan J, An Z, Krug I. Night eating syndrome in patients with obesity and binge eating disorder: A systematic review. Frontiers in Psychology. 2022;**12**:766827. DOI: 10.3389/fpsyg.2021.766827

[21] Striegel-Moore RH, Dohm FA, Hook JM, Schreiber GB, Crawford PB, Daniels SR. Night eating syndrome in young adult women: Prevalence and correlates. International Journal of Eating Disorders. 2005;**37**(3):200–206. DOI: 10.1002/eat.20128

[22] Orhan FO, UG O, Ozer A, Altunoren O, Celik M, Karaaslan MF. Night eating syndrome among patients with depression. The Israel Journal of Psychiatry and Related Sciences. 2011;**48**(3):212–217

[23] Lavery ME, Frum-Vassallo D. An updated review of night eating syndrome: An under-represented eating disorder. Current Obesity Reports. 2022;**11**(4):395–404. DOI: 10.1007/s13679-022-00487-9

[24] Carbone EA, Aloi M, Rania M, de Filippis R, Quirino D, Fiorentino TV, Segura-Garcia C. The relationship of

food addiction with binge eating disorder and obesity: A network analysis study. Appetite. 2023;**190**:107037. DOI: 10.1016/j.appet.2023.107037

[25] Lee DJ, Elias GJB, Lozano AM. Neuromodulation for the treatment of eating disorders and obesity. Therapeutic Advances in Psychopharmacology. 2018;**8**(2):73–92. DOI: 10.1177/2045125317743435

[26] Jebeile H, Baur LA, Kwok C, Alexander S, Brown J, Collins CE, Cowell CT, Day K, Garnett SP, Gow ML, Grunseit AM, Henderson M, House ET, Inkster MK, Lang S, Paxton SJ, Truby H, Varady KA, Lister NB. Symptoms of depression, eating disorders, and binge eating in adolescents with obesity: The Fast Track to Health randomized clinical trial. Journal of the American Medical Association Pediatrics. 2024;**178**(10):996–1005. DOI: 10.1001/jamapediatrics.2024.2851

[27] Liem ET, Sauer PJ, Oldehinkel AJ, Stolk RP. Association between depressive symptoms in childhood and adolescence and overweight in later life: Review of the recent literature. Archives of Pediatrics & Adolescent Medicine. 2008;**162**(10):981–988. DOI: 10.1001/archpedi.162.10.981

[28] Luppino FS, de Wit LM, Bouvy PF, Stijnen T, Cuijpers P, Penninx BW, Zitman FG. Overweight, obesity, and depression: A systematic review and meta-analysis of longitudinal studies. Archives of General Psychiatry. 2010;**67**(3):220–229. DOI: 10.1001/archgenpsychiatry.2010.2

[29] Toups MS, Myers AK, Wisniewski SR, Kurian B, Morris DW, Rush AJ, Fava M, Trivedi MH. Relationship between obesity and depression: Characteristics and treatment outcomes with antidepressant medication. Psychosomatic Medicine. 2013;**75**(9):863–872. DOI: 10.1097/PSY.0000000000000000

[30] Lamers F, de Jonge P, Nolen WA, Smit JH, Zitman FG, Beekman AT, Penninx BW. Identifying depressive subtypes in a large cohort study: Results from the Netherlands Study of Depression and Anxiety (NESDA). The Journal of Clinical Psychiatry. 2010;**71**(12):1582–1589. DOI: 10.4088/JCP.09m05398blu

[31] Goldstein BI, Liu SM, Zivkovic N, Schaffer A, Chien LC, Blanco C. The burden of obesity among adults with bipolar disorder in the United States. Bipolar Disorders. 2011;**13**(4):387–395. DOI: 10.1111/j.1399-5618.2011.00932.x

[32] Kemp DE, Gao K, Chan PK, Ganocy SJ, Findling RL, Calabrese JR. Medical comorbidity in bipolar disorder: Relationship between illnesses of the endocrine/metabolic system and treatment outcome. Bipolar Disorders. 2010;**12**(4):404–413. DOI: 10.1111/j.1399-5618.2010.00823.x

[33] Blaine B. Does depression cause obesity?: A meta-analysis of longitudinal studies of depression and weight control. Journal of Health Psychology. 2008;**13**(8):1190–1197. DOI: 10.1177/1359105308095977

[34] Mansur RB, Brietzke E, McIntyre RS. Is there a "metabolic-mood syndrome"? A review of the relationship between obesity and mood disorders. Neuroscience and Biobehavioral Reviews. 2015;**52**:89–105. DOI: 10.1016/j.neubiorev.2014.12.017

[35] Rivera M, Cohen-Woods S, Kapur K, Breen G, Ng MY, Butler AW,

Craddock N, Gill M, Korszun A, Maier W, Mors O, Owen MJ, Preisig M, Bergmann S, Tozzi F, Rice J, Rietschel M, Rucker J, Schosser A, Aitchison KJ, et al. Depressive disorder moderates the effect of the FTO gene on body mass index. Molecular Psychiatry. 2012;**17**(6):604–611. DOI: 10.1038/mp.2011.45

[36] Wojcik W, Lee W, Colman I, Hardy R, Hotopf M. Foetal origins of depression? A systematic review and meta-analysis of low birth weight and later depression. Psychological Medicine. 2013;**43**(1):1–12. DOI: 10.1017/S0033291712000682

[37] Dietze LMF, McWhinney SR, Favre P, Abé C, Alexander N, Barkhau C, Benedetti F, Berk M, Bøen E, Boye B, Brosch K, Canales-Rodríguez EJ, Cannon DM, Carruthers SP, Corkum ELV, Dannlowski U, Díaz-Zuluaga AM, Dohm K, Elvsåshagen T, Flinkenflügel K, et al. White matter microstructure in obesity and bipolar disorders: An ENIGMA bipolar disorder working group study in 2186 individuals. Molecular Psychiatry. 2025;**30**(5):1770–1779. ENIGMA BMI-X Working Group. DOI: 10.1038/s41380-024-02784-2

[38] Pickering RP, Grant BF, Chou SP, Compton WM. Are overweight, obesity, and extreme obesity associated with psychopathology? Results from the national epidemiologic survey on alcohol and related conditions. The Journal of Clinical Psychiatry. 2007;**68**(7):998–1009. DOI: 10.4088/jcp.v68n0704

[39] Cairney J, Corna LM, Veldhuizen S, Kurdyak P, Streiner DL. The social epidemiology of affective and anxiety disorders in later life in Canada. The Canadian Journal of Psychiatry. 2008;**53**(2):104–111. DOI: 10.1177/070674370805300205

[40] Sanderson K, Patton GC, McKercher C, Dwyer T, Venn AJ. Overweight and obesity in childhood and risk of mental disorder: A 20-year cohort study. Australian & New Zealand Journal of Psychiatry. 2011;**45**(5):384–392. DOI: 10.3109/00048674.2011.570309

[41] Chen L, Liu Q, Xu F, Wang F, Luo S, An X, Chen J, Tang N, Jiang X, Liang X. Effect of physical activity on anxiety, depression and obesity index in children and adolescents with obesity: A meta-analysis. Journal of Affective Disorders. 2024;**354**:275–285. DOI: 10.1016/j.jad.2024.02.092

[42] Abramovitch A, Anholt GE, Cooperman A, van Balkom AJLM, Giltay EJ, Penninx BW, van Oppen P. Body mass index in obsessive-compulsive disorder. Journal of Affective Disorders. 2019;**245**:145–151. DOI: 10.1016/j.jad.2018.10.116

[43] Cortese S, Castellanos FX. The relationship between ADHD and obesity: Implications for therapy. Expert Review of Neurotherapeutics. 2014;**14**(5):473–479. DOI: 10.1586/14737175.2014.904748

[44] Cortese S, Moreira-Maia CR, St Fleur D, Morcillo-Peñalver C, Rohde LA, Faraone SV. Association between ADHD and obesity: A systematic review and meta-analysis. American Journal of Psychiatry. 2016;**173**(1):34–43. DOI: 10.1176/appi.ajp.2015.15020266

[45] de Zwaan M, Gruss B, Müller A, Philipsen A, Graap H, Martin A, Glaesmer H, Hilbert A. Association

between obesity and adult attention-deficit/hyperactivity disorder in a German community-based sample. Obesity Facts. 2011;**4**(3):204–211. DOI: 10.1159/000329565

[46] Stice E, Presnell K, Shaw H, Rohde P. Psychological and behavioral risk factors for obesity onset in adolescent girls: A prospective study. Journal of Consulting and Clinical Psychology. 2005;**73**(2):195–202. DOI: 10.1037/0022-006X.73.2.195

[47] Quick V, Wall M, Larson N, Haines J, Neumark-Sztainer D. Personal, behavioral and socio-environmental predictors of overweight incidence in young adults: 10-yr longitudinal findings. International Journal of Behavioral Nutrition and Physical Activity. 2013;**10**:37. DOI: 10.1186/1479-5868-10-37

[48] Mougharbel F, Valois DD, Lamb M, Buchholz A, Obeid N, Flament M, Goldfield GS. Mediating role of disordered eating in the relationship between screen time and BMI in adolescents: Longitudinal findings from the Research on Eating and Adolescent Lifestyles (REAL) study. Public Health Nutrition. 2020;**23**(18):3336–3345. DOI: 10.1017/S136898002000049X

[49] Thomas M, Williams KE, Vanderwert RE. Disordered eating and internalizing symptoms in preadolescence. Brain and Behavior. 2020;**10**(11):e01865. DOI: 10.1002/brb3.1865

[50] Thamotharan S, Lange K, Zale EL, Huffhines L, Fields S. The role of impulsivity in pediatric obesity and weight status: A meta-analytic review. Clinical Psychology Review. 2013;**33**(2):253–262. DOI: 10.1016/j.cpr.2012.12.001

[51] Graziano PA, Kelleher R, Calkins SD, Keane SP, O'Brien M. Predicting weight outcomes in preadolescence: The role of toddlers' self-regulation skills and the temperament dimension of pleasure. International Journal of Obesity. 2013;**37**(7):937–942. DOI: 10.1038/ijo.2012.165

[52] Leehr EJ, Krohmer K, Schag K, Dresler T, Zipfel S, Giel KE. Emotion regulation model in binge eating disorder and obesity: A systematic review. Neuroscience and Biobehavioral Reviews. 2015;**49**:125–134. DOI: 10.1016/j.neubiorev.2014.12.008

[53] Goossens L, Braet C, Van Vlierberghe L, Mels S. Loss of control over eating in overweight youngsters: The role of anxiety, depression and emotional eating. European Eating Disorders Review. 2009;**17**(1):68–78. DOI: 10.1002/erv.892

[54] Patalay P, Hardman CA. Comorbidity, codevelopment, and temporal associations between body mass index and internalizing symptoms from early childhood to adolescence. Journal of the American Medical Association Psychiatry. 2019;**76**(7):721–729. DOI: 10.1001/jamapsychiatry.2019.0169

[55] Pryor L, Brendgen M, Boivin M, Dubois L, Japel C, Falissard B, Tremblay RE, Côté SM. Overweight during childhood and internalizing symptoms in early adolescence: The mediating role of peer victimization and the desire to be thinner. Journal of Affective Disorders. 2016;**202**:203–209. DOI: 10.1016/j.jad.2016.05.022

[56] Franklin J, Denyer G, Steinbeck KS, Caterson ID, Hill AJ. Obesity and risk of low self-esteem:

A statewide survey of Australian children. Pediatrics. 2006;**118**(6):2481–2487. DOI: 10.1542/peds.2006-0511

[57] Wang F, Wild TC, Kipp W, Kuhle S, Veugelers PJ. The influence of childhood obesity on the development of self-esteem. Health Reports. 2009;**20** (2):21–27

[58] HI K, HS K. The psychosomatic concept of obesity. The Journal of Nervous and Mental Disease. 1957;**125** (2):181–201

[59] Braden A, Flatt SW, Boutelle KN, Strong D, Sherwood NE, Rock CL. Emotional eating is associated with weight loss success among adults enrolled in a weight loss program. Journal of Behavioral Medicine. 2016;**39** (4):727–732. DOI: 10.1007/s10865-016-9728-8

[60] Burmeister JM, Hinman N, Koball A, Hoffmann DA, Carels RA. Food addiction in adults seeking weight loss treatment. Implications for psychosocial health and weight loss. Appetite. 2013;**60**(1):103–110. DOI: 10.1016/j.appet.2012.09.013

[61] Herman CP, Polivy J. Anxiety, restraint, and eating behavior. Journal of Abnormal Psychology. 1975;**84** (6):666–672

[62] Lewer M, Kosfelder J, Michalak J, Schroeder D, Nasrawi N, Vocks S. Effects of a cognitive-behavioral exposure-based body image therapy for overweight females with binge eating disorder: A pilot study. Journal of Eating Disorders. 2017;**5**:43. DOI: 10.1186/s40337-017-0174-y

[63] Pollert GA, Engel SG, Schreiber-Gregory DN, Crosby RD, Cao L, Wonderlich SA, Tanofsky-Kraff M, Mitchell JE. The role of eating and emotion in binge eating disorder and loss of control eating. International Journal of Eating Disorders. 2013;**46** (3):233–238. DOI: 10.1002/eat.22061

[64] Mitchell JE, King WC, Courcoulas A, Dakin G, Elder K, Engel S, Flum D, Kalarchian M, Khandelwal S, Pender J, Pories W, Wolfe B. Eating behavior and eating disorders in adults before bariatric surgery. International Journal of Eating Disorders. 2015;**48**(2):215–222. DOI: 10.1002/eat.22275

[65] American Psychiatric Association. Diagnostic and Statistical Manual of Mental Disorders. 5th ed. Washington, DC: American Psychiatric Publishing; 2013

[66] Gearhardt AN, Corbin WR, Brownell KD. Development of the Yale Food Addiction Scale Version 2.0. Psychology of Addictive Behaviors. 2016;**30**(1):113–121. DOI: 10.1037/adb0000136

[67] Ivezaj V, White MA, Grilo CM. Examining binge-eating disorder and food addiction in adults with overweight and obesity. Obesity (Silver Spring, Maryland). 2016;**24** (10):2064–2069. DOI: 10.1002/oby.21607

[68] Mason TB. Parental instrumental feeding, negative affect, and binge eating among overweight individuals. Eating Behaviors. 2015;**17**:107–110. DOI: 10.1016/j.eatbeh.2015.01.013

[69] Kim YR, Hwang BI, Lee GY, KH K, Kim M, KK K, Treasure J. Determinants of binge eating disorder among normal weight and overweight female college students in Korea. Eating and Weight Disorders - Studies on Anorexia,

Bulimia and Obesity. 2018;**23**(6):849–860. DOI: 10.1007/s40519-018-0574-2

[70] Naumann E, Svaldi J, Wyschka T, Heinrichs M, von Dawans B. Stress-induced body dissatisfaction in women with binge eating disorder. Journal of Abnormal Psychology. 2018;**127**(6):548–558. DOI: 10.1037/abn0000371

[71] Kristeller J, Wolever RQ, Sheets V. Mindfulness-based eating awareness training (MB-EAT) for binge eating: A randomized clinical trial. Mindfulness (New York). 2014;**5**:282–297. DOI: 10.1007/s12671-012-0179-1

[72] Öksüzoğlu ME, Okumuş HG. Impulsivity, internalizing symptoms, and disordered eating as predictors of adolescents' body mass index: A structural equation modeling study in adolescents with overweight and obesity and their mothers. Current Psychology. 2025;**44**:11170–11185. DOI: 10.1007/s12144-025-07956-z

[73] Scholten EW, Schrijvers CT, Nederkoorn C, Kremers SP, Rodenburg G. Relationship between impulsivity, snack consumption and children's weight. Public Library of Science One. 2014;**9**(2):e88851. DOI: 10.1371/journal.pone.0088851

[74] Nederkoorn C, Jansen E, Mulkens S, Jansen A. Impulsivity predicts treatment outcome in obese children. Behaviour Research and Therapy. 2007;**45**(5):1071–1075. DOI: 10.1016/j.brat.2006.05.009

[75] Bhutani S, Christian IR, Palumbo D, Wiggins JL. Reward-related neural correlates in adolescents with excess body weight. NeuroImage: Clinical. 2021;**30**:102618. DOI: 10.1016/j.nicl.2021.102618

[76] Attie I, Brooks-Gunn J. Development of eating problems in adolescent girls: A longitudinal study. Developmental Psychology. 1989;**25**(1):70–79. DOI: 10.1037/0012-1649.25.1.70

[77] Wichstrøm L. Psychological and behavioral factors unpredictive of disordered eating: A prospective study of the general adolescent population in Norway. International Journal of Eating Disorders. 2000;**28**(1):33–42. DOI: 10.1002/(SICI)1098-108X(200007)28:1<33::AID-EAT5>3.0.CO;2-H

[78] Pallister E, Waller G. Anxiety in the eating disorders: Understanding the overlap. Clinical Psychology Review. 2008;**28**(3):366–386. DOI: 10.1016/j.cpr.2007.07.001

[79] Godart NT, Perdereau F, Rein Z, Berthoz S, Wallier J, Jeammet P, Flament MF. Comorbidity studies of eating disorders and mood disorders: Critical review of the literature. Journal of Affective Disorders. 2007;**97**(1-3):37–49. DOI: 10.1016/j.jad.2006.06.023

[80] Robinson E, Sutin A, Daly M. Perceived weight discrimination mediates the prospective relation between obesity and depressive symptoms in U.S. and U.K. adults. Health Psychology. 2017;**36**(2):112–121. DOI: 10.1037/hea0000426

[81] Patalay P, Sharpe H, Wolpert M. Internalising symptoms and body dissatisfaction: Untangling temporal precedence using cross-lagged models in two cohorts. Journal of Child Psychology and Psychiatry. 2015;**56**(11):1223–1230. DOI: 10.1111/jcpp.12415

[82] Hill AJ, Oliver S, Rogers PJ. Eating in the adult world: The rise of dieting

in childhood and adolescence. British Journal of Clinical Psychology. 1992;**31**(1):95–105. DOI: 10.1111/j.2044-8260.1992.tb00973.x

[83] Polivy J, Herman CP. If at first you don't succeed: False hopes of self-change. American Psychologist. 2002;**57**(9):677–689

[84] Hemmingsson E. A new model of the role of psychological and emotional distress in promoting obesity: Conceptual review with implications for treatment and prevention. Obesity Reviews. 2014;**15**(9):769–779. DOI: 10.1111/obr.12197

[85] Keel PK, Klump KL, Miller KB, McGue M, Iacono WG. Shared transmission of eating disorders and anxiety disorders. International Journal of Eating Disorders. 2005;**38**(2):99–105. DOI: 10.1002/eat.20168

[86] Smink FRE, van Hoeken D, Dijkstra JK, Deen M, Oldehinkel AJ, Hoek HW. Self-esteem and peer-perceived social status in early adolescence and prediction of eating pathology in young adulthood. International Journal of Eating Disorders. 2018;**51**(8):852–862. DOI: 10.1002/eat.22875

[87] Favieri F, Marini A, Casagrande M. Emotional regulation and overeating behaviors in children and adolescents: A systematic review. Behavioral Sciences. 2021;**11**(1):11. DOI: 10.3390/bs11010011

[88] Pink AE, Lee M, Price M, Williams C. A serial mediation model of the relationship between alexithymia and BMI: The role of negative affect, negative urgency and emotional eating. Appetite. 2019;**133**:270–278. DOI: 10.1016/j.appet.2018.11.014

[89] de Campora G, Larciprete G, Delogu AM, Meldolesi C, Giromini L. A longitudinal study on emotional dysregulation and obesity risk: From pregnancy to 3 years of age of the baby. Appetite. 2016;**96**:95–101. DOI: 10.1016/j.appet.2015.09.012

[90] Tan Y, Xin X, Wang X, Yao S. Cognitive emotion regulation strategies in Chinese adolescents with overweight and obesity. Childhood Obesity. 2018;**14**(1):26–32. DOI: 10.1089/chi.2017.0123

[91] van Strien T, Roelofs K, de Weerth C. Cortisol reactivity and distress-induced emotional eating. Psychoneuroendocrinology. 2013;**38**(5):677–684. DOI: 10.1016/j.psyneuen.2012.08.008

[92] Willem C, Gandolphe MC, Roussel M, Verkindt H, Pattou F, Nandrino JL. Difficulties in emotion regulation and deficits in interoceptive awareness in moderate and severe obesity. Eating and Weight Disorders - Studies on Anorexia, Bulimia and Obesity. 2019;**24**(4):633–644. DOI: 10.1007/s40519-019-00738-0

[93] Young KS, Sandman CF, Craske MG. Positive and negative emotion regulation in adolescence: Links to anxiety and depression. Brain Sciences. 2019;**9**(4):76. DOI: 10.3390/brainsci9040076

[94] Book A, Berant E. The contribution of difficulties in separation–individuation and emotional regulation to obesity among adolescent girls. Asia Pacific Journal of Counseling and Psychotherapy. 2014;**5**(1):28–44. DOI: 10.1080/21507686.2013.878367

[95] Percinel I, Ozbaran B, Kose S, Simsek DG, Darcan S. Increased deficits in emotion recognition and regulation in

children and adolescents with exogenous obesity. The World Journal of Biological Psychiatry. 2018;**19**(2):112–118. DOI: 10.1080/15622975.2016.1265147

[96] Lu Q, Tao F, Hou F, Zhang Z, Ren LL. Emotion regulation, emotional eating and the energy-rich dietary pattern: A population-based study in Chinese adolescents. Appetite. 2016;**99**:149–156. DOI: 10.1016/j.appet.2016.01.011

[97] Cuesta-Zamora C, González-Martí I, García-López LM. The role of trait emotional intelligence in body dissatisfaction and eating disorder symptoms in preadolescents and adolescents. Personality and Individual Differences. 2018;**126**:1–6. DOI: 10.1016/j.paid.2017.12.021

[98] Jebeile H, Kelly AS, O'Malley G, Baur LA. Obesity in children and adolescents: Epidemiology, causes, assessment, and management. The Lancet Diabetes & Endocrinology. 2022;**10**(5):351–365. DOI: 10.1016/S2213-8587(22)00047-X

[99] Öksüzoğlu M E, Akdemir D, Akgül S, Özdemir P. Predictors of emotional eating behaviors in adolescents with overweight and obesity. Archives de Pédiatrie. 2024;**31**(8):527–532. DOI: 10.1016/j.arcped.2024.07.007

[100] Trombini E, Baldaro B, Bertaccini R, Mattei C, Montebarocci O, Rossi N. Maternal attitudes and attachment styles in mothers of obese children. Perceptual and Motor Skills. 2003;**97**(2):613–620. DOI: 10.2466/pms.2003.97.2.613

[101] Sutin AR, Terracciano A. Mother and child personality traits associated with common feeding strategies and child body mass index. Appetite. 2018;**125**:295–301. DOI: 10.1016/j.appet.2018.02.009

[102] Mahmood L, Flores-Barrantes P, Moreno LA, Manios Y, Gonzalez-Gil EM. The influence of parental dietary behaviors and practices on children's eating habits. Nutrients. 2021;**13**(4):1138. DOI: 10.3390/nu13041138

[103] Heslehurst N, Vieira R, Akhter Z, Bailey H, Slack E, Ngongalah L, Pemu A, Rankin J. The association between maternal body mass index and child obesity: A systematic review and meta-analysis. Public Library of Science Medicine. 2019;**16**(6):e1002817. DOI: 10.1371/journal.pmed.1002817

[104] Svensson V, Jacobsson JA, Fredriksson R, Danielsson P, Sobko T, Schiöth HB, Marcus C. Associations between severity of obesity in childhood and adolescence, obesity onset and parental BMI: A longitudinal cohort study. International Journal of Obesity. 2011;**35**(1):46–52. DOI: 10.1038/ijo.2010.189

[105] Zeller MH, Reiter-Purtill J, Modi AC, Gutzwiller J, Vannatta K, Davies WH. Controlled study of critical parent and family factors in the obesigenic environment. Obesity. 2007;**15**(1):126–136. DOI: 10.1038/oby.2007.517

[106] Isnard P, Quantin L, Cortese S, Falissard B, Musher-Eizenman D, Guedeney A, Frelut M-L, Mouren M-C. Bulimic behaviours and psychopathology in obese adolescents and in their parents. International Journal of Pediatric Obesity. 2010;**5**

(6):474–482. DOI: 10.3109/17477160903571987

[107] Jang M, Owen B, Lauver DR. Different types of parental stress and childhood obesity: A systematic review of observational studies. Obesity Reviews. 2019;**20**(12):1740–1758. DOI: 10.1111/obr.12930

[108] Hughes EK, Gullone E. Reciprocal relationships between parent and adolescent internalizing symptoms. Journal of Family Psychology. 2010;**24**(2):115–124. DOI: 10.1037/a0018788

[109] Wu T, Dixon WE, Dalton 3rd WT, Tudiver F, Liu X. Joint effects of child temperament and maternal sensitivity on the development of childhood obesity. Maternal and Child Health Journal. 2011;**15**(4):469–477. DOI: 10.1007/s10995-010-0601-z

[110] Zeller MH, Boles RE, Reiter-Purtill J. The additive and interactive effects of parenting style and temperament in obese youth seeking treatment. International Journal of Obesity. 2008;**32**(10):1474–1480. DOI: 10.1038/ijo.2008.125

[111] Schag K, Schönleber J, Teufel M, Zipfel S, Giel KE. Food-related impulsivity in obesity and binge eating disorder: A systematic review. Obesity Reviews. 2013;**14**(6):477–495. DOI: 10.1111/obr.12017

[112] van den Berg L, Pieterse K, Malik JA, Luman M, Willems van Dijk K, Oosterlaan J, Delemarre-van de Waal HA. Association between impulsivity, reward responsiveness and body mass index in children. International Journal of Obesity. 2011;**35**(10):1301–1307. DOI: 10.1038/ijo.2011.116

[113] Braungart-Rieker JM, Moore ES, Planalp EM, Lefever JB. Psychosocial pathways to childhood obesity: A pilot study involving a high risk preschool sample. Eating Behaviors. 2014;**15**(4):528–531. DOI: 10.1016/j.eatbeh.2014.07.004

Section 5

Utility and limitations of BMI in Specialized Clinical Practice Settings

Chapter 9

The Influence of BMI and Other Measures of Adiposity on Risks and Outcomes in Orthopaedic Traumatology

McKenna W. Box, Adam Green, John Badylak and John T. Riehl

Abstract

Obesity significantly influences risks and outcomes in orthopaedic trauma surgery, presenting unique challenges across various fracture types. This comprehensive review synthesizes current evidence on the impact of elevated body mass index (BMI) on orthopaedic trauma, highlighting epidemiological trends, perioperative considerations, surgical challenges, and postoperative complications. High BMI correlates with substantially higher intra- and post-operative risks, such as infection, nonunion, and thromboembolic events. Central adiposity further compounds fracture risks and complicates surgical management beyond BMI alone. Despite these challenges, tailored perioperative planning, vigilant postoperative management, and technical surgical adaptations can mitigate some obesity-associated risks. Future research should identify specific BMI or adiposity thresholds associated with increased risk and determine the optimal surgical techniques or interventions to improve outcomes in this growing patient population.

Keywords: obesity, orthopaedic trauma, body mass index,fracture risk,surgical complications,central adiposity, fracture healing, nonunion, thromboembolism

1. Introduction

Obesity is a growing global epidemic, affecting 16% of adults worldwide as of 2022, more than double the rate from 1990 [1]. Once limited to high-income countries, obesity now spans the globe [1, 2]. Clinical obesity is classified into Class I (BMI 30–34.9), Class II (BMI 35–39.9), Class III (BMI ≥40), and superobese (BMI ≥50) [3].

While BMI remains the standard metric in clinical practice, it fails to distinguish between fat and lean mass. Measures of central adiposity, such as waist circumference (WC), waist-to-height ratio (WtHR), and body fat percentage

IntechOpen

(BF%), offer improved risk stratification, particularly for cardiometabolic and fracture risk [4–7].

While there is evidence that obesity does not influence overall fracture risk, it does increase risk based on anatomical location and age groups [4, 8, 9]. Class III obese workers experience nearly twice the injury rate of normal-weight peers, and 85% of manufacturing-related injuries occur in overweight or obese individuals [7, 10]. Though increased weight was once thought to be protective for fractures due to increased BMD, newer evidence suggests that central adiposity (e.g., WC, WtHR) heightens fracture risk, particularly in the lower extremities [11].

Obesity also exacerbates postoperative risks through systemic inflammation and impaired bone healing. Altered cytokine profiles impair osteogenesis, contributing to delayed union and nonunion [12, 13]. Additionally, infection and thromboembolism rates are elevated, especially when obesity coexists with malnutrition [14–16]. Assessment of both adiposity and nutritional status is, therefore, essential [17].

The convergence of obesity and orthopaedic trauma presents unique perioperative and postoperative challenges. This chapter synthesizes current evidence to guide management across anatomical regions, highlighting epidemiologic patterns, surgical complexity, and complication risks in obese trauma patients.

2. Upper extremity fractures

2.1 Epidemiology and risk factors

Obesity's influence on upper extremity fracture risk varies by site. High BMI increases the likelihood of proximal humerus fractures, especially among postmenopausal women, where the risk is 30–50% higher than in non-obese peers [18, 19]. In contrast, higher BMI is associated with a lower risk of distal radius fractures [20–22]. An increased WtHR may increase fracture incidence at both the wrist and humerus, though fracture-specific WtHR analyses remain lacking [23].

Obesity may also increase fracture complexity. In distal radius and proximal humerus fractures, higher BMI is associated with greater severity, likely due to increased impact forces from ground-level falls [20, 24–26]. While data are limited in adults, overweight children demonstrate more complex radius and ulna shaft fractures [27].

2.2 Postoperative complications

In surgically managed proximal humerus fractures, overweight status raises the complication risk by 115% [28]. In addition to obesity, when patients have six or more comorbidities, this risk amplifies nearly threefold [28]. Although smaller studies have shown mixed results [26], a large database analysis of over 20,000 patients reported increased rates of shoulder stiffness, infection, and thromboembolic events following operative treatment of proximal humerus fractures in obese patients [29].

Obese patients are more likely to fail conservative management of proximal humerus fractures, with higher rates of delayed conversion to surgery [30]. Evidence on long-term outcomes is mixed; some studies report no difference in union or function [31], while others identify obesity as a predictor of adverse events or treatment failure [18]. Further research is needed to clarify optimal management strategies in this population.

In distal humerus fractures, obesity increases 90-day complication rates, including a 2.5-fold higher risk of infection and a nearly sixfold higher overall complication risk [32, 33]. Hardware-related failures, such as nonunion, implant loosening, or breakage, are more frequent in patients with a BMI > 25, particularly in bicolumnar patterns or when multiple fractures are present [34, 35]. Ulnar nerve complications are also more common, especially in those treated with total elbow arthroplasty [36].

For distal radius surgical fixation, class III obesity nearly doubles the risk of adverse outcomes, such as readmission, reoperation, and prolonged hospitalization [37]. One analysis showed a 2.3% increase in complication risk for every 1-point increase in BMI [25]. Despite these risks, radiographic and functional outcomes appear comparable between obese and non-obese patients [20, 38].

3. Ankle fractures

3.1 Epidemiology and risk factors

Obesity increases both the incidence and severity of ankle fractures, particularly in postmenopausal women. Obese women have up to three times the risk of sustaining ankle fractures from low-energy mechanisms, and postmenopausal women with obesity have a 60% higher risk compared to their non-obese peers [22, 39, 40].

Higher BMI is also associated with more complex fracture patterns. Obese patients are nearly twice as likely to sustain Weber B/C fractures with syndesmotic instability and have higher rates of open fractures [40, 41]. Preoperatively, surgeons should suspect occult syndesmotic or plafond involvement in these patients [42].

3.2 Intraoperative challenges

Ankle fracture surgery in obese patients presents technical challenges due to complex fracture patterns, requiring greater exposure and fixation [40]. While longer operative times are expected, direct comparisons between obese and non-obese individuals regarding operative time remain limited.

Increased soft tissue bulk complicates anatomic reduction and fixation. Deeper surgical planes raise the risk of soft tissue healing problems [43]. Minimally invasive options, like fibular intramedullary nailing (IMN), can reduce infection rates, especially in diabetic patients [44], but require advanced techniques and fluoroscopic guidance [45, 46]. These technical barriers raise the risk of malreduction, compounding post-traumatic complications [47].

Early surgical fixation (<24 hours) reduces the risk of wound complications and shortens hospital stays, while delays of over 7 days are associated with worse long-term functional outcomes [48–50]. However, soft-tissue swelling – not surgical delay – is the stronger predictor of wound issues [51]. Tools like the heel-pad compressibility index (ratio of weight-bearing heel pad thickness to non-weight-bearing heel pad thickness on ultrasound) can guide surgical timing in obese or high-risk patients [52].

3.3 Postoperative complications

Obesity substantially raises the risk of postoperative complications following ankle surgical fixation. In a large cohort of over 160,000 patients, obese individuals had higher 90-day complication and readmission rates [53]. At two years, nonunion and post-traumatic arthritis rates were more than doubled. Wound dehiscence and deep infections were also more frequent, often requiring reoperation or prolonged antibiotic therapy [53].

Soft-tissue condition is a stronger predictor of wound complications than BMI alone. A heel-pad index greater than 1.4 increases the odds of complications by over threefold [52]. Risk is further elevated by comorbidities (diabetes, high ASA class), age, poor function, and complex fracture patterns, which increase reoperation risk five- to sevenfold [42, 53–56].

Obese patients generally report worse functional outcomes after ankle fracture surgery, with more persistent pain, disability, and activity limitation [53, 57, 58]. Delayed weight-bearing is commonly advised postoperatively in this population due to limited BMI-specific evidence on the safety of early mobilization [59].

4. Proximal femur fractures (Hip fractures)

4.1 Epidemiology and risk factors

Hip fractures, including femoral neck and intertrochanteric types, remain high-morbidity injuries [60]. Obesity is associated with a lower overall risk of hip fracture, and a BMI > 30 reduces the risk by 25–50%, particularly in women [61–64]. However, there is evidence that obesity increases the risk of subtrochanteric femur fractures relative to femoral neck or intertrochanteric femur fractures [65]. This "obesity paradox" is thought to be due to increased BMD resulting from greater mechanical loading, which has been confirmed in multivariable models [66].

However, using BMI alone does not capture the full risk of hip fracture in obese individuals. Central adiposity, as measured by WC or WtHR, is a stronger predictor of hip fracture risk than BMI alone [67]. High baseline central obesity, utilizing WtHR, is associated with a 24% increased risk of hip fracture independent of BMI [68]. Women and men in the highest tertile of WC have an 86% and 100% higher risk of hip fracture, respectively, compared to the lowest tertile [69]. For every 0.1-unit increase in WtHR, there is an associated 16% increased risk [70]. In addition, the top tertile of BF% around the hip, measured on DEXA scans, was associated with a 32% to 68% increased risk of hip fracture [71]. Conversely, abdominal fat percentage was not associated with any increased risk regardless of the tertile. These findings indicate that the location of adiposity confers additional fracture risk beyond that captured by BMI.

Regarding fracture severity, obesity is associated with more stable Arbeitsgemeinschaft für Osteosynthesefragen/Orthopaedic Trauma Association (AO/OTA) type 31A1/A2 fracture patterns. In contrast, non-obese elderly patients are more prone to comminuted, unstable patterns (AO/OTA 31A3) [61]. However, overall data are limited on the relationship between obesity and fracture location and morphology.

4.2 Perioperative challenges

Optimizing obese patients perioperatively for hip fracture surgery is challenging. Obesity is associated with surgical delays beyond 36 hours, significantly increasing morbidity and mortality risks [72, 73]. Such delays are often due to healthcare policies requiring blanket BMI-based screenings, which can result in unnecessary delays [74–76].

During surgery, special considerations are essential for obese patients. Operating tables, such as the Hana table (Mizuho OSI) (204 kg limit) and the flat Jackson table (Mizuho OSI) (227 kg limit), typically accommodate obese patients up to a point. However, incidents of obese patients falling off tables necessitate enhanced safety measures, including the use of additional straps and supports [77–79]. When a patient's weight exceeds the capacity of a single table, the patient can be supported by taping and strapping two flat tables together in a staggered position, distributing the patient's weight across the two radiolucent tables [80].

On average, surgical duration for hip fractures is prolonged by approximately 40 minutes in obese patients (154.6 ± 54.8 min vs. 113.6 ± 44.1 min) [74]. Specifically, operative time significantly increases with obesity for femoral neck and intertrochanteric femur fractures, along with more challenging fluoroscopy and fracture reduction procedures [61, 63, 81, 82]. Subtrochanteric femur fractures, although requiring similar overall surgical time, more frequently necessitate open reductions as BMI increases, with each BMI unit increasing the odds of open exposure by 20% [83]. Yet, no significant differences were noted in blood loss or implant selection [83].

In superobese patients (BMI > 50), higher anesthetic and airway management risks were noted, though intraoperative complications remained similar to those in less obese patients. However, issues with surgical tool adequacy due to soft-tissue depth were reported, emphasizing the importance of preparing longer instruments for adequate exposure [84].

4.3 Postoperative complications

Obesity increases postoperative complication rates following hip fracture surgery, with elderly obese patients experiencing a 2.6-fold greater risk of significant complications compared to normal-weight patients [85, 86].

Patients with superobesity experience higher complication rates but not increased mortality. Studies consistently demonstrate equal or lower 30-day and 1-year mortality rates among obese patients after hip fracture surgery [84]. Conversely, underweight patients have increased short-term and long-term mortality, highlighting frailty and malnutrition as stronger predictors than obesity [87]. Additionally, extremely high or low body fat percentage (BF%), as opposed to BMI alone, is associated with increased mortality and impaired functional recovery, emphasizing limitations in using BMI alone for risk stratification [88, 89].

While the elective arthroplasty literature has identified a BMI > 35–40 as a predisposing factor for higher infection and reoperation rates, the literature on the effects of BMI on complications after femoral neck fractures treated with arthroplasty is sparse [90].

Extracapsular hip fractures (intertrochanteric and subtrochanteric) typically undergo internal fixation, and obesity significantly increases perioperative complications in these procedures. Superobese patients face major complication rates as high as 20% and minor complication rates of 33% [91]. Wound complications escalate with increasing BMI, beginning notably at a BMI of 25.6 for superficial infections and 35.5 for deep infections, with odds of wound issues nearly fivefold higher at BMI ≥ 40 [92]. However, immediate postoperative mortality rates remain similar to those of normal-weight individuals [84, 93].

Overweight and moderately obese patients demonstrate lower 30-day and 1 year mortality rates and better 1 year functional recovery compared to normal-weight and underweight individuals, showing a 34% lower early and 22% lower late mortality, termed the "obesity paradox" [93]. Patients with a BMI greater than 26 are more likely to regain independence after a pertrochanteric fracture [85, 94]. Conversely, severe obesity (BMI ≥ 40) negatively affects other outcomes, including delayed mobilization and an increased likelihood of requiring long-term nursing facility care [95]. The risk of long-term institutionalization escalates significantly with higher degrees of obesity, highlighting the adverse outcomes associated with severe obesity [95].

5. Femoral shaft and distal femur fractures

5.1 Epidemiology and risk factors

Femoral shaft fractures generally result from high-energy mechanisms, whereas distal femur fractures typically occur due to low-energy falls in older women. Obesity significantly influences the mechanism, location, and severity of femur fractures. Patients with a BMI ≥ 30 have increased odds of femoral shaft and distal femur fractures compared to normal-weight or underweight individuals, even after adjusting for confounding variables [64, 96]. Overall, obese patients are more likely to sustain femur fractures from higher-energy mechanisms [97]. When controlling for the mechanism, obese patients are more prone to femoral shaft and distal femur fractures from lower-energy incidents [62]. In contrast, normal-weight individuals typically sustain more proximal femur fractures, aligning with prior findings that obesity may confer protection against proximal femur fractures [87].

Under similar trauma mechanisms, obese patients have more severe distal femur fractures, with AO/OTA type B/C comminution in 90% versus 61% in non-obese patients [98]. Although obesity does not increase the overall incidence of femur fractures, it influences the fracture pattern and location, leading to more distal shaft involvement compared to the general population. Data remains limited regarding the relationship between other measures of adiposity (e.g., waist circumference, waist-hip ratio) and femoral fracture risk, as current literature primarily focuses on BMI-based classifications.

5.2 Perioperative challenges

Obesity complicates femoral fracture surgeries by making patient positioning and anatomical landmark identification harder to manage, often prolonging operative time. Techniques like taping the abdominal pannus up and using a reverse Trendelenburg position can enhance surgical exposure [99]. Positioning the obese patient supine on a fracture table can be problematic. The perineal post can cause soft-tissue injury or nerve palsy if excessive pressure is applied to counteract the heavy leg traction.

Lateral soft tissue may deflect instruments during antegrade IMN. Techniques such as the use of flexible reamers, more proximal incisions, and reamer extensions can help reduce this problem [100]. In addition, trochanteric entry nails may be favored over piriformis entry nails to decrease the effects of soft tissue obstruction [101]. Retrograde IMN can significantly reduce surgery duration by 40% and result in threefold lower X-ray exposure compared to antegrade nailing, on par with non-obese patients [102]. However, even though intraoperative technical challenges exist, evaluation of postoperative femoral version does not show a difference between antegrade IMN with a trochanteric or piriformis starting point versus retrograde IMN [103].

It is well-documented that associated injuries, such as ipsilateral femoral neck fractures, are common in femoral shaft fractures but are harder to detect on initial radiographs in obese individuals [104]. Evidence is lacking in evaluating the incidence of these combined injuries in obese patients. It has been recommended to perform routine advanced imaging, such as fine-cut CT scans of the hip and femur, in obese patients with femoral shaft fractures to prevent missing femoral neck fractures that may be hidden on plain radiographs [101].

Regarding distal femur fractures, finite element analysis demonstrates that increased body weight substantially increases interfragmentary strain in lateral locking plate constructs. However, shortening the working length of the plate, and thereby increasing construct rigidity, can mitigate this effect [105].

5.3 Postoperative complications

Postoperative complications are significantly increased in obese patients with femoral shaft and distal femur fractures. Morbidly obese patients with femoral shaft fractures have substantially higher complication rates (23% vs. 9% in normal-weight patients), including far greater risks of ARDS, sepsis, and even mortality [106–108]. However, obesity per se does not typically impede fracture healing. By nine months after injury, obese and non-obese patients achieve bone union at similar rates, though obesity may substantially delay early healing [102, 103]. For example, one study found that only 38% of fractures in obese patients were united at the 6-month mark, compared to 79% in non-obese patients, and all observed cases of hypertrophic nonunion in that series occurred in obese men with comminuted fractures [108, 109].

In distal femur fractures, obesity further exacerbates complications, with a 5% increase in the odds of nonunion per BMI unit increase [109]. Nonunion risk requiring additional surgery is significantly higher in obese patients (approximately 44% vs. 4% in non-obese patients) with lateral locked plating, making BMI a strong predictor of reoperation [106].

Functionally, obese patients demonstrate slower and less complete recovery compared to non-obese patients [110]. Although baseline lower-extremity function scores may be comparable, obese individuals with femoral shaft fractures often experience a prolonged period of limited mobility, potentially resulting from the combined burden of body habitus and impaired fracture healing [98, 102]. Another study focusing on distal femur fractures in elderly patients noted that being underweight (BMI < 20) was a risk factor for poor recovery of independence. In contrast, overweight patients did not differ significantly in activities of daily living recovery [111].

6. Tibial Shaft, plateau, and plafond (Pilon) fractures

6.1 Epidemiology and risk factors

Tibial fractures encompass injuries to the tibial shaft, plateau, and plafond (pilon), each characterized by distinct anatomical locations and mechanisms. Tibial shaft fractures typically follow a bimodal distribution, with high-energy trauma affecting younger individuals, predominantly males, and lower-energy fragility fractures being more common among older adults [112]. Obesity independently increases the risk of lower extremity trauma, with obese individuals demonstrating a higher incidence of tibial fractures in vehicle-related injuries (5.6% obese vs. 1.6% non-obese) [113]. As BMI rises, mechanisms shift toward low-energy ground-level falls as the primary cause of tibial shaft fractures [114]. However, fracture morphology remains dependent on injury mechanism rather than adiposity itself [115].

Central adiposity is an independent predictor of lower-limb fracture risk, even when BMI is within the normal or overweight range [116]. For every 10 cm increase in WC, the hazard of distal lower-extremity fractures increases by approximately 12%, while each standard deviation increase in WtHR is associated with a 55% greater fracture risk [117]. Remarkably, even individuals classified as overweight/obese (BMI ≥ 25 kg/m2m^2) based on BMI exhibit nearly double the fracture incidence if they possess greater central adiposity (upper tertile WtHR) [23]. Higher WtHR also correlates with lower BMD at the tibial midshaft, highlighting central adiposity as a key factor in fracture risk [23].

Specifically for tibial plateau fractures, increased body weight generates higher mechanical forces, resulting in greater fracture pattern severity, with a 1% increased risk of sustaining a bicondylar fracture per unit increase in BMI [118]. In contrast, tibial plafond fractures, which affect the distal tibial articular surface at the ankle, are not associated with increased fracture complexity due to BMI alone, but rather with a propensity toward low-energy mechanisms in obese patients [119].

6.2 Perioperative considerations

As many tibial plateau and tibial plafond fractures are secondary to high-energy mechanisms, external fixation is a common temporizing measure to allow for soft tissue swelling to dissipate [120]. BMI is not a predictor of requiring staged fixation or increased preoperative waiting times in tibial plateau or pilon fractures [118, 119].

While waiting times are not increased, intraoperative time is significantly elevated in pilon fractures in obese patients (85 vs. 61 min) [119]. For obese patients, the thicker soft tissue envelope can make implant placement more challenging due to deeper exposure and increased retraction needs. However, research has not found this to lead to larger incisions or alter implant positioning compared to non-obese patients [121].

The technical aspects of surgery, including achieving and maintaining anatomical reduction and providing adequate internal fixation, become significantly more challenging in patients with higher BMIs due to increased soft tissue depth, limited visualization, and difficulties with intraoperative fluoroscopy [122].

6.3 Postoperative complications

Obesity substantially heightens postoperative complications following tibial fractures. For tibial shaft fractures, elevated BMI significantly increases risks of infection (up to six-fold higher at BMI > 35 or 40), nonunion (2.5-fold increase), and reoperation to address these issues [115, 123–125]. In cases of nonunion, adjuncts such as circular external fixation over the existing nail combined with decortication and bone grafting have demonstrated high union rates and acceptable complication profiles [126]. Acute compartment syndrome is also notably more common in obese patients, and when present, dramatically worsens wound complications and mortality outcomes [127–129]. Despite these acute complications, factors such as open injuries, fracture severity, and smoking status remain stronger predictors of delayed union than BMI [120, 121]. In the long term, obesity is associated with joint space narrowing in the medial compartment of the knee [130]. However, while higher BMI is statistically associated with slightly lower physical function scores at one year, the difference does not exceed the minimum clinically significant difference. There is minimal evidence that other measures of adiposity have a further influence on long-term functional outcomes [131].

In tibial plateau fractures, higher BMI markedly elevates postoperative complication risks, including deep infection, wound dehiscence, and venous thromboembolism [32]. Each incremental increase in BMI corresponds to approximately a 3.8% rise in surgical complications [118]. While careful perioperative protocols may mitigate the risk of infection, obesity negatively affects long-term functional recovery, as demonstrated by significantly worse patient-reported knee function scores despite comparable radiographic union and alignment outcomes [132, 133]. Severe bicondylar plateau fractures exhibit increased nonunion risks in morbidly obese patients, likely related to vascular compromise and fixation difficulties [134].

For pilon fractures, obesity is predominantly associated with superficial wound complications [120]. In contrast, deep infection risks strongly depend on other injury characteristics, such as fracture severity and smoking status [135]. Effective staged management can mitigate deep infections, underscoring the necessity of vigilant perioperative planning [119]. Long-term functional outcomes, radiologic arthritis progression, and union times generally do not differ significantly between obese and non-obese individuals if early complications are effectively managed [119].

7. Pelvic ring and acetabulum fractures

7.1 Epidemiology and risk factors

Pelvic ring and acetabulum fractures occur at an incidence of 80 per 100,000 person-years, with pelvic ring fractures primarily affecting women in low-energy mechanisms and acetabulum fractures primarily affecting men in higher-energy mechanisms [136]. A higher BMI has been shown to have a protective effect on low-energy pelvic ring fractures in post-menopausal women and older men (22–42% risk reduction), with each 5-unit increase in BMI associated with a 35% reduction in the odds of pelvic ring fractures [39, 137]. This is most likely secondary to increased BMD and greater soft tissue padding during low-energy falls. Although a higher BMI is associated with lower abdominal injury scores in the setting of high-energy trauma [138] (potentially secondary to visceral fat dissipating force), it is not associated with a change in the risk of pelvic or acetabulum fractures [113].

There is insufficient evidence to conclude that BMI is directly associated with specific fracture morphologies or classifications, such as those defined by the Tile, Young-Burgess, or Letournel systems. Although studies have demonstrated an increase in lateral compression 1 (LC1) type fractures overall, studies have not stratified fracture patterns by BMI, which could be an area of future research.

7.2 Perioperative challenges

Obese patients present unique challenges in diagnosing pelvic ring and acetabular fractures due to limitations in imaging. Excessive soft tissue often obscures bony landmarks on standard X-rays, and obesity-related limitations, such as weight restrictions and small gantry sizes, prevent some patients from obtaining high-quality CT imaging [139]. Specialized imaging (truncated scout images, open MRI) is recommended to improve diagnostic clarity in obese patients and avoid delays in pelvic fracture management [140].

Surgical management of pelvic ring and acetabular fractures in obese patients is technically demanding due to patient positioning, exposure difficulties, and intraoperative imaging challenges. Obesity can complicate anesthetic management and head and neck positioning, increasing risks such as cardiorespiratory compromise and pressure-related injuries. The lateral decubitus position is often preferable to prone positioning for acetabular fractures in obese patients to optimize diaphragmatic movement and reduce abdominal pressure. However, additional measures, such as extensive padding and special supports, are often needed to prevent complications. Surgeons must employ techniques such as panniculus taping and adjunctive fixation methods to enhance exposure and fixation in obese patients.

Operative times and intraoperative blood loss are significantly increased in obese patients undergoing pelvic and acetabular fracture surgery [141–143]. Surgical exposure is more challenging due to substantial adipose tissue in the abdominal and gluteal regions, often necessitating longer incisions and deeper retractors [144]. Fluoroscopy imaging is less effective because scatter can obscure details, prompting reliance on tactile feedback, direct visualization, or intraoperative CT, despite logistical complexities.

Fixation constructs for pelvic and acetabular fractures in obese patients must address higher mechanical loads due to increased body weight, as obesity subjects pelvic fixation to abnormal loading forces, raising concerns for hardware failure [144, 145]. Surgeons often employ more robust fixation methods, such as additional sacroiliac screws, supplemental iliosacral bars, or larger-diameter screws. Buttress plates used for acetabular fractures may also be augmented with additional screws and thicker plates, and early weight-bearing may be recommended only after solid fixation is confirmed [146]. Despite these precautions, obese patients experience higher rates of fracture reduction loss, occurring in approximately 31% of cases compared to 6% in non-obese patients [147]. Adjunctive fixation and intraoperative stress tests can help address this issue. Percutaneous fixation techniques can reduce the rates of wound complications compared to open surgery but are technically challenging due to the difficulty of achieving clear X-ray images, accurate reductions, and implant placement through thick soft-tissue envelopes, with body mass being a significant risk factor for screw malposition during percutaneous sacroiliac fixation. External fixation alone often fails to adequately reduce pelvic ring fractures in obese patients; therefore, it is recommended to combine external fixation with internal fixation in select cases to enhance stability [145, 148].

7.3 Postoperative complications

Obese patients undergoing pelvic and acetabular fracture surgery face significantly higher postoperative complication rates compared to their non-obese counterparts [146]. Specifically, obese patients have nearly sevenfold increased odds of early complications requiring reoperation, with notably frequent deep wound infections; morbid obesity increases deep infection risk fivefold after acetabular fracture fixation [141]. Central adiposity, measured by WtHR or muscle-to-adipose ratio, independently predicts wound complications beyond BMI alone [149, 150]. Wound issues typically present as delayed healing, dehiscence, or infection, often requiring aggressive interventions such as surgical debridement or implant removal. Practical strategies to mitigate these risks include multilayered closures, strict glycemic control, and prophylactic negative-pressure wound therapy [145, 146].

Beyond wound complications, obese patients also experience significantly increased rates of systemic complications postoperatively. DVT is 2.6 times more common in obese acetabular fracture patients, and morbidly obese pelvic fracture patients face heightened risks of pneumonia, prolonged ventilatory support, and respiratory issues such as atelectasis or acute respiratory distress syndrome [146, 151–153]. Pressure ulcers are also notably more prevalent. Complication rates correlate with increasing BMI: patients with class I/II obesity exhibit about a 10% complication rate, whereas morbidly obese patients experience rates around 22%, significantly higher than non-obese patients (5.7%) [153]. Obesity negatively impacts long-term recovery, with obese patients exhibiting poorer functional outcomes, higher rates of heterotopic ossification, chronic pain, and mobility deficits at 1–2 years postoperatively [141]. Additionally, obese patients typically have more extended hospital stays and more frequently require discharge to rehabilitation or skilled nursing facilities, underscoring the necessity of proactive complication prevention strategies and the significant healthcare resource implications associated with managing obesity in this patient population [141].

8. Conclusion

Obesity substantially impacts orthopaedic trauma care, influencing fracture incidence, complexity, perioperative challenges, and postoperative outcomes across various anatomical regions. Elevated BMI, particularly central adiposity, increases risks for severe fractures, surgical complications such as infections, nonunion, thromboembolic events, and prolonged recovery periods. Despite these challenges, individualized perioperative planning, meticulous surgical techniques, and vigilant postoperative management can mitigate obesity-related complications and improve outcomes. Future research is needed to define obesity-related thresholds that clearly predict adverse outcomes and to establish optimal surgical and rehabilitative strategies tailored to this growing patient population.

Acknowledgments

The authors would like to acknowledge Dr. Michele McCarroll, Ph.D., and Devika Pavuluri, MPH, for their assistance with project organization and proofreading.

Conflict of interest

Dr. John T. Riehl, M.D., is a consultant for, and receives royalties from, Arthrex Inc. The remaining authors declare no potential conflicts of interest. There are no conflicts of interest that would potentially bias the results reported. This project received no funding. This research was supported (in whole or in part) by HCA Healthcare and/or an HCA Healthcare-affiliated entity. The views expressed in this publication represent those of the author(s) and do not necessarily represent the official views of HCA Healthcare or any affiliated entities.

Author details

McKenna W. Box*, Adam Green, John Badylak and John T. Riehl
Department of Orthopaedic Surgery, Medical City Denton, Denton, USA

*Address all correspondence to: mckenna.box.med@gmail.com

References

[1] GBD 2021 Adult BMI Collaborators. Global, regional, and national prevalence of adult overweight and obesity, 1990-2021, with forecasts to 2050: A forecasting study for the Global Burden of Disease Study 2021. Lancet. 2025;**405**(10481):813–838

[2] NCD Risk Factor Collaboration (NCD-RisC). Worldwide trends in underweight and obesity from 1990 to 2022: A pooled analysis of 3663 population-representative studies with 222 million children, adolescents, and adults. Lancet. 2024;**403**(10431):1027–1050

[3] Elmaleh-Sachs A, Schwartz JL, Bramante CT, Nicklas JM, Gudzune KA, Jay M. Obesity management in adults: A review. JAMA. 2023;**330**(20):2000–2015

[4] Jeong SM, Lee DH, Rezende LFM, Giovannucci EL. Different correlation of body mass index with body fatness and obesity-related biomarker according to age, sex and race-ethnicity. Scientific Reports. 2023;**13**(1):3472

[5] Wu Y, Li D, Vermund SH. Advantages and limitations of the Body Mass Index (BMI) to assess adult obesity. International Journal of Environmental Research and Public Health. 2024;**21**(6):757

[6] Laddu D, Neeland IJ, Carnethon M, et al. Implementation of obesity science into clinical practice: A scientific statement from the american heart association. Circulation 2024;**150**:e7–e19

[7] Ostbye T, Dement JM, Krause KM. Obesity and workers' compensation: Results from the Duke health and safety surveillance system. Archives of Internal Medicine. 2007;**167**(8):766–773

[8] Finkelstein EA, Chen H, Prabhu M, Trogdon JG, Corso PS. The relationship between obesity and injuries among U.S. adults. American Journal of Health Promotion. 2007;**21**(5):460–468

[9] Zahedi H, Atayie F, Samii Kondrud F, et al. Associations of abdominal obesity with different types of bone fractures in adults: A systematic review and dose-response meta-analysis of prospective cohort studies. Critical Reviews in Food Science and Nutrition 2024;**64**:6239–6250

[10] Pollack KM, Sorock GS, Slade MD, et al. Association between body mass index and acute traumatic workplace injury in hourly manufacturing employees. American Journal of Epidemiology 2007;**166**:204–211

[11] Evans AL, Paggiosi MA, Eastell R, Walsh JS. Bone density, microstructure and strength in obese and normal weight men and women in younger and older adulthood. Journal of Bone and Mineral Research. 2015;**30**(5):920–928

[12] Kim D, Ansari MM, Ghosh M, Heo Y, Choi KC, Son YO. Implications of obesity-mediated cellular dysfunction and adipocytokine signaling pathways in the pathogenesis of osteoarthritis. Molecular Aspects of Medicine. 2025;**103**:101361

[13] Zhao X, Wang Q, Wang W, Lu S. Increased neutrophil extracellular traps caused by diet-induced obesity delay fracture healing. FASEB Journal. 2024;**38**(20):e70126

[14] Madsen HJ, Gillette RA, Colborn KL, et al. The association between obesity and postoperative outcomes in a broad surgical population: A 7-year American college of surgeons national surgical quality improvement analysis. Surgery 2023;**173**:1213–1219

[15] Abelleyra Lastoria DA, Ogbolu C, Olatigbe O, Beni R, Iftikhar A, Hing CB. The effect of combined malnutrition and obesity on trauma and orthopaedic surgery outcomes. Bone & Joint Journal. 2024;**106**(10):1044–9

[16] Southam BR, Bowers KA, Smidt KP, et al. Obese trauma patients who sustain orthopaedic fractures experience increased length of stay, ICU admissions and mortality. Open Journal of Trauma 2020;**4**:4–11

[17] Chien SC, Chandramouli C, Lo CI, et al. Associations of obesity and malnutrition with cardiac remodeling and cardiovascular outcomes in Asian adults: A cohort study. PLoS Medicine 2021;**18**:e1003661

[18] Walter N, Szymski D, Riedl M, et al. Proximal humerus fractures in the elderly U.S. Population: A cross-sectional study of treatment trends and comparison of complication rates after joint replacement, open reduction and internal fixation, and non-surgical management. Journal of Clinical Medicine. 2023;**12**(10):3506

[19] Johansson H, Kanis JA, Odén A, et al. A meta-analysis of the association of fracture risk and body mass index in women. Journal of Bone and Mineral Research 2014;**29**:223–233

[20] Kloberdanz AL, Meyer J, Kammermeier K, et al. Impact of body mass index on fracture severity, clinical, radiological and functional outcome in distal radius fractures: A retrospective observational study after surgical treatment. Archives of Orthopaedic and Trauma Surgery 2024;**144**:2915–2923

[21] Ong T, Sahota O, Tan W, Marshall L. A United Kingdom perspective on the relationship between body mass index (BMI) and bone health: A cross sectional analysis of data from the Nottingham Fracture Liaison Service. Bone. 2014;**59**:207–210

[22] Turcotte AF, O'Connor S, Morin SN, et al. Association between obesity and risk of fracture, bone mineral density and bone quality in adults: A systematic review and meta-analysis. PLoS One. 2021;**16**(6): e0252487

[23] Cho Y, Jhee JH, Hong N, Park HS. Association between waist-to-Height Ratio Estimated Fat Mass categories and incident fractures. Journal of Cachexia, Sarcopenia and Muscle. 2025;**16**(3):e13834

[24] Ebinger T, Koehler DM, Dolan LA, McDonald K, Shah AS. Obesity increases complexity of Distal radius fracture in fall from standing height. Journal of Orthopaedic Trauma. 2016;**30**(8):450–455

[25] Goodloe JB, Traven SA, Herzog LN, Richardson CM, Daley DN, Slone HS. Elevated BMI is associated with intra-articular comminution, prolonged operative time, and postoperative complications in distal radius fractures. Injury. 2020;**51** (11):2612–2616

[26] Boadi BI, Belayneh R, Littlefield CP, Egol KA. Patient obesity is associated with severity of proximal humerus fractures, not outcomes.

Archives of Orthopaedic and Trauma Surgery. 2023;**143**(1):373–379

[27] Li Y, James C, Byl N, et al. Obese children have different forearm fracture characteristics compared with normal-weight children. Journal of Pediatric Orthopaedics 2020;**40**:e127–e30

[28] Henkelmann R, Theopold J, Kitsche J, Link PV, Mende M, Hepp P. Comorbidities, substance abuse, weight and age are independent risk factors for postoperative complications following operation for proximal humerus fractures: A retrospective analysis of 1109 patients. Archives of Orthopaedic and Trauma Surgery. 2022;**142**(10):2701–2709

[29] Werner BC, Griffin JW, Yang S, Brockmeier SF, Gwathmey FW. Obesity is associated with increased postoperative complications after operative management of proximal humerus fractures. Journal of Shoulder and Elbow Surgery. 2015;**24**(4):593–600

[30] Katthagen JC, Raschke MJ, Fischhuber K, et al. Conservative versus operative treatment of proximal humerus fractures in older individuals. Deutsches Ärzteblatt International 2024;**121**:454–460

[31] Goudie EB, MacDonald DJ, Robinson CM. Functional outcome after nonoperative treatment of a proximal humeral fracture in adults. Journal of Bone and Joint Surgery. American Volume. 2022;**104**(2):123–138

[32] Kinder F, Giannoudis PV, Boddice T, Howard A. The effect of an abnormal BMI on orthopaedic trauma patients: A systematic review and meta-analysis. Journal of Clinical Medicine. 2020;**9**(5):1302

[33] Werner BC, Rawles RB, Jobe JT, Chhabra AB, Freilich AM. Obesity is associated with increased postoperative complications after operative management of distal humerus fractures. Journal of Shoulder and Elbow Surgery. 2015;**24**(10):1602–1606

[34] Ku KH, Baek JH, Kim MS. Risk factors for non-union after open reduction and internal fixation in patients with distal humerus fractures. Journal of Clinical Medicine. 2022;**11**(10):2679

[35] Claessen FM, Braun Y, Peters RM, Kolovich GP, Ring D. Plate and screw fixation of bicolumnar distal humerus fractures: Factors associated with loosening or breakage of implants or nonunion. Journal of Hand Surgery. American Volume. 2015;**40**(10):2045–51.e2

[36] Obert L, Ferrier M, Jacquot A, et al. Distal humerus fractures in patients over 65: Complications. Orthopaedics & Traumatology: Surgery & Research 2013;**99**:909–913

[37] Vasara H, Stenroos A, Tarkiainen P, et al. Incidence and risk factors of adverse events after distal radius fracture fixation with volar locking plates: Retrospective analysis of 2,790 cases. Acta Orthopaedica. 2024;**95**:645–653

[38] Hall MJ, Ostergaard PJ, Dowlatshahi AS, Harper CM, Earp BE, Rozental TD. The impact of obesity and smoking on outcomes after Volar plate fixation of Distal radius fractures. Journal of Hand Surgery. American Volume. 2019;**44**(12):1037–1049

[39] Prieto-Alhambra D, Premaor MO, Fina Avilés F, et al. The association between fracture and obesity is

site-dependent: A population-based study in postmenopausal women. Journal of Bone and Mineral Research 2012;**27**:294–300

[40] Hjelle AM, Apalset EM, Gjertsen JE, et al. Associations of overweight, obesity and osteoporosis with ankle fractures. BMC Musculoskeletal Disorders 2021;**22**:723

[41] Chaudhry S, Egol KA. Ankle injuries and fractures in the obese patient. Orthopedic Clinics of North America. 2011;**42**(1):45–53. vi

[42] Cavo MJ, Fox JP, Markert R, Laughlin RT. Association between diabetes, obesity, and Short-term outcomes among patients surgically treated for Ankle fracture. Journal of Bone and Joint Surgery. American Volume. 2015;**97**(12):987–994

[43] Guss D, Bhattacharyya T. Perioperative management of the obese orthopaedic patient. Journal of the American Academy of Orthopaedic Surgeons. 2006;**14**(7):425–432

[44] Abdelgaid SM, Moursy AF, Elgebaly EAA, Aboelenien AM. Minimally invasive treatment of Ankle fractures in patients at high risk of soft tissue wound healing complications. Journal of Foot and Ankle Surgery. 2018;**57**(3):557–571

[45] Ottesen TD, Pathak N, Mercier MR, et al. Comparison of Differences in surgical complications between fellowship-trained orthopedic foot and ankle surgeons and all other orthopedic surgeons using the ABOS database. Orthopedics 2023;**46**: e237–e43

[46] Bazarov I, Kim J, Richey JM, Dickinson JD, Hamilton GA. Minimally invasive plate osteosynthesis for treatment of ankle fractures in high-risk patients. Journal of Foot and Ankle Surgery. 2018;**57**(3):494–500

[47] Chong HH, Hau MYT, Mishra P, Rai P, Mangwani J. Patient outcomes following ankle fracture fixation. Foot & Ankle International. 2021;**42** (9):1162–1170

[48] Edelstein A, McDonald J, Lee W. The impact of surgical timing in ankle fracture on postoperative wound complications: A critical 24-hour cutoff point through systematic review and meta-analysis. Archives of Orthopaedic and Trauma Surgery. 2025;**145**(1):269

[49] Naumann MG, Sigurdsen U, Utvåg SE, Stavem K. Associations of timing of surgery with postoperative length of stay, complications, and functional outcomes 3-6 years after operative fixation of closed ankle fractures. Injury. 2017;**48**(7):1662–1669

[50] Pilskog K, Gote TB, Odland HEJ, et al. Association of delayed surgery for ankle fractures and patient-reported outcomes. Foot & Ankle International 2022;**43**:762–771

[51] Halvachizadeh S, Klingebiel FKL, Pfeifer R, et al. The local soft tissue status and the prediction of local complications following fractures of the ankle region. Injury 2022;**53**:1789–1795

[52] Riedel MD, Parker A, Zheng M, et al. What is Too Swollen? Correlation of soft tissue swelling and timing to surgery with acute wound complications for operatively-treated lower extremity fractures. Foot & Ankle Orthopaedics. 2019;**4**(4):526–536

[53] Janghala A, Niknam K, Freshman R, Cogan CJ, Zhang AL, Lansdown D. Effect

of obesity on Short- and Long-term complications after ankle fracture fixation. Journal of Orthopaedic Trauma. 2024;**38**(9):e312–e7

[54] Basques BA, Miller CP, Golinvaux NS, Bohl DD, Grauer JN. Morbidity and readmission after open reduction and internal fixation of ankle fractures are associated with preoperative patient characteristics. Clinical Orthopaedics and Related Research. 2015;**473**(3): 1133–1139

[55] Pilskog K, Høvding P, Fenstad AM, Inderhaug E, Fevang JM, Dale H. Risk factors for fracture-related infection after ankle fracture surgery. Injury. 2023;**54**10:111011

[56] Dodd AC, Lakomkin N, Attum B, et al. Predictors of adverse events for ankle fractures: An analysis of 6800 patients. Journal of Foot and Ankle Surgery 2016;**55**:762–766

[57] Benedick A, Audet MA, Vallier HA. The effect of obesity on post-operative complications and functional outcomes after surgical treatment of torsional ankle fracture: A matched cohort study. Injury. 2020;**51**(8):1893–1898

[58] Stavem K, Naumann MG, Sigurdsen U, Utvåg SE. The association of body mass index with complications and functional outcomes after surgery for closed ankle fractures. Bone & Joint Journal. 2017;**99**(10):1389–98

[59] Khojaly R, Rowan FE, Shah V, et al. Immediate Weight-Bearing compared with Non-Weight-Bearing after operative ankle fracture fixation: Results of the INWN pragmatic, randomized, multicenter trial. JBJS. 2025;**9900**. DOI: 10.2106/ JBJS.24.00965

[60] Panula J, Pihlajamäki H, Mattila VM, et al. Mortality and cause of death in Hip fracture patients aged 65 or older: A population-based study. BMC Musculoskeletal Disorders. 2011;**12**:105

[61] Kempegowda H, Richard R, Borade A, et al. Obesity is associated with high perioperative complications among surgically treated intertrochanteric fracture of the femur. Journal of Orthopaedic Trauma 2017;**31**:352–357

[62] Gandham A, Zengin A, Bonham MP, et al. Incidence and predictors of fractures in older adults with and without obesity defined by body mass index versus body fat percentage. Bone. 2020;**140**:115546

[63] Müller M, Gutwerk A, Greve F, et al. The association between high Body Mass Index and early clinical outcomes in patients with Proximal Femur fractures. Journal of Clinical Medicine. 2020;**9**(7):2076

[64] Manirajan A, Seidel H, Bhattacharjee S, Dillman D, Shi L, Strelzow J. Effect of Body Mass Index on femur fracture location: A retrospective database study. Journal of Orthopaedic Trauma. 2022;**36**(10):519–524

[65] Maravic M, Ostertag A, Cohen-Solal M. Subtrochanteric/femoral shaft versus Hip fractures: Incidences and identification of risk factors. Journal of Bone and Mineral Research. 2012;**27** (1):130–137

[66] Shen J, Leslie WD, Nielson CM, Majumdar SR, Morin SN, Orwoll ES. Associations of Body Mass Index with incident fractures and hip structural parameters in a large canadian cohort. Journal of Clinical Endocrinology and Metabolism. 2016;**101**(2):476–484

[67] Sadeghi S, Bahrami P, Far SK, Arabi Z. Determining the diagnostic value of three clinical criteria Wells', YEARS and modified Geneva in pregnanwomen with suspected pulmonary thromboembolism. American Journal of Cardiovascular Disease. 2022;**12**(4):240–246

[68] Zheng R, Byberg L, Larsson SC, Höijer J, Baron JA, Michaëlsson K. Prior loss of body mass index, low body mass index, and central obesity independently contribute to higher rates of fractures in elderly women and men. Journal of Bone and Mineral Research. 2021;**36**(7):1288–1299

[69] Søgaard AJ, Holvik K, Omsland TK, et al. Abdominal obesity increases the risk of Hip fracture. A population-based study of 43,000 women and men aged 60-79 years followed for 8 years. Journal of Internal Medicine 2015;**277**:306–317

[70] Sadeghi O, Saneei P, Nasiri M, Larijani B, Esmaillzadeh A. Abdominal obesity and risk of Hip Fracture: A systematic review and meta-analysis of prospective studies. Advances in Nutrition. 2017;**8**(5):728–738

[71] Amin H, Khan MA, Bukhari M. Abdominal and Hip fat percentages are associated with fragility fractures: Evidence from a large cross-sectional study. Scientific Reports. 2025;**151**:23158

[72] Pedersen NSA, Mechlenburg I, Kristensen PK. Are Hip fracture patients with high or low body mass index at higher risk of missed care? A cohort study. Nursing Open. 2023;**10**(7): 4452–4460

[73] Clinkenbeard K, Bossle K, Pape T, Woltenberg LN, Saha S. Time to Hip Fracture Surgery and Mortality. Southern Medical Journal. 2023;**116** (3):274–278

[74] Akinleye SD, Garofolo G, Culbertson MD, Homel P, Erez O. The Role of BMI in Hip Fracture Surgery. Geriatric Orthopaedic Surgery & Rehabilitation. 2018;**9**:2151458517747414

[75] Solsky I, Edelstein A, Brodman M, et al. Perioperative care map improves compliance with best practices for the morbidly obese. Surgery 2016;**160**:1682–1688

[76] Yang T-I, Chen Y-H, Chiang M-H, Kuo Y-J, Chen Y-P. Inverse relation of body weight with short-term and long-term mortality following Hip fracture surgery: A meta-analysis. Journal of Orthopaedic Surgery and Research. 2022;**17**(1):249

[77] Habibi AA, Bi AS, Owusu-Sarpong S, Mahure SA, Ganta A, Konda SR. History, indications, and advantages of orthopaedic operating room tables: A review. European Journal of Orthopaedic Surgery and Traumatology. 2022;**32**(6):1207–1213

[78] McAllister RK, Lilie CJ, Garmon EH. Patient Falls in the operating room: The danger of an obese patient on an unlocked operating room table. Journal of Patient Safety. 2025;**21** (3):e18–e9

[79] Watts E, Patel D, Hoops H, Elkbuli A. Adverse events associated with disparity between patients' BMI and operating table size-A need for improved surgical innovations. American Surgeon. 2023;**89**(12): 6172–6180

[80] Bozzio AE, Gala RJ, Villasenor MA, Hao J, Mauffrey C. Orthopedic trauma surgery in the morbidly obese patient.

European Journal of Orthopaedic Surgery and Traumatology. 2014;**24**(4):421–425

[81] DeGenova DT, Passias BJ, Paulini AS, Myers PM, Dues B, Taylor BC. The Effect of obesity on hemiarthroplasty and Total Hip arthroplasty for femoral neck fractures. Journal of Long-Term Effects of Medical Implants. 2024;**34**(2):53–60

[82] Schuette HB, Durkin WM, Passias BJ, et al. The Effect of Obesity on Operative Time and Postoperative Complications for Peritrochanteric Femur Fractures. Cureus. 2020;**12**(11):e11720

[83] Merrell LA, Gibbons K, Ganta A, Konda SR, Egol KA. Subtrochanteric Femur fractures: The association between obesity and perioperative, clinical, and radiographic outcomes. Journal of Orthopaedic Trauma. 2024;**38**(7):366–372

[84] Chaudhry YP, Rao SS, Puvanesarajah V, et al. Complications and 30-Day mortality rate after hip fracture surgery in superobese patients. Journal of Orthopaedic Trauma 2021;**35**:322–328

[85] Li J, Li D, Wang X, Zhang L. The impact of body mass index on mortality rates of Hip fracture patients: A systematic review and meta-analysis. Osteoporosis International. 2022;**33**(9):1859–1869

[86] Zlowodzki M, Zelle BA, Cole PA, Jeray K, McKee MD. Treatment of acute midshaft clavicle fractures: Systematic review of 2144 fractures - on behalf of the evidence-based orthopoedic trauma working group. Journal of Orthopaedic Trauma. 2005;**19**(7):504–507

[87] Park CH, SH L, Lee R, Kim DY, Cho MR, Song SK. Effects of body mass index on mortality in elderly patients with Hip fractures. Medicine (Baltimore). 2024;**103**(31):e39157

[88] Ma Y, Wang A, Lou Y, Peng D, Jiang Z, Xia T. Effects of frailty on outcomes following surgery among patients with hip fractures: A systematic review and Meta-Analysis. Frontiers in Medicine (Lausanne). 2022;**9**:829762

[89] Fan W, Zhao Z, Wang L, Chu Q. Body fat percentage and the outcomes of Hip fractures in adults aged 50 years and above: A 1-year follow-up study. Frontiers in Medicine (Lausanne). 2025;**12**:1588069

[90] Wagner ER, Kamath AF, Fruth KM, Harmsen WS, Berry DJ. Effect of Body Mass Index on complications and reoperations after Total Hip Arthroplasty. Journal of Bone and Joint Surgery. American Volume. 2016;**98**(3):169–179

[91] Zhang JC, Matelski J, Gandhi R, Jackson T, Urbach D, Cram P. Can patient selection explain the obesity paradox in Orthopaedic Hip Surgery? An Analysis of the ACS-NSQIP Registry. Clinical Orthopaedics and Related Research. 2018;**476**(5):964–973

[92] Emara AK, Oyem PC, Ferre A, et al. Is High Body Mass Index protective or detrimental in surgical fixation of hip fractures?: A spline regression analysis of 22,388 Patients. Journal of Orthopaedic Trauma 2023;**37**:315–322

[93] Modig K, Erdefelt A, Mellner C, Cederholm T, Talbäck M, Hedström M. "Obesity Paradox" Holds True for Patients with Hip Fracture: A Registry-Based Cohort Study. Journal of Bone

and Joint Surgery. American Volume. 2019;**101**(10):888–895

[94] Flodin L, Laurin A, Lökk J, Cederholm T, Hedström M. Increased 1-year survival and discharge to independent living in overweight Hip fracture patients: A prospective study of 843 patients. Acta Orthopaedica. 2016;**87**(2):146–151

[95] Kosar CM, Thomas KS, Gozalo PL, Ogarek JA, Mor V. Effect of obesity on postacute outcomes of skilled nursing facility residents with hip fracture. Journal of the American Geriatrics Society. 2018;**66**(6): 1108–1114

[96] Soliman SS, Jordan GB, Bilaniuk JW, et al. The impact of BMI on morbidity and mortality after femoral fractures. European Journal of Trauma and Emergency Surgery 2022;**48**: 2441–2447

[97] Bryant MK, Parrish M, Roy S, et al. Inferior clinical outcomes after femur fracture in the obese are potentially preventable. Injury 2019;**50**:2049–2054

[98] Maheshwari R, Mack CD, Kaufman RP, et al. Severity of injury and outcomes among obese trauma patients with fractures of the femur and tibia: A crash injury research and engineering network study. Journal of Orthopaedic Trauma 2009;**23**: 634–639

[99] Fisher ND, Bi AS, Kirschner N, Ganta A, Konda SR. Functional Application of Tricks for Super Obese Patient Positioning: A Technical Guide for Hip Fractures on a Fracture Table With a Case Example. Cureus. 2022;**14**(2): e21932

[100] Horoz L, Kilic AI, Kircil C, Cakmak MF. Flexible reamer use to overcome entry point errors in proximal femoral nail application in severe obese intertrochanteric fracture patients. BMC Musculoskeletal Disorders. 2024;**25**(1):810

[101] Streubel PN, Gardner MJ, Ricci WM. Management of femur shaft fractures in obese patients. Orthopedic Clinics of North America. 2011;**42** (1):21–35. v

[102] Tucker MC, Schwappach JR, Leighton RK, Coupe K, Ricci WM. Results of femoral intramedullary nailing in patients who are obese versus those who are not obese: A prospective multicenter comparison study. Journal of Orthopaedic Trauma. 2007;**21** (8):523–529

[103] Koerner JD, Patel NM, Yoon RS, Gage MJ, Donegan DJ, Liporace FA. Femoral malrotation after intramedullary nailing in obese versus non-obese patients. Injury. 2014;**45** (7):1095–1098

[104] O'Toole RV, Dancy L, Dietz AR, et al. Diagnosis of femoral neck fracture associated with femoral shaft fracture: Blinded comparison of computed tomography and plain radiography. Journal of Orthopaedic Trauma 2013;**27**:325–330

[105] Shah ID, Schlauch AM, Phan L, Han J, Eng O, Farrell B. The effect of body weight on interfragmentary fracture strain in plate fixation of distal femur fractures: A finite element analysis. Orthopaedics & Traumatology: Surgery & Research. 2024;**1106**:103868

[106] Rodriguez EK, Boulton C, Weaver MJ, et al. Predictive factors of distal femoral fracture nonunion after

lateral locked plating: A retrospective multicenter case-control study of 283 fractures. Injury 2014;**45**:554–559

[107] Issace SJJ, Singh R, Sisubalasingam N, Tokgöz MA, Jaiman A, Rampal S. Does obesity affect diaphyseal femoral fracture healing treated with intramedullary locking nail? Joint Diseases and Related Surgery. 2023;**34**(1):9–15

[108] Weinlein JC, Deaderick S, Murphy RF. Morbid obesity increases the risk for systemic complications in patients with femoral shaft fractures. Journal of Orthopaedic Trauma. 2015;**29**(3):e91–5

[109] Cone R, Roszman A, Conway Y, Cichos K, McGwin G, Spitler CA. Risk factors for nonunion of distal femur fractures. Journal of Orthopaedic Trauma. 2023;**37**(4):175–180

[110] Lee C, Brodke D, O'Hara N, et al. Risk Factors for Reoperation to Promote Union in 1111 Distal Femur Fractures. Journal of Orthopaedic Trauma 2023;**37**:168–174

[111] Nishioka S, Wakabayashi H, Maeda K, et al. Body mass index and recovery of activities of daily living in older patients with femoral fracture: An analysis of a national inpatient database in Japan. Archives of Gerontology and Geriatrics. 2020;**87**:104009

[112] Anandasivam NS, Russo GS, Swallow MS, et al. Tibial shaft fracture: A large-scale study defining the injured population and associated injuries. Journal of Clinical Orthopaedics and Trauma 2017;**8**:225–231

[113] Japa JP, Shats A, Zitser P, Lakhi N. Impact of obesity on orthopedic injury and fracture patterns in motor vehicle accidents. Open Access Emergency Medicine. 2025;**17**:185–193

[114] Fakhry SM, Morse JL, Garland JM, et al. Increasing BMI is associated with higher mortality, worsening outcomes and highly specific injury patterns following trauma: A multi-institutional analysis of 191,274 patients. Journal of Trauma and Acute Care Surgery 2021;**90**:376–383

[115] Pean CA, Rivero SM, Suneja N, Weaver MJ. Severe obesity worsens 30-Day surgical outcomes and projected costs in operative femoral shaft and tibial shaft fractures. Journal of Orthopaedic Trauma. 2023;**37**(1):27–31

[116] Leslie WD, Binkley N, Schousboe JT, et al. Effect of BMI-Discordant abdominal tissue thickness on fracture probability: A Registry-based study. Journal of Bone and Mineral Research 2023;**38**:1749–1756

[117] Turcotte AF, Jean S, Morin SN, Mac-Way F, Gagnon C. Relationships between Obesity and Incidence of Fractures in a Middle-Aged Population: A Study from the CARTaGENE Cohort. JBMR Plus. 2023;7(5):e10730

[118] McGurk KM, Traven SA, McCadden A, et al. Elevated body mass index is associated with tibial plateau fracture complexity and post-operative complications. Trauma 2023;**25**:214–221

[119] Çeçen GS, Gülabi D, Yanık E, Pehlivanoğlu G, Bekler H, Elmalı N. Effect of BMI on the clinical and radiological outcomes of pilon fractures. Acta Orthopaedica Et Traumatologica Turcica. 2014;**48**(5):570–575

[120] Haller JM, Holt D, Rothberg DL, Kubiak EN, Higgins TF. Does early versus delayed spanning external

fixation impact complication rates for high-energy Tibial Plateau and Plafond Fractures? Clinical Orthopaedics and Related Research. 2016;**474**(6): 1436–1444

[121] Graves ML, Porter SE, Fagan BC, et al. Is obesity protective against wound healing complications in pilon surgery? Soft tissue envelope and pilon fractures in the obese. Orthopedics. 2010;**33**(8):01477447-20100625-27

[122] Graves ML. Periarticular tibial fracture treatment in the obese population. Orthopedic Clinics of North America. 2011;**42**(1):37–44,v–vi

[123] Zhang J, Lu V, Zhou AK, Stevenson A, Thahir A, Krkovic M. Predictors for infection severity for open tibial fractures: Major trauma centre perspective. Archives of Orthopaedic and Trauma Surgery. 2023;**143**(11):6579–6587

[124] Burrus MT, Werner BC, Yarboro SR. Obesity is associated with increased postoperative complications after operative management of tibial shaft fractures. Injury. 2016;**47**(2): 465–470

[125] Fong K, Truong V, Foote CJ, et al. Predictors of nonunion and reoperation in patients with fractures of the tibia: An observational study. BMC Musculoskeletal Disorders. 2013;**14**:103

[126] Azzam W, Gamal O, Samy A. Treatment of tibial shaft nonunion with a retained nail in morbidly obese patients. International Orthopaedics. 2022;**46**(5):1123–1131

[127] Strain R, Giannoudis P. Risk factors for acute compartment syndrome in one thousand one hundred and forty seven diaphyseal tibia fractures. International Orthopaedics. 2024;**48**(8):2211–2216

[128] Light JJ, Davis JM, Dunahoe J, Stwalley D, Miller AN, Cannada LK. Evaluation of obesity and age as a predictive factor of lower extremity compartment syndrome: A national trauma data bank analysis. American Journal of Surgery. 2024;**234**:129–135

[129] Liu Q, Wu M, Orgill DP, Bai X, Panayi AC. The effect of obesity on inpatient outcomes in lower extremity trauma: A systematic review and meta-analysis. Journal of Trauma and Acute Care Surgery. 2022;**92**(2):464–470

[130] Milner SA, Davis TR, Muir KR, Greenwood DC, Doherty M. Long-term outcome after tibial shaft fracture: Is malunion important? Journal of Bone and Joint Surgery. American Volume. 2002;**84**(6):971–980

[131] Findakli F, Busse JW, Schemitsch EH, Lonn E, Farrokhyar F, Smoking BM. Obesity, and disability benefits or litigation are not associated with clinically important reductions in physical functioning after intramedullary nailing of Tibial Shaft Fractures: A retrospective cohort study. Clinical Orthopaedics and Related Research. 2021;**479**(4):805–813

[132] Momaya AM, Hlavacek J, Etier B, et al. Risk factors for infection after operative fixation of Tibial plateau fractures. Injury 2016;**47**:1501–1505

[133] Dinçel YM, Öner A, Arikan Y, Çaglar S, Özcafer R, Güleç MA. Effect of BMI on outcomes of surgical treatment for tibial plateau fractures: A comparative retrospective case series study. Chinese Journal of Traumatology. 2018;**21**(2):104–108

[134] O'Neill DC, Sato EH, Steffenson LN, et al. Patient-reported outcomes after tibial plateau fracture: Infection confers greatest risk of poor outcome. European Journal of Orthopaedic Surgery and Traumatology 2024;**35**:34

[135] Molina CS, Stinner DJ, Fras AR, Evans JM. Risk factors of deep infection in operatively treated pilon fractures (AO/OTA: 43). Journal of Orthopaedics. 2015;**12**(Suppl 1):S7-S13

[136] Lundin N, Huttunen TT, Berg HE, Marcano A, Felländer-Tsai L, Enocson A. Increasing incidence of pelvic and acetabular fractures. A nationwide study of 87,308 fractures over a 16-year period in Sweden. Injury. 2021;**52**(6):1410–1417

[137] Compston JE, Flahive J, Hosmer DW, et al. Relationship of weight, height, and body mass index with fracture risk at different sites in postmenopausal women: The Global Longitudinal study of Osteoporosis in Women (GLOW). Journal of Bone and Mineral Research 2014; **29**:487–493

[138] Hsieh TM, Chuang PC, Liu CT, Wu BY, Liu YW, Hsieh CH. Protective role of obesity on trauma impact: A retrospective analysis of patients with surgical Blunt Bowel mesenteric injury due to road traffic accidents. Risk Management and Healthcare Policy. 2022;**15**:1533–1543

[139] Le NT, Robinson J, Lewis SJ. Obese patients and radiography literature: What do we know about a big issue? Journal of Medical Radiation Sciences. 2015;**62**(2):132–141

[140] Uppot RN. Technical challenges of imaging & image-guided interventions in obese patients. British Journal of Radiology. 2018;**91**:20170931

[141] Karunakar MA, Shah SN, Jerabek S. Body mass index as a predictor of complications after operative treatment of acetabular fractures. Journal of Bone and Joint Surgery. 2005;**87**(7):1498–1502

[142] McGee A, Obinwa C, White P, et al. Preoperative Blood Loss of Isolated Acetabular Fractures. Journal of Orthopaedic Trauma 2023;**37**:116–121

[143] Porter SE, Russell GV, Dews RC, Qin Z, Woodall Jr J, Graves ML. Complications of acetabular fracture surgery in morbidly obese patients. Journal of Orthopaedic Trauma. 2008;**22**(9):589–594

[144] Gettys FK, Russell GV, Karunakar MA. Open treatment of pelvic and acetabular fractures. Orthopedic Clinics of North America. 2011;**42**(1):69–83. vi

[145] Lazar MA, Plocher EK, Egol KA. Obesity and its relationship with pelvic and lower-extremity orthopedic trauma. American Journal of Orthopedics (Belle Mead, NJ). 2010;**39** (4):175–182

[146] Sems SA, Johnson M, Cole PA, Byrd CT, Templeman DC. Elevated body mass index increases early complications of surgical treatment of pelvic ring injuries. Journal of Orthopaedic Trauma. 2010;**24**(5): 309–314

[147] Bates P, Gary J, Singh G, Reinert C, Starr A. Percutaneous treatment of pelvic and acetabular fractures in obese patients. Orthopedic Clinics of North America. 2011;**42** (1):55–67. vi

[148] Vigdorchik JM, Esquivel AO, Jin X, Yang KH, Onwudiwe NA, Vaidya R. Biomechanical stability of a supra-acetabular pedicle screw internal fixation device (INFIX) vs external fixation and plates for vertically unstable pelvic fractures. Journal of Orthopaedic Surgery and Research. 2012;7:31

[149] Jaeblon T, Perry KJ, Kufera JA. Waist-Hip ratio surrogate is more predictive than Body Mass Index of wound complications after Pelvic and Acetabulum surgery. Journal of Orthopaedic Trauma. 2018;**32**(4): 167–173

[150] Avilucea FR, Ferreira R, Shaath MK, Haidukewych GJ. Opportunistic use of computed tomography to determine muscle-adipose ratio reliably predicts wound complications after Kocher-Langenbeck surgical exposure of the Acetabulum. Journal of Orthopaedic Trauma. 2024;**38**(1):31–35

[151] Patel M, Fairburn S, McGwin G, Spitler C. Effects of obesity on systemic complications after operative Pelvic Ring fractures. Journal of Orthopaedic Trauma. 2024;**38**(9):466–471

[152] Shaath MK, Lim PK, Andrews R, Chip Routt ML. Morbid obesity and short-term complications following acetabular fracture surgery: A comparative cohort study. Injury. 2020;**51**(11):2622–2627

[153] Morris BJ, Richards JE, Guillamondegui OD, et al. Obesity increases early complications after high-energy pelvic and acetabular fractures. Orthopedics 2015;**38**:e881–7

Chapter 10

The Influence of BMI and Other Measures of Adiposity on Risks and Outcomes in Total Joint Arthroplasty

Lachlan F. Anderson, McKenna W. Box, Andrew Chambers, Michael Muncy and John T. Riehl

Abstract

Body mass index (BMI) influences perioperative risk and outcomes in total joint arthroplasty. As obesity rates rise, surgeons must consider the impact of BMI on patient selection, surgical planning, and postoperative care. High BMI increases the risk of infection, wound issues, venous thromboembolism, prosthetic joint infection, surgical time, blood loss, and technical challenges. Evidence shows that, with proper perioperative strategies such as nutritional optimization, glycemic control, and enhanced recovery, acceptable results are achievable across a wide range of BMIs. This chapter reviews the role of BMI in preoperative, intraoperative, and postoperative management, emphasizing a risk-stratified and individualized approach to improve outcomes and reduce complications.

Keywords: total joint arthroplasty, surgical complications, postoperative outcomes, obesitybody mass index, total knee arthroplasty, total hip arthroplasty, total shoulder arthroplasty, total elbow arthroplasty, total ankle arthroplasty

1. Introduction

Obesity poses considerable challenges for orthopedic practice. Defined as excess adipose tissue that impairs health, obesity is classified by the World Health Organization (WHO) as a body mass index (BMI) of 30 kg/m^2 or greater [1]. By 2025, an estimated 2.6 billion adults worldwide will meet the criteria for overweight or obesity, continuing the dramatic rise since 1990 [2]. Over half of patients undergoing total knee arthroplasty (TKA) in the United States are obese, underscoring the direct correlation between obesity prevalence and total joint arthroplasty (TJA) [3].

Despite its widespread adoption, BMI fails to differentiate between fat and lean muscle mass, resulting in limitations to BMI as a measure for obesity. Muscular individuals, such as athletes, may exhibit a high BMI without an excess of body fat [4]. Conversely, individuals classified as having a normal BMI may possess

IntechOpen

considerable visceral fat, a condition referred to as metabolically obese, normal weight. Central (visceral) adiposity significantly increases cardiometabolic risks in comparison to peripheral (subcutaneous) fat [5]. Individuals with identical BMI values may exhibit markedly different risk profiles depending on the location of their body fat, which can influence perioperative risks due to conditions such as insulin resistance, dyslipidemia, and systemic inflammation [6]. Recent dual-energy Xray absorptiometry (DEXA) studies have revealed that, while only 36% of individuals met the criteria for obesity based on BMI, 74% were classified as obese according to DEXA-measured body fat percentage [6, 7]. Consequently, current guidelines from the American Heart Association recommend measuring waist circumference in conjunction with BMI to enhance risk stratification [5, 8].

In orthopedics, obesity contributes to joint pathology both biomechanically and systemically. Obesity magnifies mechanical strain on musculoskeletal structures. Excess weight intensifies forces across weight-bearing joints, such as the knees and hips, significantly increasing the risk of osteoarthritis (OA) [9]. Altered gait mechanics frequently accompany obesity, characterized by slower velocity, shorter stride length, wider stance, and abnormal foot biomechanics, which cumulatively exacerbate joint degeneration and increase the risk of injury [10–12].

On the cellular level, obesity has a significant impact through chronic systemic inflammation and the development of metabolic syndrome. Adipose tissue in obesity secretes inflammatory cytokines (e.g., TNF-α, IL-6) and alters adipokine levels (increased leptin, decreased adiponectin), thereby creating a persistent inflammatory state [13]. These metabolic disturbances increase bone resorption and bone marrow adiposity, manifesting as delayed bone healing and accelerated progression of OA [14–17]. Paradoxically, obesity increases bone mineral density in weight-bearing regions, particularly at the hip, spine, and tibia, due to increased mechanical loading [18].

While these biological, biomechanical, and systemic effects underscore the complexity of treating patients with obesity, an additional layer of complexity arises in surgical decision-making. The use of strict BMI thresholds for TJA candidacy remains controversial [19]. Critics argue that such limits may oversimplify risk assessment and fail to reflect the nuanced needs of individual patients. Recent literature has highlighted the importance of shared decision-making, patient-centered risk discussions, and the ethical considerations of beneficence, non-maleficence, autonomy, and justice when determining surgical eligibility [19].

Overall, an obese patient presents a complex risk profile and a higher propensity for OA, while also presenting a higher perioperative risk when surgical treatment is pursued. This chapter will explore the multifaceted impacts of BMI on TJA outcomes and outline strategies to optimize care for patients across the BMI spectrum.

2. Total knee arthroplasty

2.1 Preoperative risk assessment and optimization

Obesity is a key consideration in the preoperative evaluation for primary TKA. Obesity itself is not a contraindication for surgery, but patients with a BMI $\geq$ 40 (morbidly obese) or $\geq$ 50 (super-obese) have almost double the complication rates of those with BMIs under 40 [20–23]. Nevertheless, TKA remains highly effective in obese individuals, with numerous studies reporting comparable pain relief and functional gain in obese patients compared to non-obese patients [21, 23, 24]. In fact, because obese patients often start with worse function, their absolute improvement can be as significant or greater [25]. Current guidelines (AAOS, AAHKS/ACR 2023) state that BMI alone should not be used to deny TKA [26–28]. Rather than strict cutoffs, the emphasis is on optimization. The American Academy of Orthopaedic Surgeons (AAOS) suggests that while a BMI < 40 kg/m^2 is ideal for elective TKA, patients above this threshold can proceed with surgery after individualized risk reduction. In practice, many surgeons impose BMI thresholds (often around 40) for safety or resource reasons, but this practice remains controversial. Data show such thresholds can limit access without markedly improving outcomes [29].

Growing interest in glucagon-like peptide-1 receptor agonists (GLP-1RA) for weight loss could offer an effective way to optimize patient care preoperatively. A minimum of three months of preoperative GLP-1RA exposure appears sufficient to confer these benefits, with more prolonged exposure not showing additional risk reduction [30]. GLP-1RAs are associated with a reduced risk of periprosthetic joint infection, lower rates of postoperative medical complications, and decreased readmissions, particularly in individuals with morbid obesity (BMI ≥ 40 kg/m^2) [31–33]. With this in mind, the current American Society of Anesthesiologists (ASA) guidelines recommend a nuanced approach to managing GLP-1RA perioperatively in elective surgery based on patient risk assessment for aspiration (**Figure 1**) [34].

2.2 Intraoperative considerations

Studies show that with proper technique, proper component alignment can be achieved in morbidly obese TKA patients, and the use of modern instrumentation or computer navigation can help avoid outliers [35]. Nonetheless, the mechanical loads present in obese patients on the implant increase the risk of loosening and mechanical failure over time [36, 37]. Recent data indicate that even minor alignment deviations (like residual varus) in obese patients can predispose them to early revision [38]. Additionally, cementless fixation is suitable for obese patients when optimized through the use of newer porous baseplates, which provide improved load distribution [36, 39]. The AAOS Surgical Management of Osteoarthritis of the Knee guideline notes that while obesity poses technical challenges, BMI alone does not necessitate stemmed or constrained implants purely due to weight, nor does it justify the routine use of navigation or patient-specific guides over standard techniques [26]. Advanced technologies (navigation, patient-specific guides, robotics) may assist in complex cases but have not shown superior outcomes specifically for obese patients on a broad scale [26]. The key is meticulous execution of whichever technique is chosen.

Morbidly obese patients typically have longer operating room (OR) times for TKA (15–30 minutes longer) due to the technical complexity added by patient corpulence [40]. This prolonged exposure can increase the risk of infection, so minimizing delays is crucial [41]. Despite these longer operative times, higher estimated blood loss (EBL) transfusion rates are paradoxically lower in obese patients, possibly due to greater total blood volume and higher preoperative hemoglobin levels [42, 43]. Blood loss management strategies, such as the use of tranexamic acid (TXA), are equally effective across BMI categories [44]. TXA is

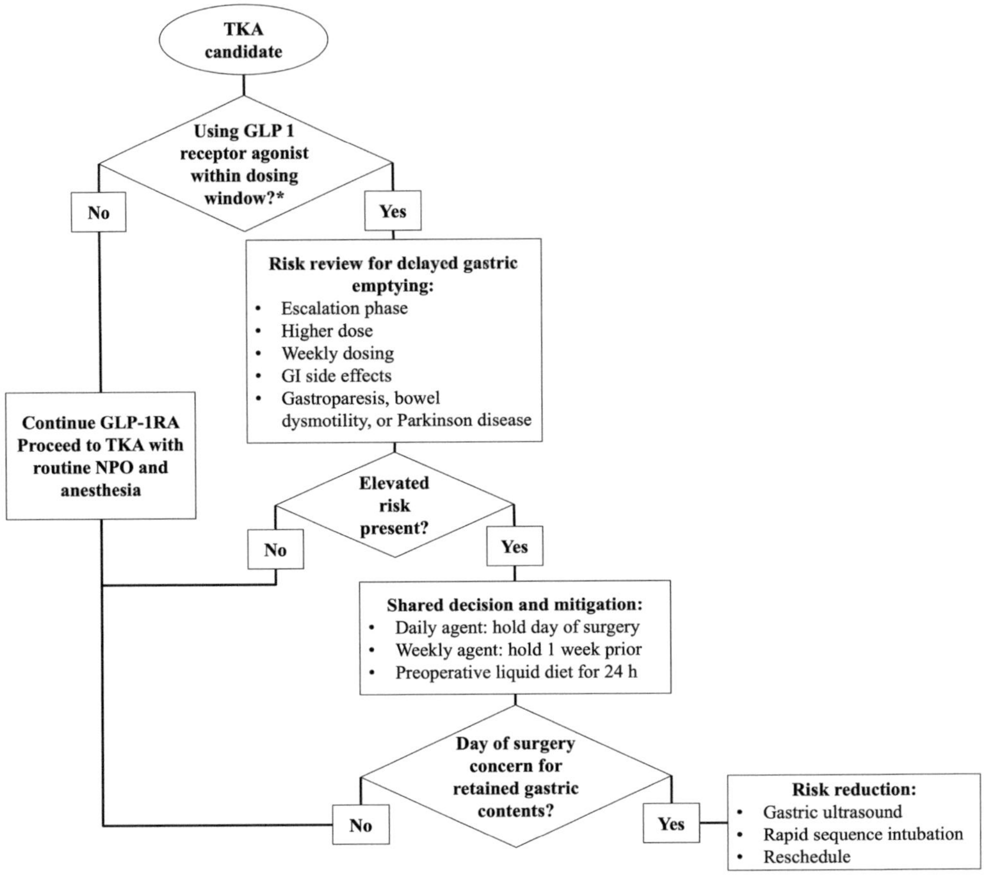

Figure 1.
Perioperative management of GLP-1RA as per American Society of Anesthesiologists recommendations [6].

strongly recommended to reduce blood loss and the need for transfusion across all BMI ranges, supported by high-quality evidence [44].

2.3 Postoperative outcomes

Obesity markedly increases the risk of periprosthetic joint infection (PJI) after TKA. Meta-analyses indicate that patients with a BMI ≥ 30 have roughly 2–3 times the odds of PJI compared to those with a BMI < 30 [22]. For morbid obesity, the odds can be 4 × higher, and super-obese patients can have a 21.3% increase in PJI risk per BMI unit beyond 50 [22, 45, 46]. Mechanisms include reduced antibiotic efficacy due to greater adipose tissue, impaired wound healing, and prolonged operative times, which can enhance bacterial exposure [21, 22]. The AAOS PJI guideline emphasizes that obesity is a moderate risk factor for PJI and recommends weight-based antibiotic dosing, extended wound surveillance, and early intervention protocols in high-risk patients [26]. Society guidelines for obese patients undergoing TKA are presented in **Table 1**.

Obese patients have increased all-cause five-year revision rates (OR = 1.15; 95% CI: 1.08–1.24; $P < 0.0001$) [47]. Studies consistently show that obesity is associated

Recommendation	Society
No difference in postoperative functional outcomes between non-obese (BMI < 30) and obese patients (BMI 30–39.9) undergoing TKA/THA. There may be an increased risk of complications in morbidly obese patients (BMI ≥ 40), particularly surgical site infections.	2022 AAOS CPG [26]
Patients with a BMI ≥ 40 have an increased perioperative risk. However, do not delay TKA solely to achieve weight loss or a target BMI. No rigid BMI cutoff should prohibit surgery, although weight loss is encouraged.	2023 ACR and AAHKS Guideline [27]
An accepted threshold for elective THA/TKA is BMI < 40 for patient safety.	AAOS (Quality Toolkit) [85]
Limited evidence suggests that elevated BMI may increase the risk of adverse events in patients undergoing THA for symptomatic hip OA.	2023AAOS CPG [86]
Limited evidence suggests that patients with elevated BMI and symptomatic OA of the hip may achieve lower absolute patient-reported outcome scores but experience a similar degree of improvement in patient satisfaction, pain, function, and quality of life after THA.	2023 AAOS CPG [86]

Table 1.
Society recommendations for TKA and THA in obese patients.

with higher hazard ratios for all-cause revision, particularly for infection and aseptic loosening [21]. Morbidly obese patients have a significantly higher risk of revision for loosening (HR = 1.39) and infection (HR = 1.72) compared to non-obese patients [21]. Morbidly obese patients also demonstrate higher rates of repeat revision, with loosening and instability being the most common causes [21].

2.4 Other measures of adiposity

For TKA, evidence consistently shows that local measures of knee adiposity outperform BMI in predicting infection and wound complications. Radiographic indices, such as the prepatellar fat thickness ratio and anterior soft-tissue depth, are independent predictors of PJI and wound breakdown [48, 49]. In contrast, BMI often loses significance once these measures are included. Increased visceral adiposity on CT is also linked to very high odds of PJI, and waist circumference better predicts severe medical complications than BMI class [50]. Additionally, sarcopenia and sarcopenic obesity confer higher risks of medical and mechanical complications [51]. These findings emphasize that fat distribution, sarcopenia, and central adiposity provide improved perioperative risk stratification for TKA compared to BMI [50].

3. Total hip arthroplasty

3.1 Preoperative risk assessment and optimization

Obesity plays a significant role in total hip arthroplasty (THA). Extensive data confirm that obese patients derive substantial improvements in pain and function from THA, similar to other patients, but morbid obesity is associated with markedly higher complication rates [47, 52, 53]. Super obesity (BMI ≥ 50) is often considered a relative contraindication due to almost three times higher rates of PJI, revision surgery, and healthcare utilization [52, 54]. Extremely low BMI (<18.5) also poses unique risks, such as increased rates of prosthetic loosening, dislocation, and periprosthetic fractures [55]. Despite this, morbidly obese patients (BMI ≥ 40) have been shown to possess the lowest preoperative function scores but exhibit the greatest improvement in perceived function postoperatively, highlighting the benefits of THA despite the potentially increased risk of complications [56].

Preoperative multidisciplinary weight-loss programs, including bariatric surgery in some studies, have been shown to significantly reduce perioperative complications. However, they do not completely mitigate longer-term risks such as revision or aseptic loosening [57, 58]. Emphasizing metabolic optimization and targeted weight reduction in high-risk THA candidates is recommended and essential for improving perioperative safety and long-term outcomes [54, 59, 60]. GLP-1RAs do not increase the risk of postoperative complications after THA in obese patients and may be associated with comparable or improved infection and readmission rates [61–63]. However, the benefits in non-diabetic obese patients are less pronounced in THA than in TKA.

3.2 Intraoperative considerations

Obesity increases intraoperative complexity during THA. Higher BMI is associated with increased difficulty in achieving optimal exposure, retractor placement, and precise component positioning, which can contribute to elevated risks of malpositioning and early loosening of prostheses, particularly in patients with morbid obesity [64, 65]. Obesity also has a negative impact on achieving adequate leg length [66]. The use of larger, high-offset femoral stems and acetabular components is recommended to restore biomechanics and accommodate increased soft tissue and mechanical loads [67]. Using a ceramic femoral head with a highly cross-linked polyethylene liner is considered the most durable option for obese patients [68]. Elevated BMI is also associated with prolonged operative times, increased intraoperative blood loss, and higher transfusion requirements [69]. These intraoperative challenges further amplify the risks of infection and postoperative complications and should be considered during operative planning [70, 71]. Referral to high-volume surgeons and specialized centers may mitigate some risks [72, 73].

3.3 Postoperative outcomes

The most consistently elevated risks after THA in obesity include PJI, wound complications, early dislocation, thromboembolic events, reoperation, revision surgery, and hospital readmission [74]. Surgical complications begin to significantly increase above a BMI of 32 kg/m^2. The risk of PJI rises exponentially above a BMI threshold of 37 kg/m^2, with morbid obesity resulting in a fourfold increased PJI risk compared to non-obese individuals [74, 75]. Super obese (BMI ≥ 50) patients also experience notably higher incidences of dislocations, aseptic loosening, and revisions within both short- and long-term follow-up periods [64, 76]. There is also a stepwise increase in medical complications [77]. Revision THA outcomes deteriorate significantly as BMI surpasses 35, with failure rates approximately doubling compared to less obese individuals [64, 78]. A low BMI also correlates with increased revision and periprosthetic fracture rates, underscoring the importance of optimal patient selection across the entire BMI spectrum [54]. Despite these risks, functional improvement after THA is still observed in obese patients, though the absolute functional scores may be slightly lower. Society recommendations for patients undergoing THA are similar to those for TKA. Both are presented in **Table 1**.

3.4 Other measures of adiposity

In THA, local fat accumulation and distribution predict complications more effectively than BMI alone [79]. Percent body fat is associated with higher rates of medical and surgical complications, lower activity scores, and increased pain after THA [80]. In contrast, BMI does not reliably predict these functional outcomes or risks [80]. Posterior hip surgical site fat thickness is a stronger predictor of postoperative wound complications and reoperations than BMI, with thresholds of approximately 50–65 mm linked to increased risk of infection [81]. BMI has only a moderate correlation with peri-incisional adiposity and may not accurately reflect the distribution or magnitude of adipose tissue relevant to surgical risk [82]. Abdominal CT studies indicate that visceral fat area strongly predicts periprosthetic joint infections. In contrast, intermuscular fat in the thigh independently doubles the risk of major complications, such as dislocation and aseptic loosening [83, 84].

4. Total shoulder arthroplasty

4.1 Preoperative optimization

Managing obese patients undergoing total shoulder arthroplasty (TSA) (both anatomic total shoulder arthroplasty (aTSA) and reverse total shoulder arthroplasty (rTSA)) warrants a tailored evaluation and optimization plan. High BMI has been linked to higher postoperative complications, yet the vast majority of obese patients still achieve significant pain relief and functional improvement [87, 88]. Optimization strategies include multidisciplinary management of comorbidities, perioperative infection prevention, and patient education regarding the increased risks associated with these conditions [89]. There is no evidence that mandatory preoperative weight loss or strict BMI cutoffs improve outcomes. In fact, using BMI thresholds as exclusion criteria would deny many patients a complication-free and beneficial procedure [90]. There are still gaps in the evidence, particularly regarding high-quality, TSA-specific randomized controlled trials on preoperative weight loss strategies, pharmacological treatments, and bariatric surgery. Therefore, a patient-centered approach that involves shared decision-making and informed consent is advised, focusing on individualized risk-benefit evaluations. Society guidelines are presented in **Table 2**.

Regarding GLP-1RA, data for TSA are mixed but trend neutral to beneficial overall. One national-cohort study reported higher 90-day medical complications

Recommendation	Source (society)
Obesity does not significantly increase the rate of early (30-day) post-operative complications after total shoulder arthroplasty.	2020 AAOS CPG [108] (Glenohumeral Joint OA)

Table 2.
Society recommendations for TSA in obese patients.

and readmissions with perioperative GLP-1RA use [91]. Several others show no increase in TSA complications [92, 93]. One study specific to semaglutide shows lower 90-day adverse event rates [94], while another study found that every measured complication was reduced in the GLP-1RA cohort in patients undergoing TSA [94].

4.2 Intraoperative considerations

The intraoperative challenges obesity presents during TSA include exposure limitations, increased complexity of alignment, and longer operative times. Specifically, excessive adipose tissue and limited visibility can hinder proper positioning of the glenoid and humeral components [95]. Notably, one study paradoxically found less scapular notching in obese rTSA patients, possibly due to altered biomechanics [95]. This finding may reflect differences in bone positioning or adapter wear patterns, though additional research is needed. Despite this, a recent study found no increase in mechanical failure or loosening in obese patients undergoing TSA during short-term follow-up, suggesting that alignment issues are manageable and not surgery-limiting in obese individuals [60].

Adiposity also poses technical difficulties due to the thicker subcutaneous tissue, which increases retraction effort, wound tension, and the potential for devascularization [96]. The soft-tissue space for humeral exposure is reduced, which can increase surgical complexity and potentially prolong the surgery [95]. Additionally, operative time is consistently prolonged in obese TSA patients by 15–45 minutes [87, 88]. Blood loss may be higher; however, multiple reports indicate no increase in transfusion rates when TXA is used, suggesting that blood-sparing protocols are effective in this population [95, 97, 98].

4.3 Postoperative complications

Obese patients undergoing TSA have been shown to have higher rates of postoperative infection, including both superficial and deep PJI, as well as an increased risk of medical complications compared to non-obese patients [89, 99, 100]. Obesity is also associated with elevated odds of dislocation (OR 2.5), periprosthetic fracture (OR 1.9), and revision surgery (OR 1.5) after TSA [101]. However, other studies have shown that when controlling for comorbidities, obesity is not an independent risk factor for long-term mechanical complications or revision at 2–5 years [89, 100]. In rTSA, higher BMI is specifically linked to an increased risk of deep infection at three years, while in aTSA, higher BMI is marginally associated with increased 90-day readmission [102]. TSA also demonstrates an "obesity paradox." Underweight patients have the highest risk of 30-day medical complications, and those with a BMI of 30–35 kg/m^2 have the lowest risk [103–105].

Despite these risks, both obese and non-obese patients experience substantial improvements in pain, function, and range of motion after aTSA and rTSA. For rTSA, obese patients with rotator cuff arthropathy or fracture achieve similar functional scores and implant survival as non-obese patients. However, they may have a slightly lower postoperative range of motion, particularly in forward flexion and internal rotation [106]. This reduction in mobility does not translate into clinically meaningful differences in overall function or satisfaction [106]. Long-term

(10-year) survival after aTSA is up to 93% in obese patients versus 96% in normal-weight patients ($P = 0.753$), and after rTSA is 92% versus 95% ($P = 0.680$), respectively [104, 105]. No significant differences in all-cause revision, aseptic loosening, or periprosthetic joint infection are observed between obese and non-obese patients at 5–10 years when comorbidities are controlled [104].

4.4 Other measures of adiposity

Local subcutaneous fat distribution at the shoulder, specifically increased tissue depth at the coracoid and bicipital groove, has been shown to correlate with higher rates of infection, instability, and stress fractures after total shoulder arthroplasty in obese patients, independent of BMI [107]. This measure is a more accurate predictor of complications than BMI alone, as it directly reflects the amount of adipose tissue encountered during surgery and its impact on wound healing and prosthetic stability.

5. Total ankle arthroplasty

5.1 Preoperative risk assessment and patient selection

Obesity is not a contraindication to total ankle arthroplasty (TAA), and multiple studies show that obese patients achieve comparable functional gains to their non-obese counterparts. Bouchard et al. noted similar improvements in pain and disability scores between obese and non-obese patients (~3.8-year follow-up) and found no significant differences in complications or revision rates [109]. Likewise, Kim et al. found no increase in short-term complications or failure rates across BMI categories [110]. However, long-term outcomes suggest diminished implant survival in obesity. Schipper et al. reported a 2.8-fold increased risk of implant failure [111], and National Korean health data ($n = 2{,}914$) supported this finding, showing that patients with a BMI ≥ 30 had a 63% increased risk of TAA failure (aHR 1.63) [112].

5.2 Intraoperative considerations

Obesity complicates surgical exposure due to increased soft-tissue depth, which can impair visualization and precise component alignment, both of which are critical for long-term implant survival [113]. While alignment metrics are infrequently reported by BMI subgroup, registry-reported higher failure rates in obese patients may reflect suboptimal component positioning over time [112]. Additional adipose tissue has also been found to increase wound tension and the risk of dehiscence [114].

Operative times are consistently prolonged by 20–45 minutes, elevating the risk of soft-tissue ischemia and infection [110, 112]. Tourniquet use beyond 90 minutes is particularly concerning in larger limbs. While BMI-specific blood loss data are limited, prolonged exposure correlates with wound issues, and evidence from other arthroplasties suggests obesity contributes to higher intraoperative bleeding [115]. Careful preoperative planning, intraoperative imaging, and meticulous soft-tissue handling are key.

5.3 Postoperative complications

Short-term outcomes are broadly similar between obese and non-obese TAA patients [110, 116]. Over longer follow-up, however, obesity is associated with an increased risk of infection and implant failure. The cumulative risk of implant failure is higher in obesity. Multiple series show cumulative implant failure odds are 1.5–2.8 × higher in patients with a BMI ≥ 30 kg/m^2 [111, 112]. Obesity-related factors, such as increased skin and wound tension and perfusion deficits, likely contribute.

5.4 Other measures of adiposity

Compared to other total joint arthroplasties, local radiographic measures of adiposity do not outperform BMI in predicting complications after TAA [117]. Recent evidence indicates that radiographic soft-tissue thickness at the tibia and talus does not significantly predict PJI or other major complications after TAA [117]. Logistic regression analyses showed no statistically significant link between these measurements and infection risk. In fact, patients with infections tended to have slightly lower soft-tissue thickness; however, this difference was neither clinically nor statistically significant.

6. Total elbow arthroplasty

6.1 Preoperative risk assessment and patient selection

As with the prior TJA procedures described, obesity is not an absolute contraindication to total elbow arthroplasty (TEA) but likely does increase perioperative risk. Collinton et al. found that 30-day complication rates were not associated with BMI in a patient cohort of 615 [118]. At 90 days, however, Werner et al. reported 2.6 times higher odds of both local complications and 4.4 times higher odds of systemic complications in obese patients [119]. Longer-term data from Baghdadi et al. demonstrated 10-year survival rates of 86% in obese patients and 76% in non-obese patients, with a BMI of 35–40 tripling the risk of revision for any cause [120]. Common complications include infection, venous thromboembolism, extensor mechanism dysfunction, and heterotopic ossification [120].

6.2 Intraoperative considerations

Obese patients pose technical difficulties in achieving optimal implant alignment and fixation due to increased soft tissue bulk and altered biomechanics. The elbow joint, although non-weight-bearing, is exposed to increased torsional loads in obese individuals [120, 121]. This elevated mechanical demand can increase stress at the cement-bone and implant-cement interfaces, potentially accelerating loosening and wear [120, 122]. Therefore, achieving precise implant positioning using robust fixation is critical in patients with a higher BMI.

The deep exposure required for TEA may also be compromised by thick adipose layers, making the visualization and protection of critical structures, such as the ulnar nerve, more challenging [82]. Excess adipose tissue further complicates retraction and increases the risk of soft-tissue trauma. Studies indicate that obese patients are 5.7% more prone to extensor mechanism dysfunction and up to 10% more prone to heterotopic ossification compared to non-obese individuals [120]. Operative time, blood loss, and the incidence of intraoperative fracture may be higher in obese patients as well [123]. Venous thromboembolism was found to be nearly four times higher in one study of obese TEA patients [122].

6.3 Postoperative complications

Obese patients undergoing TEA face substantially higher risks of infection and mechanical failure. The 90-day postoperative infection rate was 6.5% in obese patients (compared to 1.9% in non-obese patients) [122]. Multiple studies further confirm an elevated rate of mechanical failure in obese TEA patients. Baghdadi et al. reported that revision for mechanical failure is more common in obese patients, with a 10-year survival rate of 72% versus 88% in non-obese patients [120]. Morrey et al. similarly noted that loosening occurred in 26% of morbidly obese patients compared to 12% in their non-obese counterparts [120]. Periprosthetic fractures were nearly four times more frequent in morbidly obese patients, while heterotopic ossification and extensor mechanism dysfunction were also increased [120]. Systemic complications, including pneumonia, acute renal failure, and cardiovascular events, were observed in 17% of obese patients versus 4% in non-obese patients [119]. Unlike TKA, THA, TSA, and TAA, no validated measures of local adiposity beyond BMI have been studied in TEA. Evidence is, therefore, limited to BMI-based analyses.

7. Summary of other measures of adiposity

A summary of the evidence on other measures of adiposity in relation to TJA is presented in **Table 3**.

8. Conclusion

BMI remains a valuable yet imperfect tool in assessing surgical risk and guiding clinical decision-making for patients undergoing TJA. While elevated BMI is associated with increased mechanical loading, systemic inflammation, and heightened risk of complications such as infection and delayed healing, the true impact of adiposity is highly dependent on fat distribution, metabolic health, and nutritional status. Furthermore, demographic variables such as age, sex, and race can introduce additional complexity in interpreting BMI and its clinical relevance. To optimize arthroplasty outcomes, orthopedic surgeons must adopt an individualized, risk-stratified approach that integrates metabolic profiling, nutritional assessment, and functional capacity. A shift toward complication-centered obesity classification and multimodal prehabilitation strategies, including interventions such as weight management, glycemic control, and physical conditioning, can offer a path forward in minimizing complications and improving long-term function. Notably, the advent of GLP-1RA and their potential benefits were highlighted in diabetic groups in three of the arthroplasty types detailed in this chapter, presenting a promising mechanism to improve outcomes. Future research specifically looking at these medications in TJA could provide an effective optimization strategy.

Joint	Predictor (measurement)	Key evidence	Comparison to BMI
THA	Surgical site fat thickness ≥ 50–65 mm (radiographs)	Thresholds associated with wound complications in posterior approach THA [81].	Outperforms BMI predicts wound problems, even when BMI is not elevated.
	Visceral fat area (CT)	Highest quartile of VFA is strongly associated with PJI [83].	Better predictor than BMI for PJI.
	Intermuscular fat (CT)	Independently doubled the risk of major complications [84].	Captures muscle quality and fat infiltration, which BMI misses.
TKA	Prepatellar fat thickness ratio (radiographs)	Independent predictor of PJI [48].	Better predictor than BMI for PJI.
	Anterior/medial soft-tissue depth (radiographs)	Increased depth correlated with higher infection and wound complication risk [49].	Better predictor than BMI for infection.
	Waist circumference	Each cm increase is associated with higher odds of medical complications [49, 50].	Better predictor than BMI class in obese patients.
	Visceral fat area (CT)	Highest quartile has increased odds of PJI [83].	Better predictor than BMI for infection.
	Sarcopenia/sarcopenic obesity	Independently associated with longer stays, higher medical, and implant complications [51].	Captures muscle quality, which BMI entirely misses.
TAA	Anterior tibial and talar soft tissue thickness (radiographs).	Independently predicted wound complications and revision [117, 124].	More reliable than BMI – BMI is often not associated with complications.
TSA	Subcutaneous fat depth (coracoid/bicipital groove)	Independently predicted complications; BMI not significant [107].	Superior to BMI; captures local risk BMI cannot.
TEA	No validated adiposity measures beyond BMI have been studied.	Limited evidence; BMI is linked to higher medical complications and revisions [120, 122].	Only BMI data exist.

Table 3.
Summary of other measures of adiposity and outcomes in TJA.

Ultimately, acknowledging the nuanced interplay between obesity and musculoskeletal health is essential for delivering high-quality, patient-centered orthopedic care in an increasingly obese global population. Importantly, rigid BMI cutoffs may not fully capture patient needs. Incorporating shared decision-making and ethical considerations ensures that surgical candidacy decisions strike a balance between risk and individualized potential for benefit, with obesity being only one of several deciding factors.

Acronyms and abbreviations

AAOS	American Academy of Orthopaedic Surgeons
AOS	Ankle Osteoarthritis Scale
aTSA	anatomic total shoulder arthroplasty

BMD	bone mineral density
BMI	body mass index
CPG	Clinical Practice Guideline
CRP	C-reactive protein
DEXA	dual-energy Xray absorptiometry
DVT	deep vein thrombosis
EAR	early active recovery
EBL	estimated blood loss
ERAS	enhanced recovery after surgery
ESR	erythrocyte sedimentation rate
HbA1c	hemoglobin A1c
IL-6	interleukin-6
MONW	metabolically obese, normal weight
NPWT	negative-pressure wound therapy
OA	osteoarthritis
OR	operating room
OSA	obstructive sleep apnea
PJI	periprosthetic joint infection
PROs	patient-reported outcomes
rTSA	reverse total shoulder arthroplasty
SF-36	Short Form 36 Health Survey
TAA	total ankle arthroplasty
TJA	total joint arthroplasty
TKA	total knee arthroplasty
THA	total hip arthroplasty
TNF-α	tumor necrosis factor alpha
TSA	total shoulder arthroplasty
TXA	tranexamic acid
VTE	venous thromboembolism
WHO	World Health Organization

Acknowledgments

The authors would like to acknowledge Dr. Michele McCarroll, Ph.D., and Devika Pavuluri, MPH, for their assistance with project organization and proofreading.

Conflict of Interest

Dr. John T. Riehl, M.D., is a consultant for, and receives royalties from, Arthrex Inc. The remaining authors declare that they have no potential conflicts of interest. There are no conflicts of interest that would potentially bias the results reported. This project received no funding. This research was supported (in whole or in part) by HCA Healthcare and/or an HCA Healthcare-affiliated entity. The views expressed in this publication represent those of the author(s) and do not necessarily represent the official views of HCA Healthcare or any affiliated entities.

Author details

Lachlan F. Anderson[1], McKenna W. Box[2*], Andrew Chambers[2], Michael Muncy[2] and John T. Riehl[2,3]

1 Anne Burnett Marion School of Medicine at TCU, Fort Worth, USA

2 Department of Orthopaedic Surgery, Medical City Denton, Denton, United States

3 Texas Bone and Joint, Fort Worth, United States

*Address all correspondence to: mckenna.box.med@gmail.com

References

[1] Elmaleh-Sachs A, Schwartz JL, Bramante CT, Nicklas JM, Gudzune KA, Jay M. Obesity management in adults a review. JAMA. 2023;**330**(20): 2000–2015

[2] Collaborators GAB. Global, regional, and national prevalence of adult overweight and obesity, 1990-2021, with forecasts to 2050: A forecasting study for the Global Burden of Disease Study 2021. Lancet. 2025;**405** (10481):813–838

[3] George J, Klika AK, Navale SM, Newman JM, Barsoum WK, Higuera CA. Obesity epidemic: Is its impact on total joint arthroplasty underestimated? An analysis of national trends. Clinical Orthopaedics and Related Research. 2017;**475**(7):1798–1806

[4] Ode J, Pivarnik JM, Reeves MJ, Knous JL. Body mass index as a predictor of percent fat in college athletes and nonathletes. Medicine & Science in Sports & Exercise. 2007;**39** (3):403–409

[5] Laddu D, Neeland IJ, Carnethon M, Stanford FC, Mongraw-Chaffin M, Barone Gibbs B, et al. Implementation of Obesity Science Into Clinical Practice: A Scientific Statement From the American Heart Association. Circulation. 2024;**150**(1):e7–e19

[6] Wong JC, O'Neill S, Beck BR, Forwood MR, Khoo SK. Comparison of obesity and metabolic syndrome prevalence using fat mass index, body mass index and percentage body fat. PLOS ONE. 2021;**16**(1):e0245436

[7] Jeong S-M, Lee DH, Rezende LFM, Giovannucci EL. Different correlation of body mass index with body fatness and obesity-related biomarker according to age, sex and race-ethnicity. Scientific Reports. 2023;**13**:3472

[8] Atlantis E, Sahebolamri M, Cheema BS, Williams K. Usefulness of the Edmonton obesity staging system for stratifying the presence and severity of weight-related health problems in clinical and community settings: A rapid review of observational studies. Obesity Reviews: An Official Journal of the International Association for the Study of Obesity. 2020;**21**(11):e13120

[9] Messier SP, Gutekunst DJ, Davis C, DeVita P. Weight loss reduces knee-joint loads in overweight and obese older adults with knee osteoarthritis. Arthritis and Rheumatism. 2005;**52**(7):2026–2032

[10] Steinberg N, Nemet D, Pantanowitz M, Eliakim A. Gait Pattern, impact to the skeleton and postural balance in overweight and obese children: A review. Sports (Basel, Switzerland). 2018;**6**(3):75

[11] Springer BD, Carter JT, McLawhorn AS, Scharf K, Roslin M, Kallies KJ, et al. Obesity and the role of bariatric surgery in the surgical management of osteoarthritis of the hip and knee: A review of the literature. Surgery for Obesity and Related Diseases: Official Journal of the American Society for Bariatric Surgery 2017;**13**:111–118

[12] Scataglini S, Dellaert L, Meeuwssen L, Staeljanssens E, Truijen S. The difference in gait pattern between adults with obesity and adults with a normal weight, assessed with

3D-4D gait analysis devices: A systematic review and meta-analysis. International Journal of Obesity (2005). 2025;**49**(4):541–553

[13] Forte YS, Renovato-Martins M, Barja-Fidalgo C. Cellular and molecular mechanisms associating obesity to bone loss. Cells. 2023;**12**(4):521

[14] Kim D, Ansari MM, Ghosh M, Heo Y, Choi K-C, Son Y-O. Implications of obesity-mediated cellular dysfunction and adipocytokine signaling pathways in the pathogenesis of osteoarthritis. Molecular Aspects of Medicine. 2025;**103**:101361

[15] Zhao X, Wang Q, Wang W, Lu S. Increased neutrophil extracellular traps caused by diet-induced obesity delay fracture healing. The FASEB Journal. 2024;**38**(20):e70126

[16] Oliveira MC, Vullings J, van de Loo FAJ. Osteoporosis and osteoarthritis are two sides of the same coin paid for obesity. Nutrition (Burbank, Los Angeles County, Calif.). 2020;**70**:110486

[17] Cao JJ. Effects of obesity on bone metabolism. Journal of Orthopaedic Surgery and Research. 2011;**6**:30

[18] Evans AL, Paggiosi MA, Eastell R, Walsh JS.Bone density, microstructure and strength in obese and normal weight men and women in younger and older adulthood. Journal of Bone and Mineral Research: The Official Journal of the American Society for Bone and Mineral Research. 2015;**30**(5):920–928

[19] Lachance AD, Steika R, Lutton J, Chessa F. Total joint arthroplasty in patients who are obese or morbidly obese: An ethical analysis. The Journal of Bone and Joint Surgery American Volume. 2024;**106**(7):659–664

[20] Onggo JR, Onggo JD, De Steiger R, Hau R. Robotic-assisted total knee arthroplasty is comparable to conventional total knee arthroplasty: A meta-analysis and systematic review. Archives of Orthopaedic and Trauma Surgery. 2020;**140**(10):1533–1549

[21] Wall CJ, Vertullo CJ, Kondalsamy-Chennakesavan S, Lorimer MF, de Steiger RN. A prospective, longitudinal study of the influence of obesity on total knee arthroplasty revision rate: Results from the Australian orthopaedic association national joint replacement registry. The Journal of Bone and Joint Surgery American Volume. 2022;**104**(15):1386–1392

[22] Telang S, Yoshida B, Burdick GB, Palmer R, Ball JR, Lieberman JR, et al. Body mass index and the risk of postoperative complications after total knee arthroplasty. Journal of the American Academy of Orthopaedic Surgeons 2025;**33**:e36–e45

[23] Uvodich ME, Dugdale EM, Pagnano MW, Berry DJ, Abdel MP, Bedard NA. Outcomes of obese patients undergoing primary total knee arthroplasty: Trends over 30 years. The Journal of Bone and Joint Surgery American Volume. 2024;**106**(21):1963–1970

[24] Mulford JS, Ackerman I, Holder C, Cashman KS, Graves SE, Harris IA. The association between body mass index and patient-reported outcome measures before and after primary total hip or knee arthroplasty: A registry. ANZ Journal of Surgery. 2023;**93**(6):1665–1673

[25] Bosler AC, Deckard ER, Buller LT, Meneghini RM. Obesity is associated

with greater improvement in patient-reported outcomes following primary total knee arthroplasty. The Journal of Arthroplasty. 2023;**38**(12):2484–2491

[26] Srivastava AK. American academy of orthopaedic surgeons clinical practice guideline summary of surgical management of osteoarthritis of the knee. Journal of the American Academy of Orthopaedic Surgeons. 2023;**31**(24):1211–1220

[27] Hannon CP, Goodman SM, Austin MS, Yates Jr A, Guyatt G, Aggarwal VK, et al. 2023 American college of rheumatology and American association of hip and knee surgeons clinical practice guideline for the optimal timing of elective hip or knee arthroplasty for patients with symptomatic moderate-to-severe osteoarthritis or advanced symptomatic osteonecrosis with secondary arthritis for whom nonoperative therapy is ineffective. The Journal of Arthroplasty 2023;**38**:2193–2201

[28] Giesinger JM, Loth FL, MacDonald DJ, Giesinger K, Patton JT, Simpson AHRW, et al. Patient-reported outcome metrics following total knee arthroplasty are influenced differently by patients' body mass index. Knee Surgery, Sports Traumatology, Arthroscopy 2018;**26**:3257–3264

[29] Orr SV, Pereira GC, Christiansen BA. Justification of body mass index cutoffs for hip and knee joint arthroplasty among California orthopedic surgeons. Journal of Orthopaedic Surgery and Research. 2025;**20**(1):125

[30] Seddio AE, Vasudevan RS, Gouzoulis MJ, Ansah-Twum JK, Grauer JN, Rubin LE. As few as three months of preoperative semaglutide exposure prior to total knee arthroplasty is associated with reduced postoperative adverse events in patients with type II diabetes. The Journal of Arthroplasty. 2025;**40**(12):3089–3096.e1

[31] Kim BI, LaValva SM, Parks ML, Sculco PK, Della Valle AG, Lee GC. Glucagon-like peptide-1 receptor agonists decrease medical and surgical complications in morbidly obese patients undergoing primary TKA. The Journal of Bone and Joint Surgery American Volume. 2025;**107**(4):348–355

[32] Magruder ML, Yao VJH, Rodriguez AN, Ng MK, Sasson V, Erez O. Does semaglutide use decrease complications and costs following total knee arthroplasty? The Journal of Arthroplasty. 2023;**38**(11):2311–5e1

[33] Ramanathan R, Lee JY, Dalton JF, Lin RT, Lee I, Gonzalez Jr C, et al. GLP-1 receptor agonists in orthopaedic surgery: Implications for perioperative and outcomes: An orthopaedic surgeon's perspective. The Journal of Bone & Joint Surgery. 2021. DOI: 10.2106/JBJS.24.01287

[34] Kindel TL, Wang AY, Wadhwa A, Schulman AR, Sharaiha RZ, Kroh M, et al. Multisociety clinical practice guidance for the safe use of glucagon-like peptide-1 receptor agonists in the perioperative period. Clinical Gastroenterology and Hepatology 2024;**39**:180–183

[35] Ojard C, Habashy A, Meyer M, Chimento G, Ochsner JL. Effect of obesity on component alignment in total knee arthroplasty. Ochsner Journal. 2018;**18**(3):226–229

[36] Goh GS, Wells Z, Ong CB, Small I, Ciesielka K-A, Fillingham YA. Does

body mass index influence the outcomes and survivorship of modern cementless total knee arthroplasty? The Journal of Arthroplasty. 2022;**37**(11):2171–2177

[37] Wan Q, Zhang A, Liu Y, Chen H, Zhang J, Xue H, et al. The influence of body weight index on initial stability of uncemented femoral knee protheses: A finite element study. Heliyon 2023;**9**: e13819

[38] Lai Y-H, Cao J, Li Z-X, Feng W, Xu H, Zhou Z-K. Effect of body mass index on postoperative mechanical alignment and long-term outcomes after total knee arthroplasty: A retrospective cohort study of 671 knees. Annals of Translational Medicine. 2022;**10**(15):829

[39] Moya-Angeler J, Akkaya M, Innocenti M, Bergadano D, Martin-Alguacil J, León-Muñoz V. Fixation options for total knee arthroplasty: A comprehensive literature review. Journal of Orthopaedic Surgery and Research. 2024;**19**(1):463

[40] Abbas Z, Hafeez S, Naseem A, Habib Y, Mumtaz H. Effect of body mass index on duration of total knee replacement surgery: A prospective cross sectional study. Annals of Medicine and Surgery. 2022;**82**:104637

[41] Shin KH, Kim JH, Han SB. Greater risk of periprosthetic joint infection associated with prolonged operative time in primary total knee arthroplasty: Meta-analysis of 427,361 patients. Journal of Clinical Medicine. 2024;**13** (11):3046

[42] Evans JT, Mouchti S, Blom AW, Wilkinson JM, Whitehouse MR, Beswick A, et al. Obesity and revision surgery, mortality, and patient-reported outcomes after primary knee replacement surgery in the national joint registry: A UK cohort study. PLoS Medicine 2021;**18**:e1003704

[43] Frisch N, Wessell NM, Charters M, Peterson E, Cann B, Greenstein A, et al. Effect of body mass index on blood transfusion in total hip and knee arthroplasty. Orthopedics. 2016;**39**(5):e844–e849

[44] Meftah M, White PB, Siddiqi A, Siddappa VH, Kirschenbaum I. Tranexamic acid reduces transfusion rates in obese patients undergoing total joint arthroplasty. Surgical Technology International. 2019;**34**:451–455

[45] Xu J-L, Liang Z-R, Xiong B-L, Zou Q-Z, Lin T-Y, Yang P, et al. Correlation between body mass index and periprosthetic joint infection following total joint arthroplasty: A protocol for systematic review and meta analysis. Medicine 2020;**99**:e20549

[46] Righolt CH, Armstrong ML, Turgeon TR, Bohm ER, Sniderman J. Primary total knee arthroplasty in patients with BMI of ≥50 kg/m 2: A cohort study with long-term follow-up. The Journal of Bone and Joint Surgery American Volume. 2025;**107** (13):1472–1479

[47] Onggo JR, Ang JJM, Onggo JD, de Steiger R, Hau R. Greater risk of all-cause revisions and complications for obese patients in 3 106 381 total knee arthroplasties: A meta-analysis and systematic review. ANZ Journal of Surgery. 2021;**91**(11): 2308–2321

[48] Wagner RA, Hogan SP, Burge JR, Bates CM, Sanchez HB. The radiographic prepatellar fat thickness ratio correlates with infection risk after total knee arthroplasty. The Journal of Arthroplasty. 2018;**33**(7):2251–2255

[49] Vahedi H, Ward DT, Lee YS, Shohat N, Chen AF. Greater knee soft tissue thickness predisposes patients to subsequent periprosthetic joint infection after total knee arthroplasty. The Journal of Arthroplasty. 2020;**35** (7):1924–1927

[50] Gordon AM, Nian PP, Hameed D, Vakharia RM, Mont MA. Increased waist circumference is associated with severe postoperative medical complications following total knee arthroplasty: Understanding waist circumference and relation to body mass index. The Journal of Arthroplasty. 2025;**40**(7s1):S188–s93

[51] Ardeljan AD, Polisetty TS, Palmer J, Vakharia RM, Roche MW. Comparative analysis on the effects of sarcopenia following primary total knee arthroplasty: A retrospective matched-control analysis. The Journal of Knee Surgery. 2022;**35** (2):128–134

[52] Issa K, Harwin SF, Malkani AL, Bonutti PM, Scillia A, Mont MA. Bariatric orthopaedics: Total hip arthroplasty in super-obese patients (those with a BMI of ≥50 kg/m2). The Journal of Bone and Joint Surgery American Volume. 2016;**98**(3):180–185

[53] Chammout G, Kelly-Pettersson P, Hedbeck C-J, Stark A, Mukka S, Sköldenberg O. HOPE-trial: Hemiarthroplasty compared with total hip arthroplasty for displaced femoral neck fractures in octogenarians: A randomized controlled trial. JBJS Open Access. 2019;**4**(2):e0059

[54] Meller MM, Toossi N, Johanson NA, Gonzalez MH, Son M-S, Lau EC. Risk and cost of 90-day complications in morbidly and superobese patients after total knee arthroplasty. The Journal of Arthroplasty. 2016;**31**(10):2091–2098

[55] McDonald CL, Alsoof D, Johnson KG, Kuczmarski A, Lemme NJ, Testa EJ, et al. Underweight patients are at increased risk for complications following total hip arthroplasty. The Journal of Arthroplasty 2023;**38**: 1559–64.e1

[56] Huffman N, Pasqualini I, Redfern RE, Murray TG, Deren ME, Israelite CL, et al. Patient satisfaction and patient-reported outcomes do not vary by BMI class in total hip arthroplasty. European Journal of Orthopaedic Surgery & Traumatology 2024;**34**:1979–1985

[57] Smith TO, Aboelmagd T, Hing CB, MacGregor A. Does bariatric surgery prior to total Hip or knee arthroplasty reduce post-operative complications and improve clinical outcomes for obese patients? Systematic review and meta-analysis. The Bone & Joint Journal. 2016;**98-B**(9):1160–1166

[58] LaValva SM, Grubel J, Ong J, Chiu Y-F, Lyman S, Mandl LA, et al. Is preoperative weight reduction in patients who have body mass index ≥ 40 associated with lower complication rates after primary total hip arthroplasty? The Journal of Arthroplasty 2024;**39**:S73–S9

[59] Seward MW, Briggs LG, Bain PA, Chen AF. Preoperative nonsurgical weight loss interventions before total hip and knee arthroplasty: A systematic review. The Journal of Arthroplasty. 2021;**36**(11):3796–806.e8

[60] Mayfield CK, Abu-Zahra MS, Yensen K, Kotlier JL, Bolia IK, Hwang NM, et al. Effect of body mass index on complications following total

shoulder arthroplasty: A population-wide analysis. Journal of Shoulder and Elbow Surgery 2025;**34**:33–42

[61] Verhey JT, Austin RP, Tarabichi S, Paul B, Deckey DG, Christopher ZK, et al. GLP-1 agonists for weight loss: Do they increase complications in non-diabetic patients undergoing primary total hip arthroplasty? The Journal of Arthroplasty 2025;**40**:S101–s7

[62] Chan YC, Chuang SH, Kuo YJ, Lian YZ, Chen YP. The association between glucagon-like peptide-1 receptor agonists and postoperative complications after arthroplasty: A systematic review and meta-analysis. The Journal of Arthroplasty. 2025;**40** (12):3080–3088.e7

[63] Magruder ML, Miskiewicz MJ, Rodriguez AN, Mont MA. Semaglutide use prior to total hip arthroplasty results in fewer postoperative prosthetic joint infections and readmissions. The Journal of Arthroplasty. 2024;**39** (3):716–720

[64] Jeschke E, Citak M, Günster C, Halder AM, Heller K-D, Malzahn J, et al. Obesity increases the risk of postoperative complications and revision rates following primary total hip arthroplasty: An analysis of 131,576 total hip arthroplasty cases. The Journal of Arthroplasty 2018;**33**:2287–92.e1

[65] DeMik DE, Bedard NA, Dowdle SB, Elkins JM, Brown TS, Gao Y, et al. Complications and obesity in arthroplasty-a hip is not a knee. The Journal of Arthroplasty 2018;**33**:3281–3287

[66] Al-Amiry B, Pantelakis G, Mahmood S, Kadum B, Brismar TB, Sayed-Noor AS. Does body mass index affect restoration of femoral offset, leg length and cup positioning after total hip arthroplasty? A prospective cohort study. BMC Musculoskeletal Disorders. 2019;**20**(1):422

[67] Boisgard S, Descamps S, Bouillet B. Complex primary total hip arthroplasty. Orthopaedics & Traumatology, Surgery & Research. 2013;**99**(1 Suppl):S34–42

[68] Su J, Wang JJ, Yan ST, Zhang M, Wang HZ, Zhang NZ, et al. In vitro analysis of wearing of hip joint prostheses composed of different contact materials. Materials (Basel). 2021;**14**(14):3805

[69] Liu W, Wahafu T, Cheng M, Cheng T, Zhang Y, Zhang X. The influence of obesity on primary total hip arthroplasty outcomes: A meta-analysis of prospective cohort studies. Orthopaedics & Traumatology, Surgery & Research. 2015;**101**(3): 289–296

[70] Haynes J, Nam D, Barrack RL. Obesity in total Hip arthroplasty: Does it make a difference? The Bone & Joint Journal. 2017;**99-B**(1 Supple A):31–36

[71] Houdek MT, Wagner ER, Watts CD, Osmon DR, Hanssen AD, Lewallen DG, et al. Morbid obesity: A significant risk factor for failure of two-stage revision total hip arthroplasty for infection. The Journal of Bone and Joint Surgery American Volume 2015;**97**:326–332

[72] Ashkenazi I, Thomas J, Lawrence KW, Meftah M, Rozell JC, Schwarzkopf R. The impact of obesity on total hip arthroplasty outcomes when performed by high-volume surgeons-a propensity matched analysis from a high-volume urban center. The Journal of Arthroplasty. 2024;**39**(6):1412–1418

[73] Charalambous A, Pincus D, High S, Leung FH, Aktar S, Paterson JM, et al. Association of surgical experience with risk of complication in total hip arthroplasty among patients with severe obesity. JAMA Network Open 2021;**4**: e2123478

[74] Orringer M, Palmer RC, Ball JR, Telang S, Lieberman JR, Heckmann ND. Effect of BMI on the risk of postoperative complications following total hip arthroplasty. The Bone & Joint Journal. 2025;**107-b**(5 Supple A):47–54

[75] Lee K-J, Goodman SB. Identification of periprosthetic joint infection after total hip arthroplasty. Journal of Orthopaedic Translation. 2014;**3** (1):21– 25

[76] Barrett M, Prasad A, Boyce L, Dawson-Bowling S, Achan P, Millington S, et al. Total hip arthroplasty outcomes in morbidly obese patients: A systematic review. EFORT Open Reviews 2018;**3**:507–512

[77] Sayed-Noor AS, Mukka S, Mohaddes M, Kärrholm J, Rolfson O. Body mass index is associated with risk of reoperation and revision after primary total hip arthroplasty: A study of the Swedish hip arthroplasty register including 83,146 patients. Acta Orthopaedica. 2019;**90**(3):220–225

[78] Bongers J, Smulders K, Nijhof MW. Severe obesity increases risk of infection after revision total hip arthroplasty. The Journal of Arthroplasty. 2019;**34** (12):3023–9e2

[79] Heifner JJ, Fox YM, Sakalian PA, Corces A. The use of local adiposity as a proxy for obesity in primary total Hip arthroplasty: A systematic review. Journal of Orthopaedics. 2023;**38**:79–84

[80] Ledford CK, Ruberte Thiele RA, Appleton Jr JS, Butler RJ, Wellman SS, Attarian DE, et al. Percent body fat more associated with perioperative risks after total joint arthroplasty than body mass index. The Journal of Arthroplasty 2014;**29**:150–154

[81] Song BM, Adil SA, Schneider AM, Bendich I. Surgical site fat thickness is more predictive of postoperative wound complications than body mass index following posterior approach total hip arthroplasty. The Journal of Arthroplasty. 2025;**40**(12):3215–3220

[82] Heifner JJ, Pannu TS, Gomez O, Sakalian PA, Corces A. Body mass index is not an appropriate proxy for the condition of peri-incisional adiposity in primary total joint arthroplasty patients. The Journal of Arthroplasty. 2025;**40** (2):346–351

[83] Blackburn AZ, Katakam A, Roberts T, Humphrey TJ, Salimy MS, Egan CR, et al. Visceral fat as a risk factor for periprosthetic joint infection after total hip and knee arthroplasty. The Journal of Arthroplasty 2023;**38**:1839–45.e1

[84] Yu J, Wang M, Shen H. Intermuscular fat, but not subcutaneous fat, correlated with major complications after primary total hip arthroplasty. Academic Radiology. 2023;**30**(7): 1367–1373

[85] American Academy of Orthopaedic S. Obesity. 2024.

[86] Hannon CP, Delanois RE, Nandi S, Fillingham Y. American academy of orthopaedic surgeons clinical practice guideline summary management of osteoarthritis of the hip. Journal of the American Academy of Orthopaedic Surgeons. 2024;**32**(20):e1027–e34

[87] Werner BC, Burrus MT, Begho I, Gwathmey FW, Brockmeier SF. Early revision within 1 year after shoulder arthroplasty: Patient factors and etiology. Journal of Shoulder and Elbow Surgery. 2015;**24**(12):e323–30

[88] Jiang J, Yang C-H, Lin Q, Yun X-D, Xia Y-Y. Does arthroplasty provide better outcomes than internal fixation at mid- and long-term followup? A meta-analysis. Clinical Orthopaedics and Related Research. 2015;**473**(8):2672–2679

[89] Cogan CJ, Flores SE, Freshman RD, Chi HM, Feeley BT. Effect of obesity on short- and long-term complications of shoulder arthroplasty. Journal of Shoulder and Elbow Surgery. 2023;**32**(2):253–259

[90] Saini S, Bono O, Li L, MacAskill M, Chilton M, Ross G, et al. Investigating a potential limit to access to care: Preoperative cutoff values for body mass index for shoulder arthroplasty. Journal of the American Academy of Orthopaedic Surgeons 2022;**30**:e67–e73

[91] Lawand JJ, Tansey PJ, Ghali A, Tye C, Hantouly A, Fares MY, et al. Glucagon-like peptide-1 receptor agonist use is associated with increased risk of perioperative complication and readmission following shoulder arthroplasty. Journal of Shoulder and Elbow Surgery 2025;**34**:1152–1157

[92] Elsabbagh Z, Haft M, Murali S, Best M, McFarland EG, Srikumaran U. Does use of glucagon-like peptide-1 agonists increase perioperative complications in patients undergoing shoulder arthroplasty? Journal of Shoulder and Elbow Surgery. 2025;**34**(4):997–1006

[93] Omurzakov A, Omurzakov AM, Reddy RP, Megerian M, White AE, Miller M, et al. Perioperative glucagon-like peptide-1 receptor agonist use is not associated with increased complications in obese patients undergoing total shoulder arthroplasty: a propensity-matched large database study. In: Seminars in Arthroplasty: JSES. 2025;**35**(4):604–611

[94] Seddio AE, Wilhelm CV, Gouzoulis MJ, Islam W, Vasudevan RS, Halperin SJ, et al. Improved total shoulder arthroplasty outcomes associated with semaglutide utilization in patients with type II diabetes: A promising new addition to preoperative optimization. JSES International 2025;**9**:735–740

[95] Eichinger JK, Rao MV, Lin JJ, Goodloe JB, Kothandaraman V, Barfield WR, et al. The effect of body mass index on internal rotation and function following anatomic and reverse total shoulder arthroplasty. Journal of Shoulder and Elbow Surgery 2021;**30**:265–272

[96] De Martino I, Gulotta LV. The effect of obesity in shoulder arthroplasty outcomes and complications. Orthopedic Clinics of North America. 2018;**49**(3):353–360

[97] Wu KA, Helmkamp J, Levin JM, Hurley ET, Goltz DE, Cook CE, et al. Association between radiographic soft-tissue thickness and increased length of stay, operative time, and infection rate after reverse shoulder arthroplasty. Journal of Shoulder and Elbow Surgery 2024;**33**:1267–1275

[98] Pecold J, Al-Jeabory M, Krupowies M, Manka E, Smereka A, Ladny JR, et al. Tranexamic acid for shoulder arthroplasty: A systematic review and meta-analysis. Journal of Clinical Medicine 2021;**11**:48

[99] Werner BC, Burrus MT, Browne JA, Brockmeier SF. Superobesity (body mass index >50 kg/m2) and complications after total shoulder arthroplasty: An incremental effect of increasing body mass index. Journal of Shoulder and Elbow Surgery. 2015;**24**(12):1868–1875

[100] Theodoulou A, Krishnan J, Aromataris E. Risk of poor outcomes in patients who are obese following total shoulder arthroplasty and reverse total shoulder arthroplasty: A systematic review and meta-analysis. Journal of Shoulder and Elbow Surgery. 2019;**28**(11):e359–e76

[101] Werner BC, Griffin JW, Yang S, Brockmeier SF, Gwathmey FW. Obesity is associated with increased postoperative complications after operative management of proximal humerus fractures. Journal of Shoulder and Elbow Surgery. 2015;**24**(4):593–600

[102] Anakwenze O, Fokin A, Chocas M, Dillon MT, Navarro RA, Yian EH, et al. Complications in total shoulder and reverse total shoulder arthroplasty by body mass index. Journal of Shoulder and Elbow Surgery 2017;**26**:1230–1237

[103] Reid JJ, Kunkle BF, Kothandaraman V, Roche C, Eichinger JK, Friedman RJ. Effects of obesity on clinical and functional outcomes following anatomic and reverse total shoulder arthroplasty. Journal of Shoulder and Elbow Surgery. 2022;**31**(1):17–25

[104] Katayama ES, Durisek GR, Bustamante GC, Barry LW, Wilson S, Barnett JS, et al. The role of body mass index in survivorship and clinical outcomes in total shoulder arthroplasty. Journal of Shoulder and Elbow Surgery 2024;**33**:1980–1989

[105] Hones KM, Hao KA, Cueto RJ, Wright JO, King JJ, Wright TW, et al. The obesity paradox: A nonlinear relationship between 30-day postoperative complications and body mass index after total shoulder arthroplasty. Journal of the American Academy of Orthopaedic Surgeons 2023;**31**:1165–1172

[106] Miralles-Muñoz FA, Sebastia-Forcada E, Albero-Catala L, Ruiz-Martínez M. The obese patient undergoing reverse shoulder arthroplasty for a fracture has similar postoperative functional outcomes as the non-obese patient, but with a lower range of motion. Archives of Orthopaedic and Trauma Surgery. 2025;**145**(1):183

[107] Haase LR, Piper MM, Sinkler MA, Strony JT, Smith KL, Gillespie RJ, et al. Local subcutaneous fat depth is associated with increased complications after total shoulder arthroplasty. Journal of the American Academy of Orthopaedic Surgeons 2025;**33**:787–792

[108] Khazzam MS, Pearl ML. AAOS clinical practice guideline: Management of glenohumeral joint osteoarthritis. Journal of the American Academy of Orthopaedic Surgeons. 2020;**28**(19):790–794

[109] Bouchard M, Amin A, Pinsker E, Khan R, Deda E, Daniels TR. The impact of obesity on the outcome of total ankle replacement. The Journal of Bone & Joint Surgery. 2015;**97**(11):904

[110] Kim BI, Anastasio AT, Wixted CM, DeOrio JK, Nunley JA, Easley ME, et al. Total ankle

arthroplasty: Does obesity matter? Foot & Ankle International 2023;**44**:587–595

[111] Schipper ON, Denduluri SK, Zhou Y, Haddad SL. Effect of obesity on total ankle arthroplasty outcomes. Foot & Ankle International. 2016;**37**(1):1–7

[112] Suh DH, Han K, Lee JW, Kim HJ, Kim B, Koo BM, et al. Risk factors associated with failure of total ankle arthroplasty: A nationwide cohort study. Scientific Reports 2021;**11**:2878

[113] Maktouf W, Ferhi H, Boyas S, Beaune B, Chortane SG, Portero P, et al. The influence of obesity and fat distribution on ankle muscle coactivation during gait. PLOS ONE 2024;**19**:e0294692

[114] Sansosti LE, Van JC, Meyr AJ. Effect of obesity on total ankle arthroplasty: A systematic review of postoperative complications requiring surgical revision. The Journal of Foot and Ankle Surgery: Official Publication of the American College of Foot and Ankle Surgeons. 2018;**57**(2):353–356

[115] Gross CE, Hamid KS, Green C, Easley ME, DeOrio JK, Nunley JA. Operative wound complications following total ankle arthroplasty. Foot & Ankle International. 2017;**38**(4): 360–366

[116] Bakaes Y, Gonzalez T, Hardin JW, Benjamin Jackson Iii J. Effect of body mass index on acute postoperative complications following Total Ankle Arthroplasty (TAA). Foot and ankle surgery. Official Journal of the European Society of Foot and Ankle Surgeons. 2024;**30**(3):226–230

[117] Wu KA, Anastasio AT, Kutzer KM, Krez AN, DeOrio JK, Nunley JA, et al. Radiographic soft tissue thickness is not a risk factor for infection after primary total ankle arthroplasty. Journal of Foot and Ankle Surgery 2025;**64**:408–413

[118] Colliton E, Clippinger B, Jonczyk MM, Coccoluto N, Cassidy C. Total elbow arthroplasty complications and relation to body mass index: An American college of surgeons national surgery quality improvement program database study. Seminars in Arthroplasty: JSES. 2022;**32** (3):532–538

[119] Werner BC, Rawles RB, Jobe JT, Chhabra AB, Freilich AM. Obesity is associated with increased postoperative complications after operative management of distal humerus fractures. Journal of Shoulder and Elbow Surgery. 2015;**24**(10): 1602–1606

[120] Baghdadi YMK, Veillette CJH, Malone AA, Morrey BF, Sanchez-Sotelo J. Total elbow arthroplasty in obese patients. The Journal of Bone and Joint Surgery American Volume. 2014;**96**(9): e70

[121] Wall JC, Wall HP, Osemwengie BO, MacKay BJ. The impact of obesity on orthopedic upper extremity surgery. The Orthopedic Clinics of North America. 2018;**49** (3):345–351

[122] Morrey ME, Hevesi M. The influence of obesity on total elbow arthroplasty. Orthopedic Clinics. 2018;**49**(3):361–370

[123] Kamineni S, Morrey BF. Proximal ulnar reconstruction with strut allograft in revision total elbow arthroplasty. The Journal of Bone and Joint Surgery American Volume. 2004;**86**(6): 1223–1229

[124] Raikin SM, Kane J, Ciminiello ME. Risk factors for incision-healing complications following total ankle arthroplasty. The Journal of Bone and Joint Surgery American Volume. 2010;**92**(12):2150–2155

Chapter 11

Body Mass Index and Optimizing Physical Activity Levels in Rehabilitation Patients

Roxana Nartea and Gavril Gheorghievici

Abstract

Obesity represents a global health issue that leads to long-term repercussions for all organ systems, thereby causing negative health outcomes, higher healthcare costs, and disability. Although bariatric surgery and pharmacological treatment remain the primary courses of action, rehabilitation programs can make a significant contribution to addressing functional impairment. Optimal rehabilitation programs require tailored physical exercise prescriptions, adapted environments, and interdisciplinary coordination. Physical activity remains a central element, with international guidelines recommending between 150 and 300 minutes of moderate-intensity activity per week. Emerging approaches, such as aquatic therapy for cardiovascular and metabolic improvement, in combination with nutritional interventions focusing on macronutrient intake and adequate hydration, need to be implemented in a personalized plan.

Keywords: weight management, rehabilitation, physical activity, obesity, endurance training

1. Introduction

Obesity represents a global health issue that determines long-term repercussions for all organ systems, thus leading to negative health outcomes, higher healthcare costs, and disability. Over the last decade, bariatric surgery has been viewed as an efficient intervention for patients with severe obesity. At the same time, the ongoing development of pharmaceuticals can help close the gap between surgical treatment and lifestyle changes. These new drugs can contribute to an increase in the therapeutic range and offer further treatment options for these patients. This is why the increasing prevalence of obesity requires rapid and coordinated planning by all healthcare specialists. Physicians in rehabilitation medicine are often at the forefront of managing the functional impairments associated with obesity. Patients frequently present with reduced exercise tolerance, compromised respiratory capacity, pain, diminished strength and balance, and an elevated risk of falls – factors that independently contribute to disability. Furthermore, obesity exacerbates a range of comorbid conditions, including type 2 diabetes, cardiovascular disease, nonalcoholic fatty liver disease (NAFLD), sarcopenia, sleep apnea, and dermatological disorders, all of which further impair independence and quality of life.

Despite these challenges, the impact of obesity on rehabilitation outcomes is frequently overlooked. Many rehabilitation facilities, optimized for normal-weight populations, remain structurally, organizationally, and technologically ill-prepared to meet the complex needs of individuals with severe obesity. This mismatch compromises care quality and patient safety. Compounding this issue, the number of obese individuals requiring postacute rehabilitation continues to rise, underscoring the urgency of specialized care.

Effective rehabilitation for this population requires comprehensive assessment and individualized protocols, delivered by professionals trained in obesity-specific considerations. Care must be provided in ergonomically adapted environments that ensure safety while promoting functional recovery. Addressing these gaps is essential to improve outcomes, reduce disability, and ultimately mitigate the growing burden of obesity within healthcare systems worldwide.

2. Optimal level of physical activity

2.1 What does "optimal physical activity" mean?

For adults, "optimal" physical activity (PA) is the weekly dose shown to yield substantial health benefits (lower cardiometabolic risk, better function, reduced mortality) with acceptable risk and high feasibility. Current international guidelines converge on 150–300 minutes per week of moderate-intensity aerobic activity (or 75–150 minutes per week of vigorous activity), ideally spread across the week, plus muscle-strengthening activities on ≥2 days per week. More activity confers additional benefits; older adults should add balance training. For weight-loss maintenance and greater cardiometabolic benefits, totals toward the upper end (≥300 min/week) are advantageous [1].

2.2 How to quantify "dose"

There are various compatible approaches to calculate PA dose:

a) Minutes at a given intensity

- Moderate intensity: breathing faster but able to talk (not sing).
- Vigorous intensity: only a few words before pausing for breath [2].

b) MET-minutes (energy cost)

1 MET ≈ resting energy use; moderate = 3.0–5.9 METs, vigorous ≥6 METs.

- Weekly 500–1,000 MET-min corresponds roughly to guideline targets (e.g., 150 min at ~ 4 METs = 600 MET-min). Use the Compendium of Physical Activities to look up MET values (e.g., brisk walking ~ 3.5–4.5 METs, cycling ~4–8 METs) [3].

c) Heart-rate–based zones

- Percentage heart-rate reserve (HRR; Karvonen): target HR = ([HR_max − HR_rest] × %intensity) + HR_rest. Moderate ≈ 40–59% HRR; vigorous ≈ 60–89% HRR. Use age-predicted HR_max (e.g., 208 − 0.7 × age) or, ideally, measured values [4].

d) Perceived exertion (RPE, Borg 6–20)

- Light ≤; intermediate 12–14; intense 15–17 – can be of use when on rate-limiting medication (e.g., β-blockers) [5].

e) Steps/day

- New research data express the fact that the therapeutic benefit starts well below 10,000 steps. Risk reductions are obvious between 6000 and 9000 steps/day in age-dependent patients. It is necessary to concentrate on increasing the baseline [6].

2.3 Adaptation of physical exercise for adults with obesity

Main principles

- Begin at a slow intensity (increase by 5–10% weekly)
- Focus on joint-sparing modes (cycling, walking on soft surfaces, deep-water running) and then associate combinations between them.
- Combine aerobic + resistance training (≥2 days/week, 1–3 sets, 8–12 reps for major muscle groups) to preserve or augment lean mass, glycemic control, and function.
- Include balance and mobility work, especially for individuals with fall risk or osteoarthritis (OA) [7].

2.3.1 Aerobic dose for weight and metabolic health

For weight loss and long-term weight-loss maintenance, accumulating ≥200–300 minutes per week of moderate physical activity (or equivalent) is supported; combine this with nutrition therapy for clinically meaningful weight reduction [8].

2.3.2 Strength training specifics

Two to three nonconsecutive days/week; emphasize multijoint movements (sit-to-stand/squats to a box, step-ups, rowing/pulling, presses), tempo control, and machines/cables for stability. Progress resistance when two to three extra reps are possible above the target range [9].

2.3.3 If a musculoskeletal condition or pain is present

Prefer low-impact modes; use graded exposure (shorter bouts, more frequent rests), assistive devices, and appropriate footwear. For knee/hip OA, combine aerobic, strengthening, and neuromotor/balance exercises; walking aids and home/work adaptations can reduce pain and enable adherence [7].

2.3.4 If using antiobesity medications (AOMs) or postbariatric

Maintain exercise for independent health benefits (fitness, glycemic control, bone/muscle). Emphasize resistance training to counter fat-free mass (FFM) loss during rapid weight reduction; coach expectations away from "calorie-burn only" toward function and well-being. Coordinate with the prescribing team for GI symptom days and hydration/electrolytes [10].

2.3.5 Environment and safety

Use properly rated equipment (benches, treads, bikes, plinths), safe patient-handling aids, and more expansive spaces for transfers when available – key in rehab or clinical gyms. Screen for sleep apnea, cardiovascular disease, diabetes complications, and heat sensitivity; prefer RPE or talk test when HR is unreliable [11].

2.4 Putting it together: A practical framework

Assess: medical clearance as indicated; resting HR and BP; mobility, pain, balance; baseline steps; goals that matter (function, stamina, glucose control, mood) [8].

Prescribe (initial 4–6 weeks):

- Aerobic: 3–5 days/week, 20–40 min/bout (can be 10-min blocks), RPE 12–13 (or 40–59% HRR). Choose joint-sparing modes.

- Steps: find baseline (e.g., 4,000/day) and add + 500–1,000 steps/day every 1–2 weeks toward 6,000–9,000 +.

- Strength: 2–3 days/week, full-body, 1–2 sets × 8–12 reps, RPE 13–15 by last reps; emphasize technique, use machines if balance is limited.

- Balance/mobility: 10–15 minutes/session (e.g., tandem stance, sit-to-stand, ankle/hip mobility).

Progress (weeks 6–12):

- Build toward ≥ 150–300 min/week of moderate activity (or equivalents), then – if weight-loss maintenance is a priority – aim for ≥200–300 min/week. Add intervals (e.g., 1–3 minutes at RPE 14–16, with equal easy recovery) if joint-tolerant. Increase strength training to 2–3 sets, include hip/knee extensors, and place emphasis on pulling [12].

Monitor and adapt:

- Use RPE and the talk test day-to-day; adjust for pain flares, illness, and medication changes. Protect skin (friction/moisture), hydrate, and favor cooler environments if heat-intolerant. If persistent pain or swelling occurs more than 24–48 hours after a session, reduce the next dose by ~ 10–20%.

2.5 Key takeaways

- "Optimal" for most adults = 150–300 min/week moderate (or 75–150 vigorous) + strength ≥2 days/week; ≥300 min/week and regular resistance training are especially valuable for people with obesity, particularly for weight-loss maintenance and function [9, 12].

- Quantify dose via minutes, MET-minutes, HRR, RPE, or steps – choose the method that best fits the person and context [3, 6].

- Adaptation matters: joint-sparing modes, gradual progression, resistance training to preserve lean mass, balance work, and attention to equipment and safety yield better adherence and outcomes.

3. Endurance training modalities: Evidence and perspectives

Endurance training has evolved over the years. Stepping away from the classic long-slow distance (LSD) paradigm, this type of training combines high-intensity interval formats with structured intensity distributions and data-guided personalization. In this section, we analyze the most recent evidence regarding primary modalities – moderate-intensity continuous training (MICT), high-intensity interval training (HIIT), sprint-interval training (SIT), and emerging distribution models (pyramidal, polarized, threshold, and lactate-guided) – and determine the practical implications and future directions regarding health and performance.

3.1 MICT and HIIT: Complementary, not competing

Large comparative syntheses show that both MICT (typically 40–70% of VO_2max for ≥20–30 min) and HIIT (repeated bouts at ~ 85–100% VO_2max interspersed with recovery) improve cardiorespiratory fitness (CRF) and cardiometabolic health. Across adults, HIIT tends to produce equal or greater gains in VO_2max and vascular function with smaller time commitments. At the same time, MICT remains effective and highly tolerable – particularly valuable for building aerobic base, durability, and adherence. In cardiovascular and metabolic populations, several recent meta-analyses suggest HIIT is at least as safe as MICT under supervision and often superior for CRF and selected risk factors. Together, these data support a "both-and" approach in which HIIT augments, rather than replaces, continuous training [13].

3.2 Low-volume HIIT and SIT: Time-efficiency with caveats

Low-volume HIIT (LV-HIIT; ≤5 minutes of work above vigorous intensity per session) and SIT (supramaximal ~ 20–30-second "all-out" efforts) have attracted interest as time-efficient strategies. Meta-analyses indicate LV-HIIT meaningfully improves CRF and blood pressure, and SIT can enhance performance in trained athletes over four to eight weeks. However, heterogeneity is high, effect sizes are sensitive to study design, and some reviews caution against overinterpreting small trials. In practice, LV-HIIT or SIT blocks can be potent "spices" in a broader plan, especially when logistics limit volume. Still, they should be dosed judiciously for musculoskeletal tolerance and recovery [14].

3.3 Molecular adaptations: Intensity and volume both matter

At the cellular level, endurance work upregulates mitochondrial biogenesis and angiogenesis via pathways centered on PGC-1α. Recent human data suggest both interval and continuous modalities stimulate these adaptations; high-intensity efforts robustly activate acute signaling, while accumulated volume supports sustained remodeling of mitochondrial content and capillarity. This helps explain why mixed programs – adequate volume of low-to-moderate work plus a judicious dose of high intensity – reliably raise VO_2max and endurance economy [15–17].

3.4 Training-intensity distribution (TID): Polarized, pyramidal, threshold

How best to allocate time across easy, moderate/threshold, and hard zones remains debated. Short-term interventions (≤12 weeks) often find polarized distributions (high volume at low intensity with a small but distinct high-intensity dose) yield larger VO_2peak gains than alternative models. However, superiority for other performance surrogates (e.g., time-trial, lactate thresholds) is inconsistent. Over longer interventions, differences between distributions tend to converge, and individual context – event demands, training age, injury risk – matters. Pyramidal models (mostly low, some moderate, a few high) are common in successful programs and may be functionally similar across seasons. Meanwhile, threshold-heavy approaches can work for some athletes but risk accumulating fatigue if not periodized. Altogether, data from the literature supports low-intensity volume with targeted high-intensity "peaks" which allows the midzone to expand or contract depending on needs and response [18, 19].

3.5 Lactate-guided threshold interval training (LGTIT): A pragmatic delivery

A notable development is the incorporation of lactate-guided threshold intervals within a high-volume, low-intensity background, mirroring practices employed by some world-class runners. By titrating work to a lactate "ceiling" (often ~2–3 $mmol \cdot L^{-1}$), LGTIT aims to accumulate large quantities of high-aerobic work without incurring undue autonomic or neuromuscular strain. Although the literature is early and primarily descriptive, it offers a physiologically coherent method for increasing quality volume in athletes who tolerate higher workloads [20].

3.6 Durability: Beyond peak tests

Traditional profiling emphasizes VO_2max and fresh-state thresholds, but the durability construct – resilience of physiological variables over prolonged efforts – has gained traction. Recent studies show that both low- and high-intensity training can improve durability (delaying the drift in heart rate, oxygen cost, and lactate at given workloads), which likely mediates late-race performance. Practically, building durability argues for substantial, easy-to-moderate volume, strategic fueling, and periodic long sessions that create fatigue-resistant adaptations [21].

3.7 Personalization: HRV-guided loading and wearables

Another trend is day-to-day heart-rate variability (HRV)-guided programming, which adjusts intensity based on autonomic recovery. RCTs in athlete runners have evidenced that HRV-guided groups can match or even outperform fixed plans for improving VO_2max, while at the same time particularizing the evolution of easy vs. hard days and therefore potentially reducing nonfunctional fatigue. Although methods and data present variations across different studies, HRV guidance represents a reasonable instrument for modulating load in high-stress contexts. The provided determinations are standardized, and the interpretation is made in a conservative manner [22].

3.8 Clinical and aging populations: Translating performance science to health

In people with overweight/obesity and older adults, both MICT and HIIT improve CRF, glycemic control, and functional capacity. Recent meta-analyses indicate that HIIT can be particularly efficient for raising VO_2peak and walking endurance in older adults and can outperform MICT for CRF in overweight populations, with careful screening and supervision. For routine care, blending modalities – progressive MICT to build base and tolerance, plus small amounts of intervals tailored to joint health and confidence – maximizes adherence and safety [23, 24].

3.9 Programming implications

For most endurance goals, focus on three pillars:

- Volume at low intensity to enhance durability, peripheral adaptations, and technical economy.

- Targeted intensity (HIIT or longer threshold work) to raise VO_2max stroke volume, and glycolytic/oxidative interplay.

- Intelligent distribution – often polarized or pyramidal over a season – is shaped by constraints (time, injury history), event specificity, and responsiveness (e.g., via HRV, session RPE, or lactate checks). Periodize across mesocycles: build extensive capacity, layer intensity, then sharpen race-specific tolerance;

interleave recovery microcycles to manage autonomic and musculoskeletal load [13].

3.10 Unresolved questions and future directions

First, who benefits most from polarized versus pyramidal versus threshold-heavy models remains unsettled; head-to-head trials with adequate duration and standardized metrics are needed. Second, the dose-response of LV-HIIT and SIT beyond six to eight weeks – and their long-term injury and adherence profiles – requires clarification. Third, integrating molecular markers (e.g., PGC-1α expression, citrate synthase activity) with field performance may improve individualization, but translating lab signals into weekly prescriptions is nascent. Lastly, broader adoption of durability-focused testing (late-exercise thresholds, critical speed/power drift) may yield programs that better reflect real-world racing and long-duration work [15, 21, 25].

3.11 Conclusion

The last decade has reframed endurance training as a palette rather than a single color. MICT builds foundational capacity; HIIT and SIT deliver potent stimuli when time or performance ceilings demand; and contemporary distribution models and guidance tools refine how we sequence and dose these elements. The clearest throughline is not the supremacy of any one modality, but the strategic combination of volume and intensity – tuned to the athlete or patient, the event or health target, and the response observed week by week. As evidence accumulates, an agile, data-informed blending of modalities appears to be the most reliable path to durable fitness, robust performance, and cardiometabolic resilience [18, 26].

4. Latest techniques

4.1 Aquatic exercise for obesity and rehabilitation: Physiological principles and clinical applications

Aquatic exercise (AQE) offers a unique and effective environment for rehabilitation and physical conditioning, particularly for individuals with obesity, musculoskeletal disorders, or reduced exercise tolerance. The therapeutic benefits of immersion stem from fundamental hydrodynamic principles, including density, hydrostatic pressure, buoyancy, viscosity, and thermodynamic properties [27].

4.2 Physical properties of water and biological effects

The density of water provides vertical thrust that reduces body weight load, facilitating movement and joint protection. Hydrostatic pressure increases with immersion depth, enhancing venous return, stroke volume, and peripheral circulation while reducing edema and modulating hormonal pathways, such as the renin-angiotensin-aldosterone system. Buoyancy allows up to 90% body weight support depending on immersion depth, enabling vigorous aerobic exercise with minimal joint stress. Water viscosity provides resistance proportional to movement velocity, allowing safe, controlled strengthening exercises within the patient's comfort range. Thermodynamically, water transfers heat efficiently, enabling both cooling and warming interventions for muscle recovery or rehabilitation [28].

4.3 Pool characteristics and environmental guidelines

Optimal pool conditions are crucial for effective AQE. Water temperatures of 28–30°C are ideal for aerobic and resistance exercises, while 32–35.5°C is recommended for therapy sessions, accommodating longer immersion without discomfort. Air temperature should not exceed 29–30°C, with 50–60% humidity. Pool depth determines weight offloading: immersion to the neck provides ~ 90% support, while hip-level immersion provides ~ 50%. Shallow-water areas of 1–1.4 m depth are suitable for most rehabilitative activities [29].

4.4 Clinical applications and program design

AQE is broadly applicable, supporting cardiovascular, musculoskeletal, neurological, respiratory, metabolic, geriatric, and psychiatric rehabilitation, as well as conditions such as pregnancy, osteoporosis, and lymphedema. Programs typically include warm-up (5–15 min), conditioning (20–120 min), and cool-down (5–15 min). Evidence indicates that 8–12 weeks of thrice-weekly sessions can produce significant improvements in CRF, body composition, and metabolic health. Familiarization with buoyancy, viscosity, and aquatic proprioception is essential before introducing resistance equipment or higher-intensity training [30].

4.5 Resistance and aerobic training in water

Aquatic resistance exercises utilize water drag and equipment to adjust intensity. Resistance can be manipulated through acceleration, frontal surface area, and limb positioning, producing "isokinetic" contractions and enhancing muscle strength safely. Aquatic bikes and treadmills provide variable resistance and are well-tolerated in obese patients, though external power output is recommended to guide exercise intensity due to water-induced changes in heart rate and VO_2max [31].

4.6 High-intensity interval training (HIIT) in water

HIIT protocols, consisting of short, intense bouts interspersed with recovery, have been shown to improve oxidative capacity, vascular function, and fat metabolism in obese individuals. Aquatic HIIT allows patients to achieve higher heart rate ranges safely than on land, with reduced cardiac stress and joint loading. Short bouts of 15–60 seconds are recommended, progressing gradually in frequency and volume over 15 weeks [27].

4.7 Progression strategy

AQE progression begins with familiarization and motor adaptation in water, followed by aerobic conditioning, incremental resistance training, circuit exercises, and finally low-volume HIIT. Heart rate and perceived exertion monitoring guide intensity and ensure safety [32].

4.8 Conclusion

AQE leverages the physical properties of water to enable safe, effective, and adaptable training for obese and rehabilitative populations. When properly prescribed and progressed, aquatic exercise enhances CRF, strength, metabolic health, and adherence, making it a vital component of modern rehabilitation strategies.

5. Nutrition and exercise

5.1 Nutrition and exercise strategies for obese and sarcopenic individuals: Macronutrient, micronutrient, and hydration considerations

Carbohydrates are the primary energy substrate during moderate-intensity exercise (50–70% VO_2max), particularly in the first 30 minutes [33–35]. Muscle glycogen, comprising 70–79% of total body glycogen, supports prolonged activity, while hepatic glycogen (20%) and circulating glucose (<1%) contribute to systemic energy availability [35]. Glycogen depletion leads to muscular fatigue, limiting exercise performance. The recommended daily carbohydrate intake ranges from 5–12 g/kg/day, with higher intakes recommended for athletes or individuals performing at least 70% of their VO_2max for more than 12 hours per week. Postexercise, carbohydrate timing can accelerate glycogen resynthesis, particularly when combined with protein (0.2–0.4 g/kg/h), which concurrently stimulates muscle protein synthesis [36].

5.2 Lipids and dietary fats

Dietary lipids provide concentrated energy and support the absorption of fat-soluble vitamins. Balanced intake, with an emphasis on unsaturated fatty acids, particularly omega-3 polyunsaturated fatty acids (PUFAs), is associated with reduced inflammation, improved cardiovascular function, and enhanced musculoskeletal health [37–39]. Mediterranean diet patterns, rich in monounsaturated and polyunsaturated fats, are particularly effective in reducing obesity-related inflammation, hepatic fat, and OA symptoms [38, 40].

5.3 Water and micronutrients

Hydration is essential for exercise performance and recovery. Dehydration of even 1–5% body weight reduces physical and cognitive function, while greater losses may precipitate heat-related illnesses [41]. Recommended fluid intake includes 300 mL of water 2 hours before exercise and 250 mL every 20–30 minutes during prolonged activity, with adjustments based on environmental conditions and exercise intensity [42]. Electrolytes, including sodium, potassium, and magnesium, are lost through sweat and require replacement, particularly in high-intensity or prolonged exercise. Micronutrient sufficiency is best achieved through a varied diet rich in fruits, vegetables, and whole grains, which also provide antioxidants like polyphenols to mitigate oxidative stress from exercise. Vitamins C and E have demonstrated benefits in reducing fatigue and supporting cardiovascular health in obese adults during moderate exercise [12, 43, 44].

5.4 Exercise and macronutrient interactions

Aerobic and resistance exercises improve insulin sensitivity, mitochondrial content, and muscle oxidative capacity, thereby enhancing glucose and fatty acid metabolism. Exercise also protects against lean mass loss during weight reduction, particularly when combined with adequate protein intake. Resistance training promotes muscle protein synthesis, increasing skeletal muscle mass and function, while aerobic activity reduces fat mass and improves CRF. HIIT further enhances metabolic adaptations, including hepatic fat reduction in patients with NAFLD [28, 45, 46].

5.5 Special considerations in obesity-related comorbidities

Patients with obesity often present with insulin resistance, NAFLD, chronic kidney disease, obstructive sleep apnea, OA, and heart failure. Nutritional interventions must account for these comorbidities. For example, low-protein diets are indicated in early-stage chronic kidney disease, whereas higher protein intake is necessary postbariatric surgery or during weight loss to preserve lean mass [11]. Carbohydrate management is critical in diabetes prevention and glycemic control, and exercise intensity and duration must be tailored to avoid hypoglycemia in insulin-treated patients. Weight loss of 3–7% of initial body weight improves glycemic control, hepatic steatosis, and sleep apnea severity, with additional benefits observed when exercise is integrated [15, 47].

5.6 Sarcopenic obesity and older adults

Sarcopenic obesity is characterized by the coexistence of excess fat mass and inadequate muscle mass and function, often exacerbated by aging. Protein intake of 1.0–1.2 g/kg/day, combined with aerobic and resistance exercise, supports muscle protein synthesis, mitigates FFM loss, and enhances physical performance. Even distribution of protein intake across meals maximizes anabolic responses. Moderate-intensity PA reduces intermuscular fat, improves muscle quality, and promotes functional independence. Resistance training increases strength, preserves skeletal muscle mass, and decreases fat mass in sarcopenic obese adults [48–51].

6. Conclusion

Optimal management of obesity and sarcopenic obesity requires integrated nutritional and exercise strategies. Adequate carbohydrate, protein, and lipid intake, along with hydration and micronutrient sufficiency, supports energy metabolism, preserves lean mass, and enhances exercise performance. Structured aerobic and resistance exercise programs synergize with diet to improve body composition, insulin sensitivity, hepatic health, and musculoskeletal function (see **Table 1**). Personalized interventions, considering comorbidities, age, and functional status,

Category	Target/recommendation	Exercise type and frequency	Expected outcomes
Carbohydrates	5–12 g/kg/day (higher end for ≥70% VO_2max >12 h/wk); postexercise: 0.8 g/kg/h with 0.2–0.4 g/kg/h protein	Aerobic (50–70% VO_2max), duration: 30–60 min/d	Maintain glycogen stores, delay fatigue, and support exercise performance
Proteins	1.0–1.6 g/kg/day (for older adults or during energy restriction: 1.2–1.6 g/kg/d); spread across meals every 3–4 h	Resistance training 2–3x/wk, combined with aerobic exercise	Preserve lean mass, stimulate muscle protein synthesis, and maintain strength
Lipids/fats	Emphasize unsaturated fats, omega-3 PUFAs (1 g/d); Mediterranean diet patterns	Combined with aerobic and resistance exercise	Reduce inflammation, improve cardiovascular and musculoskeletal health
Water and electrolytes	300 mL 2 h preexercise; 250 mL every 20–30 min; replace sodium, potassium, and magnesium as needed	All exercise modalities	Prevent dehydration, maintain performance, and reduce the risk of heat stress
Micronutrients	Adequate intake via fruits, vegetables, cereals; Vitamin C/E, calcium 1,200 mg/d, magnesium 320 mg/d, vitamin D 800 IU/d, fiber 25 g/d	Supports exercise recovery and overall health	Reduce oxidative stress, support bone/muscle health, and improve fatigue perception
Aerobic exercise	Moderate intensity: ≥150 min/wk; high-intensity: >250 min/wk for hepatic fat reduction	Walking, cycling, elliptical, swimming	Improve cardiorespiratory fitness, reduce fat mass, enhance insulin sensitivity, and reduce liver fat
Resistance training	2–3 sessions/wk; progressive overload, 3 sets/exercise	Free weights, resistance bands, machines	Maintain/increase skeletal muscle mass, enhance strength, and preserve FFM during weight loss
Combined exercise	Aerobic + resistance 3x/wk, 60– 90 min/session	Circuit training, interval sessions	Maximize fat loss, improve lean mass, and enhance functional performance
Special populations	Sarcopenic obesity: high-protein intake, leucine supplementation, resistance exercise	Tailored progressive training 2–3x/wk	Preserve muscle mass, improve strength and physical function, and reduce frailty risk
Obesity with comorbidities	Adjust protein, carbs, and calories according to CKD, HF, NAFLD, diabetes	Individualized aerobic/resistance programs	Improve glycemic control, reduce hepatic fat, manage blood pressure, and maintain functional capacity

Table 1.
Recommendations regarding optimal physical exercise for metabolic patients.

are essential for maximizing long-term health outcomes in obese and sarcopenic populations.

Acknowledgments

This manuscript has been edited for language issues using AI-assisted tools.

Conflict of Interest

The authors declare no conflict of interest.

Author details

Roxana Nartea[1,2]* and Gavril Gheorghievici[1,2]

1 Carol Davila, University of Medicine and Pharmacy, Bucharest, Romania

2 National Institute of Rehabilitation, Physical Medicine and Balneology, Bucharest, Romania

*Address all correspondence to: nartea.roxana@yahoo.com

References

[1] RECOMMENDATIONS. In: WHO Guidelines on Physical Activity and Sedentary Behaviour [Internet]. World Health Organization; 2020. Available from: https://www.ncbi.nlm.nih.gov/books/NBK566046/ [Accessed: 2025-August-27]

[2] Measuring Physical Activity Intensity | Physical Activity | CDC [Internet]. 2022. Available from: https://www.cdc.gov/physicalactivity/basics/measuring/index.html [Accessed: 2025August-27]

[3] Ainsworth BE, Haskell WL, Herrmann SD, Meckes N, Bassett DRJ, Tudor-Locke C, et al. 2011 compendium of physical activities: A second update of codes and MET values. Medicine and Science in Sports and Exercise 2011;**43**:1575

[4] ACSM CPT chapter 15: Cardiorespiratory training programs [Internet]. Available from: https://www.ptpioneer.com/personal-training/certifications/acsm/acsm-cpt-chapter-15/?utm_source=chatgpt.com [Accessed: 2025-August-27]

[5] Cleveland Clinic [Internet]. 2025. Rate of perceived exertion (RPE) scale. Available from: https://my.clevelandclinic.org/health/articles/17450-rated-perceived-exertion-rpe-scale [Accessed: 2025-August-27]

[6] Paluch AE, Bajpai S, Bassett DR, Carnethon MR, Ekelund U, Evenson KR, et al. Daily steps and all-cause mortality: A meta-analysis of 15 international cohorts. The Lancet Public Health 2022;7:e219–28

[7] Moseng T, Vlieland TPMV, Battista S, Beckwée D, Boyadzhieva V, Conaghan PG, et al. EULAR recommendations for the non-pharmacological core management of hip and knee osteoarthritis: 2023 update. Annals of the Rheumatic Diseases 2024;**83**:730–740

[8] Donnelly JE, Blair SN, Jakicic JM, Manore MM, Rankin JW, Smith BK, et al. American College of Sports Medicine position stand. Appropriate physical activity intervention strategies for weight loss and prevention of weight regain for adults. Medicine and Science in Sports and Exercise 2009;**41**:459–471

[9] Piercy KL, Troiano RP, Ballard RM, Carlson SA, Fulton JE, Galuska DA, et al. The physical activity guidelines for Americans. Jama 2018;**320**:2020–2028

[10] Jakicic JM, Rogers RJ. Association of eating behaviors with variability in weight change in response to physical activity interventions in adults with overweight. Nutrients. 2023;**15**(15):3452

[11] McClean K, Cross M, Reed S. Risks to healthcare organizations and staff who manage obese (bariatric) patients and use of obesity data to mitigate risks: A literature review. Journal of Multidisciplinary Healthcare. 2021;**14**:577–588

[12] Bull FC, Al-Ansari SS, Biddle S, Borodulin K, Buman MP, Cardon G, et al. World Health Organization 2020 guidelines on physical activity and sedentary behaviour. British Journal of Sports Medicine 2020;**54**:1451–1462

[13] Oliveira R, Brito J, editors. Exercise Testing and Prescription Strategies to Improve Quality of Life. MDPI; 2024. Available from: https://

www.mdpi.com/books/reprint/9515 [Accessed: 2025-September-27]

[14] Stavrinou PS, Astorino TA, Giannaki CD, Aphamis G, Bogdanis GC. Customizing intense interval exercise training prescription using the "frequency, intensity, time, and type of exercise" (FITT) principle. Frontiers in Physiology. 2025;**16**:1553846. DOI: 10.3389/fphys.2025.1553846

[15] Lim AY, Chen YC, Hsu CC, Fu TC, Wang JS. The effects of exercise training on mitochondrial function in cardiovascular diseases: A systematic review and meta-analysis. International Journal of Molecular Sciences. 2022;**23**(20):12559

[16] Abrego-Guandique DM, Rojas NMA, Chiari A, Luciani F, Cione E, Cannataro R. The impact of exercise on mitochondrial biogenesis in skeletal muscle: A systematic review and meta-analysis of randomized trials. Biomolecular Concepts. 2025;**16**(1). Available from: DOI: 10.1515/bmc-2025-0055/html?lang=en&srsltid=AfmBOoqS97wb8FqyV4vs6W_0r8GZy_0cgH58g7sg8VEIqGm_pqFWSqgQ&utm_source=chatgpt.com

[17] Siddall B, Ram A, Jones MD, Booth J, Perriman D, Summers SJ. Short-term impact of combining pain neuroscience education with exercise for chronic musculoskeletal pain: A systematic review and meta-analysis. Pain. 2022;**163**(1):e20–30

[18] Olivieri F, Biscetti L, Pimpini L, Pelliccioni G, Sabbatinelli J, Giunta S. Heart rate variability and autonomic nervous system imbalance: Potential biomarkers and detectable hallmarks of aging and inflammaging. Ageing Research Reviews. 2024;**101**:102521. DOI: 10.1016/j.arr.2024.102521

[19] Röhrken G, Held S, Donath L. Six weeks of polarized versus moderate intensity distribution: A pilot intervention study. Frontiers in Physiology. 2020;**11**:534688. Available from: https://www.frontiersin.org/journals/physiology/articles/10.3389/fphys.2020.534688/full. DOI: 10.3389/fphys.2020.534688

[20] Casado A, Foster C, Bakken M, Tjelta LI. Does lactate-guided threshold interval training within a high-volume low-intensity approach represent the "next step" in the evolution of distance running training? International Journal of Environmental Research and Public Health. 2023;**20**(5):3782

[21] Maunder E, Seiler S, Mildenhall MJ, Kilding AE, Plews DJ. The importance of "durability" in the physiological profiling of endurance athletes. Sports Medicine. 2021;**51**(8):1619–1628

[22] Carrasco-Poyatos M, González-Quílez A, Altini M, Granero-Gallegos A. Heart rate variability-guided training in professional runners: Effects on performance and vagal modulation. Physiology and Behavior. 2022;**244**:113654

[23] Sanca-Valeriano S, Espinola-Sánchez M, Caballero-Alvarado J, Canelo-Aybar C. Effect of high-intensity interval training compared to moderate-intensity continuous training on body composition and insulin sensitivity in overweight and obese adults: A systematic review and meta-analysis. Heliyon. 2023;**9**(10):e20402

[24] Sert H, Gulbahar Eren M, Gurcay B, Koc F. The effectiveness of a high-intensity interval exercise on cardiometabolic health and quality of

life in older adults: A systematic review and meta-analysis. BMC Sports Science, Medicine and Rehabilitation. 2025;**17**(1):128

[25] Yin M, Li H, Bai M, Liu H, Chen Z, Deng J, et al. Is low-volume high-intensity interval training a time-efficient strategy to improve cardiometabolic health and body composition? A meta-analysis. Applied Physiology, Nutrition, and Metabolism 2024;**49**:273–292

[26] Yu H, Zhao X, Wu X, Yang J, Wang J, Hou L. High-intensity interval training versus moderate-intensity continuous training on patient quality of life in cardiovascular disease: A systematic review and meta-analysis. Scientific Reports. 2023;**13**(1):13915

[27] Depiazzi JE, Forbes RA, Gibson N, Smith NL, Wilson AC, Boyd RN, Hill K. The effect of aquatic high-intensity interval training on aerobic performance, strength and body composition in a non-athletic population: Systematic review and meta-analysis. Clinical Rehabilitation. 2019;**33**(2):157–170. DOI: 10.1177/0269215518792039

[28] Tedeschi R, Giorgi F, Donati D. Harnessing the power of water: A scoping review of hydrokinesiotherapy as a game-changer in knee osteoarthritis management. Journal of Clinical Medicine. 2024;**13**(19):5811. DOI: 10.3390/jcm13195811

[29] Schets FM, van den Berg HHJL, Lynch G, de Rijk S, de Roda Husman AM, Schijven JF. Evaluation of water quality guidelines for public swimming ponds. Environment International. 2020;**137**:105516. DOI: 10.1016/j.envint.2020.105516

[30] Faíl LB, Marinho DA, Marques EA, Costa MJ, Santos CC, Marques MC, Izquierdo M, Neiva HP. Benefits of aquatic exercise in adults with and without chronic disease-a systematic review with meta-analysis. Scandinavian Journal of Medicine and Science in Sports. 2022;**32**(3):465–486. DOI: 10.1111/sms.14112

[31] Costa RR, Buttelli ACK, Coconcelli L, Pereira LF, Vieira AF, Fagundes AO, Farinha JB, Reichert T, Stein R, Kruel LFM. Water-based aerobic and resistance training as a treatment to improve the lipid profile of women with dyslipidemia: A randomized controlled trial. Journal of Physical Activity and Health. 2019;**16**(5):348–354. DOI: 10.1123/jpah.2018-0602

[32] Murray L, Kennedy M, Malone M, Mair L, Alexander L. Aquatic exercise interventions in the treatment of musculoskeletal upper extremity disorders: A scoping review. Clinical Rehabilitation. 2025;**39**(5):565–579. DOI: 10.1177/02692155251315078

[33] Coyle EF. Substrate utilization during exercise in active people. The American Journal of Clinical Nutrition. 1995;**61**(4):968S–979S

[34] Mitoiu BI, Nartea R, Miclaus RS. Impact of resistance and endurance training on ghrelin and plasma leptin levels in overweight and obese subjects. International Journal of Molecular Sciences. 2024;**25**(15):8067

[35] Jeukendrup A. A step towards personalized sports nutrition: Carbohydrate intake during exercise. Sports Medicine. 2014;**44**(Suppl S1):25–33

[36] Cao W, He Y, Fu R, Chen Y, Yu J, He Z. A review of carbohydrate supplementation approaches and strategies for optimizing performance in elite long-distance endurance. Nutrients. 2025;**17**(5):918

[37] Zou P, Wang L. Dietary pattern and hepatic lipid metabolism. Liver Research. 2023;7(4):275–284

[38] Lal S, Gunji S, Ahluwalia P, Kolhe R, Bollag WB, Hill WD, et al. Lipid metabolism in age-related musculoskeletal disorders: Insights into sarcopenia and osteoporosis. BMC Biology 2025;**23**:265

[39] Otelea MR, Nartea R, Popescu FG, Covaleov A, Mitoiu BI, Nica AS. The pathological links between adiposity and the carpal tunnel syndrome. Current Issues in Molecular Biology. 2022;**44**(6):2646–2663

[40] Effect of the Mediterranean diet supplemented with olive oil versus the low-fat diet on serum inflammatory and endothelial indexes among adults: A systematic review and meta-analysis of clinical controlled trials | Nutrition Reviews | Oxford Academic [Internet]. 2025. Available from: https://academic.oup.com/nutritionreviews/article-abstract/83/7/e1421/7895737?redirectedFrom=fulltext [Accessed: 2025-August-29]

[41] Latzka WA, Montain SJ. Water and electrolyte requirements for exercise. Clinics in Sports Medicine. 1999;**18**(3):513–524

[42] Nobari H, Saedmocheshi S, Chung LH, Suzuki K, Maynar-Mariño M, Pérez-Gómez J. An overview on how exercise with green tea consumption can prevent the production of reactive oxygen species and improve sports performance. International Journal of Environmental Research and Public Health. 2021;**19**(1):218

[43] Nartea R, Mitoiu BI, Ghiorghiu I. The link between magnesium supplements and statin medication in dyslipidemic patients. Current Issues in Molecular Biology. 2023;**45**(4):3146–3167

[44] Dioaguardi FS. Use of amino acids as supplements for matching nutrition, training, and rehabilitation-focusing on some questions. Nutrients. 2025;**17**(16):2667

[45] Colleluori G, Aguirre L, Phadnis U, Fowler K, Armamento-Villareal R, Sun Z, et al. Aerobic plus resistance exercise in obese older adults improves muscle protein synthesis and preserves myocellular quality despite weight loss. Cell Metabolism 2019;**30**:261–273.e6

[46] Colberg SR, Sigal RJ, Yardley JE, Riddell MC, Dunstan DW, Dempsey PC, et al. Physical activity/exercise and diabetes: A position statement of the American Diabetes Association. Diabetes Care 2016;**39**:2065–2079

[47] Office of Dietary Supplements - Omega-3 fatty acids [Internet]. 2025. Available from: https://ods.od.nih.gov/factsheets/Omega3FattyAcids-Consumer/ [Accessed: 2025-August-29]

[48] Moon J, Koh G. Clinical evidence and mechanisms of high-protein diet-induced weight loss. Journal of Obesity and Metabolic Syndrome. 2020;**29**(3):166–173

[49] Deer RR, Volpi E. Protein intake and muscle function in older adults.

Current Opinion in Clinical Nutrition and Metabolic Care. 2015;**18**(3):248–253

[50] Drummen M, Tischmann L, Gatta-Cherifi B, Adam T, Westerterp-Plantenga M. Dietary protein and energy balance in relation to obesity and co-morbidities. Frontiers in Endocrinology. 2018;**9**:443

[51] Lal S, Gunji S, Ahluwalia P, Kolhe R, Bollag WB, Hill WD, McGee-Lawrence ME, Isales CM, & Fulzele S. Lipid metabolism in age-related musculoskeletal disorders: Insights into sarcopenia and osteoporosis. BMC Biology. 2025;**23**(1). DOI: 10.1186/s12915-025-02383-9

Section 6

Obesity in the Age of Artificial Intelligence: A Look into the Future

Chapter 12

From Metrics to Meaning: LLM-Driven Lifestyle Intelligence for Personalized Obesity Prevention

Heewon Kim and Hannah Kim

Abstract

This chapter redefines obesity prevention through the lens of whole-person health and recent advances in large language models (LLMs). While body mass index (BMI) remains a useful population-level marker, its limitations in capturing nuanced behavioral, psychological, and contextual health factors have led to growing interest in complementary approaches. Similarly, traditional machine learning (ML) models built on structured lifestyle surveys suffer from rigid variable definitions, lack of contextual depth, and poor adaptability to individual lived experiences. Without understanding the root causes embedded in real-life behaviors, any intervention risks being superficial or short-lived. We explore how unstructured, real-world health narratives can be transformed into clinically meaningful signals through LLM-driven analysis. By bridging preventive medicine and modern artificial intelligence (AI), this chapter positions LLMs not merely as assistants but as interpretive engines capable of understanding the psychological, behavioral, and social context that surrounds lifestyle-related risk. We examine cutting-edge developments such as EntroLLM, which embeds latent health concepts from free-form text, and contrast them with earlier ML approaches that relied heavily on structured survey data. These innovations support more personalized, context-aware, and adaptive interventions – aligned with the principles of whole-person care. Concrete applications include Noom's LLM-guided behavior coaching, Welli's AI wellness journaling tools, and emerging LLM integrations in insurance-based health nudging platforms. We evaluate their potential for stratifying obesity risk even in the absence of BMI, and their limits in terms of evidence, trust, and regulatory fitness. The aim is a paradigm that enriches BMI with narrative insight and makes obesity care more human-centered.

Keywords: real-world health narratives, unstructured health data, whole-person health, LLM-driven analysis, AI wellness, behavioral vector modeling, AI for preventive medicine

1. Introduction: The limits of metrics – Why body mass index and structured surveys fall short in lifestyle understanding

Body Mass Index (BMI) has long played a central role in epidemiology and public health as a practical and scalable population-level indicator. At the same time, a substantial body of evidence has firmly established its limitations in capturing individual-level health risk and lifestyle complexity. In particular, its usefulness declines sharply when applied to personalized lifestyle assessment. As many expert reviews have noted, BMI is fundamentally an "imperfect clinical measure" that collapses physiologically distinct constructs—fat mass, lean mass, bone density, and visceral adiposity—into a single number. This flattening effect produces widespread misclassification: muscular individuals, older adults with sarcopenic obesity, and people across diverse ethnic groups can share the same BMI despite markedly different metabolic risk profiles.

Because BMI cutoffs were historically derived from White, non-Hispanic cohorts, the metric fails to reflect racial and ethnic variation in body composition and cardiometabolic risk – a limitation recognized by major organizations such as the American Medical Association, which explicitly warns that BMI "loses predictability when applied on the individual level." To address these discrepancies, complementary measures such as percent body fat, Fat Mass Index (FMI), waist circumference, and imaging-based assessments like DEXA and MRI – along with newer indices such as relative fat mass (RFM) – are increasingly used to provide more accurate estimates of adiposity and cardiometabolic risk across diverse populations [1–7].

1.1 Measurement biases in structured lifestyle surveys

The limitations observed in BMI reflect a broader challenge in preventive health measurement: the tendency to compress complex lived realities into simplified, standardized proxies. This pattern extends beyond anthropometric metrics to other commonly used instruments for lifestyle assessment, including structured self-report surveys. Structured self-report surveys – commonly used to assess physical activity, diet, and stress – are consistently shown to introduce significant biases. Participants tend to overestimate physical activity and underestimate sedentary behaviors, with discrepancies especially pronounced in certain groups (e.g., males, obese individuals). Social desirability bias further distorts self-reports, as individuals often report healthier behaviors than they actually perform, which can confound associations with health outcomes. Underreporting of unhealthy behaviors and overreporting of healthy ones are well-documented, and these biases can be exacerbated by declining participation rates and non-representative samples [8–11].

1.2 Loss of context and narrative in health assessment

By reducing complex behaviors to rigid categories, structured surveys erase important contextual factors such as cultural practices, emotional triggers, and environmental constraints. For example, barriers like cost, lack of time, or social support are often underrepresented or mischaracterized, especially in marginalized or rural populations. This narrative loss can lead to the misinterpretation of nonadherence as individual failure, rather than as a reflection of broader social or environmental challenges [12–14].

1.3 Implications for machine learning and predictive models

Machine learning (ML) models trained on these structured, biased metrics inherit their limitations. While such models may achieve high predictive accuracy, they often function as "black boxes" with limited interpretability, making it difficult to understand or address the underlying causes of risk. This lack of transparency undermines clinical trust and can reinforce structural biases, especially when models rely on flawed proxies like BMI or self-reported activity [15, 16].

Consequently, even advanced predictive models built on these biased, low-resolution metrics remain constrained by the limitations of their inputs. To address these issues, efforts have shifted toward integrating genomic data (e.g., polygenic risk scores), behavioral measures (e.g., structured surveys), and multimodal longitudinal lifestyle data – such as photo-based dietary records and wearable-derived activity signals – laying the foundation for the richer, narrative-based approaches explored in the next chapter [17]. In this sense, multimodal integration represented a natural progression within existing measurement frameworks.

For obesity prevention, this loss is not merely methodological – it is clinical. When we cannot understand the contextual reasons why individuals eat, move, or cope the way they do, interventions become generic, short-lived, and misaligned with real-world behavior. BMI may capture population-level patterns, and structured surveys may reflect coarse behavioral trends, but neither can account for the granular, situational factors that drive individual variation or enable sustainable, personalized change. Bridging this fidelity gap requires complementing traditional quantitative metrics with richer, narrative-based contextual data – a direction that the following sections examine in detail.

2. Real-world health narratives as data: Unlocking context, motivation, and lived experience

2.1 Effective obesity prevention requires understanding both behaviors and their context, not just outcomes

Given that one of the central goals of BMI use in clinical practice is obesity prevention, the metric must be evaluated not only for its ability to classify weight status, but also for its capacity to inform meaningful preventive action. Traditional metrics like BMI, step counts, and food-frequency questionnaires quantify behaviors but fail to capture the emotional, social, and environmental contexts that drive those behaviors. This lack of contextual data—termed the "narrative gap"—limits the personalization and effectiveness of preventive care.

2.2 Why context matters in obesity prevention

Emotional and psychological factors play a critical role in obesity risk and management. Emotional eating—often triggered by stress, depression, or anxiety—serves as a key behavioral mechanism linking psychological distress to weight gain. Addressing these emotional drivers is therefore essential for both prevention and treatment.

Beyond individual psychology, social vulnerabilities such as low socioeconomic status, limited social support, and adverse life experiences independently contribute to obesity risk. Neighborhood environments—including levels of social capital and collective efficacy—can either undermine or enhance the effectiveness of clinical interventions.

Moreover, the lived experience of obesity is frequently shaped by stigma, discrimination, and psychosocial stress. When unaddressed, these experiences can lead to disengagement from health-promoting behaviors and ultimately worsen clinical outcomes.

2.3 The role of patient-generated narratives and digital tools

Patient-generated narratives—including journals, chat logs, and counseling notes—provide rich insight into individual motives, stressors, and perceived barriers. By capturing subjective experience, such narrative data help bridge the "narrative gap" and enable more personalized and context-sensitive care.

Digital tools, including mobile applications, social media platforms, and conversational agents, can further support self-monitoring, personalized feedback, and social connection. However, their effectiveness depends not merely on technological sophistication, but on empathetic, context-aware design and the meaningful integration of narrative data.

In addition, group-based interventions that foster shared social identity and psychological connection have been shown to enhance motivation and sustain behavior change over time [18–28].

2.4 Why context matters: Moving beyond decontextualized metrics

Contextual data, including patient narratives, provide critical insights that structured metrics often miss. Context helps patients and clinicians make sense of complex health data, supports action planning, and builds trust in data-driven decisions. Without context, trends may be unclear or counterintuitive, limiting the usefulness of health information for both patients and providers.

2.5 Defining narrative real-world data

Narrative real-world data (NRWD) encompasses unstructured, free-form accounts of patient experiences, often captured in electronic health records (EHRs), web-based platforms, or participatory storytelling. These narratives serve as behavioral and emotional sensors, revealing patient perspectives, emotional states, and social determinants that structured data may overlook. Integrating narrative with digital tools enhances empathy, communication, and professional identity among healthcare providers.

2.6 Narrative RWD versus structured RWD: Complementary strengths

While structured RWD (e.g., lab results, claims data) offers standardization and scalability, NRWD provides depth, context, and meaning. Combining both enables a more holistic view of patient health, supporting both evidence-based and person-centered care. Narrative data can contextualize quantitative findings, making them more actionable and relatable (see **Table 1**).

Data type	Strengths	Limitations
Structured RWD	Standardized, scalable, easy to analyze	Lacks context, may miss nuances
Narrative RWD	Rich context, emotional/behavioral insight	Harder to standardize/analyze

Table 1.
Complementary strengths of narrative and structured RWD.

2.7 The equity imperative: Narratives for minority and under-represented populations

Narrative approaches are especially powerful for amplifying the voices of minority and under-represented groups, addressing health disparities, and promoting equity. Storytelling and critical narrative interventions foster empathy, reduce stigma, and support culturally grounded health communication and behavior change [29–39].

2.8 From narrative insight to preventive action

Narratives – stories grounded in lived experience – are increasingly recognized as powerful tools for motivating preventive health behaviors. Unlike traditional fact-based messages, narratives enhance engagement and personal relevance, reduce resistance, and strengthen self-efficacy by allowing individuals to identify with characters and contexts similar to their own. Culturally tailored and community-informed storytelling has been shown to improve motivation, intention, and uptake of health-promoting actions – from cancer screening to chronic disease management – particularly in populations underserved or skeptical of conventional health messaging. Though effect sizes are generally modest in controlled trials, evidence consistently demonstrates that narrative approaches can meaningfully support sustained lifestyle modification when they complement, rather than replace, traditional information-based strategies [32, 40–51].

Narrative real-world data brings essential clinical perspective, emotional insight, and equity considerations into healthcare decision-making, complementing structured metrics. Integrating both data types enables more patient-centered context-responsive, and equitable care, guiding proactive clinical action and improving health outcomes for all populations.

3. Large language models as interpretive engines: From unstructured text to clinically meaningful signals

Recent advances in large language models (LLMs) are transforming obesity prevention by enabling the extraction of clinically meaningful signals from unstructured health narratives, moving beyond the limitations of BMI and structured survey data.

3.1 Converting narratives into structured clinical signals

LLMs excel at extracting complex behavioral, psychological, and social determinants of health (SDoH) from free-text sources such as EHRs, patient journals, and chat transcripts. Fine-tuned LLMs have shown that they can accurately identify

SDoH categories like employment, housing, and social support. They do better than traditional pattern-matching and earlier ML methods, and they can capture nuanced, context-rich information that structured data fields often miss. Tools like SBDH-Reader and open-source LLMs have achieved F1 scores above 0.94 in extracting SDoH, supporting scalable, real-time patient-level data collection [52–55].

3.2 Behavioral vector modeling and latent health embeddings

LLMs can embed latent health concepts from free-form text, enabling the modeling of psychosocial–behavioral phenotypes and contextual risk factors. By identifying subgroups with similar behavioral and psychological profiles, these embeddings can link obesity risk and inform personalized interventions. Contextual word embeddings and topic modeling further enhance the ability to capture the interplay between lifestyle, environment, and health outcomes [53, 56, 57], which can lead to more effective strategies for addressing obesity and improving overall health by tailoring interventions to specific subgroups.

3.3 Habit–emotion–context extraction from narratives

LLMs are capable of extracting patterns of habits, emotions, and contextual factors from patient narratives, supporting reflective self-monitoring and personalized feedback. Artificial intelligence (AI)-driven journaling systems leverage LLMs to provide real-time, context-aware insights, fostering patient engagement and health literacy while maintaining privacy and transparency. These systems can identify early warning signs, such as changes in mood or behavior, and support proactive health management by alerting patients and healthcare providers to potential issues before they escalate[58–60].

3.4 Case study: EntroLLM and latent temporal structure

While specific mention of EntroLLM is not found, similar LLM-based frameworks demonstrate the ability to model temporal health patterns and latent structures from longitudinal data, such as wearable sensor streams and daily health logs. These models outperform traditional ML in predicting health outcomes and generating personalized recommendations [61].

3.5 LLM-driven features versus traditional feature engineering

LLMs surpass traditional feature engineering by automatically generating interpretable, clinically relevant features from unstructured data, reducing reliance on rigid variable definitions and enhancing adaptability to individual lived experiences. This shift enables more personalized, context-aware, and adaptive interventions that can be tailored to meet the specific needs of patients based on their unique health profiles and circumstances. [53, 62, 63].

3.6 Explainability: What the LLM "reads" and how it can be traced

Despite their power, LLMs present challenges in interpretability and transparency. Efforts to improve explainability include prompt engineering, attention mechanisms, and clinician-facing summarization tools, which help trace model reasoning and build trust in AI-driven insights. However, concerns remain regarding data privacy, algorithmic bias, and the need for robust ethical frameworks [53, 58, 59, 62, 64].

LLMs are redefining obesity prevention by transforming unstructured health narratives into actionable, personalized insights. While they offer significant advantages over traditional methods, challenges in explainability, fairness, and regulatory compliance must be addressed for safe and effective clinical integration.

4. LLM-driven lifestyle intelligence in obesity prevention: Case-based applications and the shift to whole-person healthcare

This section explores how LLMs are transforming obesity prevention by enabling more personalized, context-aware, and adaptive interventions. The focus is on real-world applications—AI coaching, which uses artificial intelligence to provide personalized guidance; journaling, the practice of recording daily activities and thoughts; digital phenotyping, the collection and analysis of data from digital sources to understand behavior; and behavioral profiling, the assessment of individual behaviors to tailor interventions—culminating in a holistic approach to health.

4.1 Converting narratives into structured clinical signals

4.1.1 Case examples: From AI coaching to digital phenotypes

4.1.1.1 Personal AI coach: Nuli

LLM-powered coaching systems, such as those modeled after Noom and similar platforms, deliver personalized, motivational, and context-sensitive guidance for weight management. Studies show that LLM-generated coaching messages can match human coaches in helpfulness and empathy, especially after prompt refinement, though users sometimes perceive them as formulaic or overly data-driven. These systems offer scalable, cost-effective support and can increase access to care but require ongoing improvements in authenticity and trustworthiness [60, 65, 66].

4.1.1.2 Simplified health journaling: Luji

AI-assisted journaling tools leverage LLMs to transform unstructured, user-generated narratives into actionable health insights. Such systems encourage reflective self-monitoring, enhance health literacy, and provide real-time, context-aware feedback. Key design principles include transparency, adaptive consent, and clinician-facing data summarization. Early prototypes demonstrate improved patient engagement and the potential to bridge patient-generated data with clinical care, though rigorous trials are needed to confirm long-term benefits [58].

4.2 Digital phenotyping and behavioral profiling

LLMs and advanced AI models can extract nuanced behavioral, psychological, and social determinants of health from free-text data, such as EHRs and patient narratives. These models are better at finding risk factors and social determinants than traditional pattern-matching and structured survey methods. This helps with more accurate risk stratification and targeting of interventions [52, 54, 67]. Explainable AI models that focus on lifestyle factors – rather than BMI alone – achieve high accuracy in predicting obesity risk and highlight the importance of meal frequency, technology use, and other daily behaviors [68].

4.3 Toward whole-person healthcare

The integration of LLM-driven tools supports a shift from population-level metrics like BMI to individualized, narrative-based insights. This aligns with the principles of whole-person care, emphasizing psychological, behavioral, and social context in obesity prevention. LLMs facilitate adaptive, human-centered interventions that can be tailored to diverse lived experiences, potentially improving both engagement and outcomes [69, 70, 71], by providing personalized recommendations and support that consider each individual's unique circumstances and challenges in managing obesity.[69–71].

5. Opportunities and risks: Evidence, trust, bias, and regulatory readiness

5.1 Opportunities and challenges of introducing medical AI

LLMs demonstrate high potential for innovation in clinical document summarization, decision support, and patient communication, enabling patient-centered care through the utilization of unstructured data [72, 73].

However, key risks also exist, including regulatory uncertainty, lack of reliability, fairness issues, and ambiguity regarding accountability.

5.2 Global regulatory environment

5.2.1 U.S. Food and Drug Administration

The U.S. Food and Drug Administration (FDA) regulates AI medical devices through its SaMD (Software as a Medical Device) framework, classifying them into Class I–III and applying certification procedures based on risk levels [74, 75] (see **Table 2**).

Because AI/ML-based devices (including LLMs) evolve continuously, the FDA manages the safety of dynamic algorithms through PCCP (Predetermined Change Control Plan) and GMLP (Good Machine Learning Practices) [76, 77].

5.2.2 EU AI act

The EU AI Act classifies medical AI systems as high-risk and mandates dataset representativeness, risk-management systems, transparency, and human oversight [78, 79] (see **Table 2**).

In particular, data-governance requirements aimed at reducing bias represent strong obligations for market entry into the EU.

Regulatory country	FDA SaMD (United States)	EU AI Act (Europe)	MFDS/NHI (Korea)
Risk Classification Criteria	Class I, II, III (based on clinical risk) [76]	High-risk (based on intended use and personal profiling) [80]	Medical device classes (based on risk level and dependency) [83].
Core Regulatory Framework	PCCP, GMLPs, RWP monitoring [78]	Risk management system, data governance, human oversight [81]	MFDS approval, followed by New Health Technology Assessment (NHI reimbursement) [83].
Bias Management Obligations	Specified within the AI/ML action plan, supporting evaluation and mitigation [79].	Obligations for representativeness and error minimization in datasets for high-risk systems [80].	Data control under PIPA (Personal Information Protection Act) and the requirement for Institutional Review Board (IRB) review [83].

Table 2.
Comparison of major regulations and medical AI (LLM SaMD) requirements by country.

5.2.3 Insurance and reimbursement systems

In the United States, CPT Category III codes are used to pilot reimbursement for innovative technologies [80]. Germany's DiGA system requires clinical evidence and health-economic evaluations [81]. In Korea, reimbursement decisions are made through the New Health Technology Assessment following MFDS approval [82] (see **Table 2**).

5.3 Technical requirements for trustworthy AI (explainability, auditability, and reproducibility)

For clinical use of LLMs, explainability, auditability, and reproducibility are critical. Due to the opacity of LLM reasoning processes, hallucinations and factual errors pose risks, making calibrated confidence-score reporting essential for controlling these risks. A further limitation is that LLMs remain highly sensitive to dataset and context shifts. Models that perform well on benchmark datasets or curated pilot populations may degrade substantially when exposed to new demographic groups, evolving lifestyle trends, or different documentation styles, even if their surface-level fluency appears unchanged. For lifestyle and obesity prevention, this gap is critical: models may capture language patterns without fully reflecting cultural norms, food environments, or health system constraints. XAR in this sense is not only about "opening the black box," but about making the operational boundaries of the model – its valid use-cases, populations, and data regimes – explicit and continuously revisited [84–86].

5.4 Legal and ethical uncertainties

5.4.1 Accountability

When LLM errors occur, responsibility among clinicians, institutions, and developers is unclear, raising the issue of a "liability chasm" [87].

This is attributed to the black-box nature of LLMs and the difficulty of error tracing [86].

5.4.2 Privacy and consent issues

When clinical data are used for LLM training, existing de-identification techniques have limitations [88], and many studies have failed to implement adequate patient-consent procedures – an issue regarded as a significant ethical concern [83].

5.5 Conclusion and strategic recommendations

This analysis highlights that, although LLM-based medical AI has great innovative potential, regulatory, technical, and ethical foundations are essential for safe adoption.

The following strategies are proposed:

(1) International standardization of PCCP and GMLP [76].

(2) Representative data governance and mandatory bias audits to minimize bias [78, 89].

(3) Establishment of reimbursement systems centered on demonstrating economic value [81].

(4) Mandatory reporting of LLM confidence scores [86].

(5) Long-term technological strategy focused on multimodal AI [72].

6. Conclusion

BMI is not a good way to understand someone's lifestyle on an individual level because it doesn't take into account differences in body composition, age, race and ethnicity, and lived context. Similar constraints recur in structured survey data and conventional ML models, where decontextualized metrics often lead to interpretations and interventions misaligned with real-world behavior, resulting in ineffective health strategies that do not address the unique needs of individuals. Against this backdrop, the importance of narrative data and LLMs capable of interpreting such context has emerged, leading to new practical attempts such as AI coaching, health journaling, and digital phenotyping in real-world settings. From the perspective of working directly with data in practice, one lesson becomes consistently clear: data are always incomplete. No dataset can fully represent reality, and models inevitably inherit these imperfections. The critical task, therefore, is not to build increasingly complex models, but to recognize the limits of the data and to distinguish what can – and cannot – be meaningfully interpreted. In lifestyle and obesity prevention, LLMs should not be viewed as tools for producing definitive answers, but rather as supportive interpretive systems that help surface context and enable dialogue. In the end, the usefulness of medical AI in the real world depends not only on how well it works, but also on how clear its purpose and responsibility are.

The author acknowledges the use of LLM solely for language polishing and minor grammatical refinement of the manuscript. All conceptualization, methodology, analysis, and final content decisions were conducted independently by the author. The author takes full responsibility for the integrity and accuracy of the work.

Author details

Heewon Kim[1*] and Hannah Kim[2]

1 Independent Researcher, Incheon, South Korea

2 Independent Researcher, Seoul, South Korea

*Address all correspondence to: work.wonniey@gmail.com

References

[1] Wu Y, Li D, Vermund SH. Advantages and limitations of the body mass index (BMI) to assess adult obesity. International Journal of Environmental Research and Public Health. 2024;**21**(6):757. DOI: 10.3390/ijerph21060757

[2] Potter AW, Chin GC, Looney DP, Friedl KE. Defining overweight and obesity by percent body fat instead of body mass index. Journal of Clinical Endocrinology & Metabolism. 2025;**110**(4):e1103–e1107. DOI: 10.1210/clinem/dgae341

[3] Katzmarzyk PT, Bray GA, Greenway FL, Johnson WD, RL Jr N, Ravussin E, Ryan DH, Bouchard C. Ethnic-specific BMI and waist circumference thresholds. Obesity (Silver Spring). 2011;**19**(6):1272–1278. DOI: 10.1038/oby.2010.319

[4] Taylor Jr HA, Coady SA, Levy D, Walker ER, Vasan RS, Liu J, Akylbekova EL, Garrison RJ, Fox C. Relationships of BMI to cardiovascular risk factors differ by ethnicity. Obesity (Silver Spring). 2010;**18**(8):1638–1645. DOI: 10.1038/oby.2009.407

[5] Santorelli G, West J, Yang T, Wright J, Bryant M, Lawlor DA. Differences in total and regional body fat and their association with BMI in UK-born White and South Asian children: Findings from the Born in Bradford birth cohort. Wellcome Open Research. 2022;**6**:65. DOI: 10.12688/wellcomeopenres.16659.3

[6] Suthahar N, Lau ES, Savarese G. Relative fat mass: Refining adiposity measurement in the era beyond body mass index. Current Heart Failure Reports. 2025;**22**(1):22. DOI: 10.1007/s11897-025-00709-w

[7] Ricardo RR, Tamayo M, Correa R, Burguera B, Griebeler ML. Body composition changes in latino population: Longitudinal associations of fat and muscle mass indices. Obesity Science & Practice. 2025;**11**(3):e70077. DOI: 10.1002/osp4.70077

[8] Klesges RC, Eck LH, Mellon MW, Fulliton W, Somes GW, Hanson CL. The accuracy of self-reports of physical activity. Medicine & Science in Sports & Exercise. 1990;**22**(5):690–697. DOI: 10.1249/00005768-199010000-00022

[9] Klesges LM, Baranowski T, Beech B, Cullen K, Murray DM, Rochon J, Pratt C. Social desirability bias in self-reported dietary, physical activity and weight concerns measures in 8- to 10-year-old African-American girls: Results from the Girls Health Enrichment Multisite Studies (GEMS). Preventive Medicine. 2004;**38**:S78–87. DOI: 10.1016/j.ypmed.2003.07.003

[10] Ghaneapur M, Ezati Asar M, Belji Kangarlou M, Saleh E. Comparison of two methods of measuring physical activity and its related components among middle age women: Pedometer versus self-report. PLoS One. 2025;**20**(2):e0319288. DOI: 10.1371/journal.pone.0319288

[11] Latkin CA, Edwards C, Davey-Rothwell MA, Tobin KE. The relationship between social desirability bias and self-reports of health, substance use, and social network factors among urban substance users in

Baltimore, Maryland. Addictive Behaviors. 2017;**73**:133–136. DOI: 10.1016/j.addbeh.2017.05.005

[12] Pelletier CA, White N, Duchesne A, Sluggett L. Barriers to physical activity for adults in rural and urban Canada: A cross-sectional comparison. SSM - Population Health. 2021;**16**:100964. DOI: 10.1016/j.ssmph.2021.100964

[13] Trujillo-Garrido N, Santi-Cano MJ. Motivation and limiting factors for adherence to weight loss interventions among patients with obesity in primary care. Nutrients. 2022;**14**(14):2928. DOI: 10.3390/nu14142928

[14] Manyanga T, White N, Sluggett L, Duchesne A, Anekwe D, Pelletier C. Perceived barriers to physical activity among youth living in rural and urban canadian communities: A nationally representative cross-sectional study. Journal of Physical Activity & Health. 2024;**21**(7):645–656. DOI: 10.1123/jpah.2023-0254

[15] Gallucci D, Ecy H, Geraci J, Loren J, Pani L. Respondents of health survey powered by the innovative NURO app exhibit correlations between exercise frequencies and diet habits, and between stress levels and sleep wellness. Frontiers in Psychiatry. 2022;**13**:945780. DOI: 10.3389/fpsyt.2022.945780

[16] Liu T, Krentz AJ, Huo Z, Ćurčin V. Opportunities and challenges of cardiovascular disease risk prediction for primary prevention using machine learning and electronic health records: A systematic review. Reviews in Cardiovascular Medicine. 2025;**26**(4):37443. DOI: 10.31083/RCM37443

[17] Kang JH, Kim H, Kim J, Seo JH, Cha S, Oh H, Kim K, Sj P, Kim E, Kong S, Lee JH, Bae JS, Won HH, Joung JG, Yj Y, Kim J, Park WY. Interaction of genetic and environmental factors for body fat mass control: Observational study for lifestyle modification and genotyping. Scientific Reports. 2021;**11**(1):13180. DOI: 10.1038/s41598-021-92229-5

[18] Konttinen H. Emotional eating and obesity in adults: The role of depression, sleep and genes. Proceedings of the Nutrition Society. 2020;**79**(3):283–289. DOI: 10.1017/S0029665120000166

[19] Hemmingsson E. A new model of the role of psychological and emotional distress in promoting obesity: Conceptual review with implications for treatment and prevention. Obesity Reviews. 2014;**15**(9):769–779. DOI: 10.1111/obr.12197

[20] Spinosa J, Christiansen P, Dickson JM, Lorenzetti V, Hardman CA. From socioeconomic disadvantage to obesity: The mediating role of psychological distress and emotional eating. Obesity (Silver Spring). 2019;**27**(4):559–564. DOI: 10.1002/oby.22402

[21] Iguacel I, Gasch-Gallén Á, Ayala-Marín AM, De Miguel-Etayo P, Moreno LA. Social vulnerabilities as risk factor of childhood obesity development and their role in prevention programs. International Journal of Obesity (London). 2021;**45**(1):1–11. DOI: 10.1038/s41366-020-00697-y

[22] Flint SW, Vázquez-Velázquez V, Le Brocq S, Brown A. The real-life experiences of people living with overweight and obesity: A psychosocial perspective. Diabetes, Obesity and Metabolism. 2025;**27**(Suppl 2):35–47. DOI: 10.1111/dom.16255

[23] Luig T, Keenan L, Campbell-Scherer DL. Transforming health experience and action through shifting the narrative on obesity in primary care encounters. Qualitative Health Research. 2020;**30**(5):730–744. DOI: 10.1177/1049732319880551

[24] Chatterjee A, Prinz A, Gerdes M, Martinez S. Digital interventions on healthy lifestyle management: Systematic review. Journal of Medical Internet Research. 2021;**23**(11):e26931. DOI: 10.2196/26931

[25] Virtanen M, Kerimaa H, Männikkö N, Männistö M, Paalimäki-Paakki K, Lahtinen M, Jansson M, Kivelä K, Oikarinen A, Rajala M, Vanhanen M, Kääriäinen M, Kaakinen P. Digital components and interaction types in counseling interventions for childhood and adolescent obesity: A systematic review. International Journal of Nursing Sciences. 2025;**12**(2):123–129. DOI: 10.1016/j.ijnss.2025.02.014

[26] Saadi A, Fellrath JM, Bec-Moussally J, Papastathi-Boureau C, Blanc C, Courtine V, Vanini L, Marechal M, Authier F, Curty B, Fournier P, Diana M, Saillant S. Using patient-reported outcome measures to assess the effectiveness of social media networking programs for people living with overweight and obesity to adopt a healthier lifestyle. Frontiers in Public Health. 2023;**11**:1161851. DOI: 10.3389/fpubh.2023.1161851

[27] Noh E, Won J, Jo S, Hahm DH, Lee H. Conversational agents for body weight management: Systematic review. Journal of Medical Internet Research. 2023;**25**:e42238. DOI: 10.2196/42238

[28] Tarrant M, Khan SS, Farrow CV, Shah P, Daly M, Kos K. Patient experiences of a bariatric group programme for managing obesity: A qualitative interview study. British Journal of Health Psychology. 2017;**22**(1):77–93. DOI: 10.1111/bjhp.12218

[29] Raj S, Lee JM, Garrity A, Newman MW. Clinical data in context: Towards sensemaking tools for interpreting personal health data. Proceedings of the ACM on Interactive, Mobile, Wearable and Ubiquitous Technologies. 2019;**3**(1):20. DOI: 10.1145/3314409

[30] Costa V, Custodio MG, Gefen E, Fregni F. The relevance of the real-world evidence in research, clinical, and regulatory decision making. Frontiers in Public Health. 2025;**13**:1512429. DOI: 10.3389/fpubh.2025.1512429

[31] Liu F, Panagiotakos D. Real-world data: A brief review of the methods, applications, challenges and opportunities. BMC Medical Research Methodology. 2022;**22**(1):287. DOI: 10.1186/s12874-022-01768-6

[32] Shaffer VA, Focella ES, Hathaway A, Scherer LD, Zikmund-Fisher BJ. On the usefulness of narratives: An interdisciplinary review and theoretical model. Annals of Behavioral Medicine. 2018;**52**(5):429–442. DOI: 10.1093/abm/kax008

[33] Efthymiou E. Integrating digital and narrative medicine in modern healthcare: A systematic review. Medical Education Online. 2025;**30**(1):2475979. DOI: 10.1080/10872981.2025.2475979

[34] Drewniak D, Glässel A, Hodel M, Biller-Andorno N. Risks and benefits of web-based patient narratives: Systematic review. Journal of Medical

Internet Research. 2020;**22**(3):e15772. DOI: 10.2196/15772

[35] Bastarache L, Brown JS, Cimino JJ, Dorr DA, Embi PJ, Payne PRO, Wilcox AB, Weiner MG. Developing real-world evidence from real-world data: Transforming raw data into analytical datasets. Learning Health Systems. 2021;**6**(1):e10293. DOI: 10.1002/lrh2.10293

[36] Fiddian-Green A, Gubrium A. Critical narrative intervention for health equity research and practice: Editorial commentary introducing the health promotion practice. Critical Narrative Intervention Special Collection. Health Promotion Practice. 2021;**22**(2_suppl):2S–7S. DOI: 10.1177/15248399211046185

[37] Lee H, Fawcett J, DeMarco R. Storytelling/narrative theory to address health communication with minority populations. Applied Nursing Research. 2016;**30**:58–60. DOI: 10.1016/j.apnr.2015.09.004

[38] Taborda C, Sofer N, Beard J, Wang M. Identifying and dismantling racist narratives to promote health equity. HPHR Journal. 2023. DOI: 10.54111/0001/TTT3

[39] Blonde L, Khunti K, Harris SB, Meizinger C, Skolnik NS. Interpretation and impact of real-world clinical data for the practicing clinician. Advances in Therapy. 2018;**35**(11):1763–1774. DOI: 10.1007/s12325-018-0805-y

[40] Nagarkar A, Martin G, Sadaniantz K, Iyengar S, Wisniewski HC, Denu MK, Chiriboga G, Forrester SN, Allison JJ, Kovell LC. Storytelling for health promotion: A scoping review. American Journal of Health Promotion. 2025;8901171251365366. DOI: 10.1177/08901171251365366

[41] Xin M, Coulson NS, Jiang CL, Sillence E, Chidgey A, Kwan NNM, Mak WWS, Goggins W, Lau JTF, Pkh M. Web-based behavioral intervention utilizing narrative persuasion for hiv prevention among chinese men who have sex with men (hehe talks project): Intervention development. Journal of Medical Internet Research. 2021;**23**(9):e22312. DOI: 10.2196/22312

[42] Frank LB, Murphy ST, Chatterjee JS, Moran MB, Baezconde-Garbanati L. Telling stories, saving lives: Creating narrative health messages. Health Communication. 2015;**30**(2):154–163. DOI: 10.1080/10410236.2014.974126

[43] Sitto K, Lubinga E, Geya M.The power of narrative health communication: Exploring possible effects of first-hand experiential stories on cancer awareness amongst university students. The Journal for Transdisciplinary Research in Southern Africa. 2021;**17**(1):10

[44] Chen M, Taylor LD, Bell RA. Persuasive narratives about osteoporosis: Effects of protagonist competence, narrator point of view, and subjective risk. Health Education & Behavior. 2024;**51**(3):446–456. DOI: 10.1177/10901981231158412

[45] Lillie HM, Jensen JD, Krakow M. The importance of structural elements in narrative persuasion: Using the narrative immersion model to promote melanoma prevention. Risk Analysis. 2025;**45**(9):2895–2907. DOI: 10.1111/risa.70063

[46] Shin Y, Miller-Day M, Pettigrew J, Hecht ML. Does narrative quality

matter during implementation of a school-based prevention intervention? A Test of Narrative Engagement Theory. Journal of Health Communication. 2023;**28**(8):526–538. DOI: 10.1080/10810730.2023.2231886

[47] Guan M, Chiang SC, Murray RM, Lo WJ, Hill LT, Klassen AC, Manganello JA, Leader AE, Massey PM. Narratives or not? Examining the roles of message format and individuals' stages of change in the context of HPV vaccination promotion. Health Education Research. 2025;**40**(3): cyaf015. DOI: 10.1093/her/cyaf015

[48] Shen F, Sheer VC, Li R. Impact of narratives on persuasion in health communication: A meta-analysis. Journal of Advertising. 2015;**44**(2): 105–113. DOI: 10.1080/00913367.2015.1018467

[49] Xu J. A meta-analysis comparing the effectiveness of narrative vs. Statistical Evidence: Health Vs. Non-Health Contexts. Health Communication. 2023;**38**(14): 3113–3123. DOI: 10.1080/10410236.2022.2137750

[50] Martell R, Reade M, Boesch L, Kaur DP, Kumar S, McArthur M, Maar MA. The role of narratives in promoting vaccine confidence among Indigenous peoples in Canada, the United States, Australia, and New Zealand: A scoping review. International Journal for Equity in Health. 2025;**24**(1):63. DOI: 10.1186/s12939-025-02424-3

[51] Butsch Kovacic M, Gertz SE. Leveraging stories to promote health and prevent cancer. Cancer Prevention Research (Philadelphia). 2022;**15**(7):419–422. DOI: 10.1158/1940-6207.CAPR-22-0199

[52] Guevara M, Chen S, Thomas S, Chaunzwa TL, Franco I, Kann BH, Moningi S, Qian JM, Goldstein M, Harper S, Aerts HJWL, Catalano PJ, Savova GK, Mak RH, Bitterman DS. Large language models to identify social determinants of health in electronic health records. NPJ Digital Medicine. 2024;**7**(1):6. DOI: 10.1038/s41746-023-00970-0

[53] Farrag A, Soliman A, Hatef E, Goodin A, Rouhizadeh M Beyond Metrics to Methods: A Scoping Review of Large Language Models for Detection of Social Drivers of Health in Clinical Notes. medRxiv. 2025. DOI: 10.1101/2025.07.04.25330866

[54] Gu B, Shao V, Liao Z, Carducci V, Brufau SR, Yang J, Desai RJ. Scalable information extraction from free text electronic health records using large language models. BMC Medical Research Methodology. 2025;**25**(1):23. DOI: 10.1186/s12874-025-02470-z

[55] Gu Z, He L, Naeem A, Chan PM, Mohamed A, Khalil H, Guo Y, Huang J, Villanueva-Miranda I, Ding Y, Shi W, Dupre ME, Xiao G, Peterson ED, Xie Y, Navar AM, Yang DM. SBDH-Reader: A large language model-powered method for extracting social and behavioral determinants of health from clinical notes. Journal of the American Medical Informatics Association. 2025;**32**(10):1570–1580. DOI: 10.1093/jamia/ocaf124

[56] Burgermaster M, Rodriguez VA. Psychosocial-behavioral phenotyping: A novel precision health approach to modeling behavioral, psychological, and social determinants of health using machine learning. Annals of Behavioral Medicine. 2022;**56**(12):1258–1271. DOI: 10.1093/abm/kaac012

[57] Yeruva VK, Junaid S, Lee Y. Contextual word embeddings and topic modeling in healthy dieting and obesity. Journal of Healthcare Informatics Research. 2019;**3**(2):159–183. DOI: 10.1007/s41666-019-00052-5

[58] Moëll B, Sand Aronsson F. Journaling with large language models: A novel UX paradigm for AI-driven personal health management. Frontiers in Artificial Intelligence. 2025;**8**:1567580. DOI: 10.3389/frai.2025.1567580

[59] Guo Z, Lai A, Thygesen JH, Farrington J, Keen T, Li K. Large language models for mental health applications: Systematic review. JMIR Mental Health. 2024;11e57400. DOI: 10.2196/57400

[60] Huang Z, et al Comparing large language model AI and human-generated coaching messages for behavioral weight loss. Journal of Technology in Behavioral Science. 2025;**10**:1–12

[61] Kim Y, et al. "Health-LLM: Large language models for health prediction via wearable sensor data, arXiv." arXiv preprint arXiv:2401. 06866 (2024)

[62] McInerney D, et al. CHiLL: Zero-shot custom interpretable feature extraction from clinical notes with large language models. Findings of the Association for Computational Linguistics: EMNLP 2023. 2023; 8477–8494. DOI: 10.18653/v1/2023. findings-emnlp.568

[63] Khan AZ. Extraction of normalized symptom mentions from clinical narratives using large language models. AMIA Annual Symposium Proceedings. 2025;**2024**:600–609

[64] Thirunavukarasu AJ, et al. Large language models in medicine. Nature Medicine 2023;**29**:1930–1940

[65] Talay L, Lagesen L, Yip A, Vickers M, Ahuja N. ChatGPT-4o and 4o1 preview as dietary support tools in a real-world medicated obesity program: A prospective comparative analysis. Healthcare. 2025;**13**. DOI: 10.3390/healthcare13060647

[66] Meywirth S. Designing a Large Language Model-Based Coaching Intervention for Lifestyle Behavior Change. Cham, Switzerland: Springer; 2024. DOI: 10.1007/978-3-031-61175-9_6

[67] Liu S, Wang X, Hou Y, Li G, Wang H, Xu H, Xiang Y, Tang B. Multimodal data matters: Language model pre-training over structured and unstructured electronic health records. IEEE Journal of Biomedical and Health Informatics. 2022;**27**. DOI: 10.1109/jbhi.2022.3217810

[68] Khater T, Tawfik H, Singh B. Explainable artificial intelligence for investigating the effect of lifestyle factors on obesity. Intelligent Systems with Applications. 2024;**23**. DOI: 10.1016/j.iswa.2024.200427

[69] Li C, Zhao Y, Bai Y, Zhao B, Tola Y, Chan C, Zhang M, Fu X. Unveiling the potential of large language models in transforming chronic disease management: Mixed methods systematic review. Journal of Medical Internet Research. 2024;**27**. DOI: 10.2196/70535

[70] An R, Shen J, Xiao Y. Applications of Artificial Intelligence to obesity research: Scoping review of methodologies. Journal of Medical Internet Research. 2022;**24**. DOI: 10.2196/40589

[71] Liu M, Zhang W, Wang J, Bao K, Fu Z, Wang B. Promoting active health with AI technologies: Current status and prospects of high-altitude therapy, simulated hypoxia, and LLM-driven lifestyle rehabilitation approaches. Bioscience Trends. 2025. DOI: 10.5582/bst.2025.01105

[72] Meng X, Yan X, Zhang K, Liu D, Cui X, Yang Y, Zhang M, Cao C, Wang J, Wnag X, Gao J, Wang Y, Ji J, Qiu Z, Li M, Qian C, Guo T, Ma S, Wang Z, Guo Z, Lei Y, Shao C, Wnag W, Fan H, Tang Y. The application of large language models in medicine: A scoping review. iScience. 2024;**27**(5):109713. DOI: 10.1016/j.isci.2024.109713

[73] Nassiri K, Akhloufi M. Recent advances in large language models for healthcare. BioMedInformatics. 2024;**4**(2):1097–1143. DOI: 10.3390/biomedinformatics4020062

[74] FDA. Classify your medical device [internet]. Available from: https://www.fda.gov/medical-devices/overview-device-regulation/classify-your-medical-device [Accessed: 2025-December-9]

[75] FDA. How to study and market your device [internet]. Available from: https://www.fda.gov/medical-devices/device-advice-comprehensive-regulatory-assistance/how-study-and-market-your-device [Accessed: 2025-December-9]

[76] FDA. Releases action plan for Artificial Intelligence/Machine Learning-Enabled Software as a medical device [internet]. Available from: https://www.akingump.com/en/insights/alerts/fda-releases-action-plan-for-artificial-intelligencemachine-learning-enabled-software-as-a-medical-device-providing-another-iterative-step-forward-on-the-long-road-ahead [Accessed: 2025-December-9]

[77] Artificial Intelligence/machine learning (AI/ML)-based. Jf/U.S. FOOD & DRUG. 2021

[78] EU Artificial Intelligence Act. High-level summary of the AI Act[internet]. Available from: https://artificialintelligenceact.eu/high-level-summary [Accessed: 2025-December-9]

[79] Wilmerhale. What are high-risk ai systems within the meaning of the EU's AI act, and what requirements apply to them? [internet]. What Are High-Risk AI Systems Within the Meaning of the EU's AI Act, and What Requirements Apply to Them? 2024

[80] Dogra S, Silva E, Rajpurkar P. Reimbursement in the age of generalist radiology artificial intelligence. NPJ Digital Medicine. 2024;7:350. DOI: 10.1038/s41746-024-01352-w

[81] DELLE Techology. How: Germany's reimbursement systems [internet]. Available from: https://odelletechnology.com/the-g-ba-scientific-governance-and-reimbursement-authority-in-the-german-healthcare-system/ [Accessed: 2025-December-9]

[82] Lee W. Regulating artificial intelligence in medical care in South Korea Barfield W Pagallo U. In Research Handbook on Health, AI and the Law Cheltenham, UK. Edward Elgar Publishing Ltd; 2024. p. 392–407. DOI: 10.4337/9781802205657.ch22

[83] Zhong X, Li S, Chen Z, Ge L, Yu D, Wang S, You L, Shang H. Considerations for patient privacy of large language models in health care:

scoping review. Journal of Medical Internet Research. 2025;**27**:e76571. DOI: 10.2196/76571

[84] Kim M, Sohn H, Choi S, Kim S. Requirements for trustworthy Artificial Intelligence and its application in healthcare. Healthcare Informatics Research. 2023;**29**(4):315–322. DOI: 10.4258/hir.2023.29.4.315

[85] Xu H, Wang Y, Xun Y, Shao R, Jiao Y. Artificial intelligence for clinical reasoning: The reliability challenge and path to evidence-based practice. QJM: An International Journal of Medicine. 2025;hcaf114. DOI: 10.1093/qjmed/hcaf114

[86] Kim Y, Jeong H, Chen S, Li S, Lu M, Alhamound K, Mun J, Grau C, Jung M, Gameiro R, Fan L, Park E, Lin T, Yoon J, Yoon W, Sap M, Tsvetkov Y, Lang P, Xu X, Liu X, McDuff D, Lee H, Park H, Tulebaev S, Breazeal C. Medical hallucination in foundation models and their impact on healthcare. medRxiv. 2025. DOI: 10.1101/2025.02.28.25323115

[87] Artsi Y, Sorin V, Glicksberg B, Korfiatis P, Freeman R, Nadkarni G, Klang E. Challenges of implementing llms in clinical practice: Perspectives. Journal of Clinical Medicine. 2025;**14**(17):6169. DOI: 10.3390/jcm14176169

[88] Sarkar A, Chuang Y, Jiang X, Mohammed N. Not fully synthetic: LLM-based hybrid approaches towards privacy-preserving clinical note sharing. AMIA Joint Summits on Translational Science Proceedings. 2025;**2025**:441–450

[89] Norori N, Hu Q, Aellen F, Faraci F. Tzovara A.Addressing bias in big data and AI for health care: A call for open science. Patterns (New York). 2021;**2**(10):100347. DOI: 10.1016/j.patter.2021.100347